Introduction to
Hematology

Introduction to
Hematology

Second Edition

Samuel I. Rapaport, M.D.

Professor of Medicine and Pathology
Hematology/Oncology Division
UCSD Medical Center
San Diego, California

J.B. LIPPINCOTT COMPANY
Philadelphia · London · Mexico City · New York
St. Louis · São Paulo · Sydney

Acquisitions Editor: Lisa Biello
Sponsoring Editor: Sanford J. Robinson
Manuscript Editor: Helen Ewan
Indexer: Catherine Battaglia
Design Director: Tracy Baldwin
Design Coordinator: Don Shenkle
Designer: Patricia Pennington
Production Manager: Kathleen P. Dunn
Production Coordinator: George V. Gordon
Compositor: Ruttle, Shaw & Wetherill, Inc.
Printer/Binder: R. R. Donnelley & Sons Company

Second Edition

6 5 4 3

Library of Congress Cataloging-in-Publication Data

Rapaport, Samuel I., 1921–
    Introduction to hematology.

    Includes bibliographies and index.
    1. Hematology. I. Title. [DNLM: 1. Hematologic
Diseases. WH 100 R216i]
RB145.R28 1987   616.1'5   86-21313
ISBN 0-397-50838-7

The author and publisher have exerted every effort to
ensure that drug selection and dosage set forth in this
text are in accord with current recommendations and
practice at the time of publication. However, in view of
ongoing research, changes in government regulations,
and the constant flow of information relating to drug
therapy and drug reactions, the reader is urged to check
the package insert for each drug for any change in
indications and dosage and for added warnings and
precautions. This is particularly important when the
recommended agent is a new or infrequently employed
drug.

Dedicated to the memory
of Hyman Rapaport, M.D.

Preface

In the second edition of *Introduction to Hematology,* as in the first, I have sought to relate clinical findings and treatment to physiologic and pathologic processes, in the belief that this is the way to build a clinical foundation that withstands the stress of difficult diagnostic problems. I began writing with the goal of making the second edition no longer than the first. I failed in this. Much more is now known about the mechanisms and manifestations of hematologic diseases than was known at the beginning of the 1970s. Consequently, the second edition is longer than the first. All of us must learn and use more information than previously to provide the best of care for our patients.

I wish to acknowledge colleagues with whom I have worked in the past at the University of Southern California School of Medicine—particularly Dr. Thomas Brem, who taught me how high one aims to become a good internist, Dr. Gurth Carpenter, my first teacher in hematology, and Dr. Robert J. Lukes, from whom I learned much about the biology of the lymphomas. I have benefited from continuing contacts with Drs. Donald Feinstein, Alexandra Levine, and Carol Kasper, who have provided material helpful in preparing this second edition.

I also wish to acknowledge my debt to colleagues, too many to name individually, with whom I currently work at the UCSD School of Medicine and from whom I continue to learn hematology, pathology, and internal medicine. I want, however, to mention the names of two—Drs. Helen Anderson and Raymond Taetle—with whom I have worked very closely in the care of patients and the teaching of house officers and fellows.

I also wish to thank those who provided me with illustrations for the book: Mrs. Kathy Donnelly for preparing the electroimmunoassay and crossed immunoelectrophoresis gels of von Willebrand factor used in Figures 26-3 and 26-4 and for the radioautographs of multimers of von Willebrand factor shown in Figure 26-5; Dr. Robert J. Lukes for providing the microphotographs of diffuse large cell lymphoma and B cell-immunoblastic lymphoma shown in Figure 18-7 and for making available to me the originals of the microphotographs of immunoblastic lymphadenopathy shown in Figure 18-8; Dr. Ivor Royston for the microphotographs of immunofluorescence of lymphocytes shown in Figure 17-8; and Dr. James G. White for the electron micrographs of platelets shown in Figure 23-1. I am also grateful to Mrs. Frances Otto-Depner, who took several of the new microphotographs of blood cells used in the second edition. I am also indebted to Drs. Serapheim Masourides and Thomas Lane, who reviewed Chapter 30, Transfusion Therapy, to Dr. Mark Hyman Rapaport, who read early drafts of many of the chapters, to Ms. Michelle Lambert for assistance with the illustrations, and to Ms. Angela Wakeham for expert editorial and secretarial assistance.

Writing the second edition used up most of my spare time for 3 years—evenings, weekends, and vacations. With grace and good humor, my wife accepted "working on the damn book" as my overriding preoccupation. For this, dear Joyce—heartfelt gratitude and love.

SAMUEL I. RAPAPORT, M.D.
San Diego, California

Preface to the First Edition

A knowledge of basic hematology is invaluable to the student, house officer, and practicing physician caring for patients with problems in internal medicine. In this book, I have sought to relate clinical findings and treatment to physiologic and pathologic processes, in the belief that this is the way to build a clinical foundation that withstands the stress of difficult diagnostic problems.

Writing a short book has necessitated a somewhat dogmatic and selective approach. In choosing the clinical material to be included, I imposed two requirements: (1) Is the condition common or important enough that most doctors should know something about it (e.g., iron deficiency anemia, the major causes of abnormal bleeding, drug-induced agranulocytosis)? (2) If rare, does it illustrate an important pathogenetic mechanism of disease, a principle of diagnosis or treatment, or how study of an "experiment of nature" has increased our basic knowledge of biology?

For those who might wish to pursue certain topics in greater detail, a few selected references have been listed: review articles or monographs, new material that I thought important at this writing, and a few books on special aspects of hematology. The standard reference texts, which can be found on the shelves of every good medical library, have not been included.

I wish to acknowledge my debt to those colleagues from whom I have learned much hematology, pathology, and internal medicine: Drs. Thomas Brem, Gurth Carpenter, Donald Feinstein, Clement Finch, Peter Hjort, Robert Lukes, William McGehee, Paul Owren, and Jesse Steinfeld.

I also wish to thank those who helped me to write this book: Dr. Helen Martin, whose course in Survey of Diseases at the University of Southern California School of Medicine inspired the approach of this book; Dr. George Anday, for the karyogram and karyotype shown in Figure 16-3; Dr. Joseph Goodman, for the electron microscopic picture of a platelet shown in Figure 25-1; Mr. Lloyd Matlovsky, for taking the microphotographs; Mrs. Lynda Dümmel and Miss Mary Jane Patch, for preparing the figures; Mrs. Ruth Crandall, for helping to prepare the blood and bone marrow slides; and Mrs. Arlene Sherman, for superb secretarial assistance.

Preparation of this book consumed the spare time of many evenings, weekends, and holidays over the past few years. To my wife, Joyce, and my sons, Mark and Bruce, from whom this time was taken, my gratitude and love.

S.I.R.
Los Angeles, California

Contents

Introduction to
Hematology

1

Erythropoiesis

STAGES OF DIFFERENTIATION

The marrow contains *pluripotent stem cells* possessing two functional properties: an ability to give rise to new stem cells (i.e., self-renewal), and an ability to differentiate into any one of the blood cell lines. With beginning differentiation a stem cell loses its pluripotent potential and becomes directed toward the production of one or more cell lines. Its capacity for self-renewal is also lost, and the stem cell becomes a *progenitor cell.* Although committed to a given blood cell line, a progenitor cell has not yet acquired distinctive features permitting its recognition as a member of that cell series by conventional morphologic techniques. Rather, it is recognized by its ability to give rise to a colony of differentiated progeny of that series in in vitro cultures.

The stages of red blood cell (red cell, RBC) differentiation (Fig. 1-1) may be divided as follows:

1. *Progenitor cells*
   a. Burst forming units-erythroid (BFU-E). BFU-E are the most primitive erythroid progenitor cells. They form very large colonies of thousands of nucleated erythroid percursors in culture.
   b. Intermediate forms (see below).
   c. Colony forming units-erythroid (CFU-E). CFU-E are the most differentiated erythroid progenitor cells. They form small colonies of up to 64 nucleated erythroid precursors on culture.
2. *Morphologically recognizable nucleated precursors.* These are

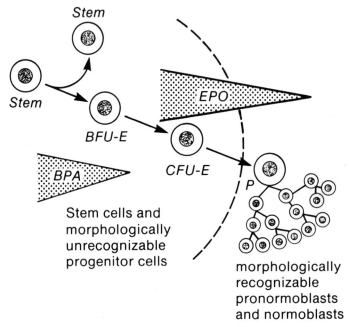

Fig. 1-1. A diagram illustrating stages of erythropoiesis and their regulation. Amplification of erythropoiesis occurs through proliferation of progenitor cells, but for simplicity of illustration a single BFU-E is shown differentiating into a single CFU-E and a single CFU-E into a single pronormoblast. Abbreviations are: BFU-E, burst forming unit-erythroid; BPA, burst-promoting activity; CFU-E, colony forming unit-erythroid; EPO, erythropoietin; P, pronormoblast.

categorized from their appearance on an aspirate smear of bone marrow stained with a methylene blue-eosin stain (e.g., Wright's stain) as follows:

a. *Pronormoblast.* This earliest recognizable RBC precursor is a large cell with blue cytoplasm and a nucleus that occupies most of the cell. The nucleus has fine punctate chromatin and contains one to several small blue nucleoli.

b. *Normoblast.* Three stages of increasing differentiation are recognized:

    (1) *Basophilic.* The cell has lost its nucleoli, and early clumping of nuclear chromatin is seen. The cytoplasm is still deep blue because of its high RNA content.

    (2) *Polychromatophilic.* The cell and its nucleus are smaller. Large clumps of nuclear chromatin are seen. The color of the cytoplasm varies from gray-purple to purple-pink, re-

flecting a decreasing RNA content and an increasing hemoglobin content.

(3) *Orthrochromatic.* The cell is still smaller, and the nucleus has shrunk into a solid black ball. The cytoplasm is definitely pink.

3. *Reticulocyte.* The cell, now almost mature, has extruded its nucleus. However, it still contains residual RNA in its cytoplasm, which can be precipitated into a reticulin network by certain supravital stains (see Fig. 2-11). This gives the cell its name, reticulocyte. Staining for the reticulin network is used to distinguish the reticulocyte from a fully mature RBC.

After fetal life, the human normally makes RBCs only in the bone marrow. In certain disorders, RBCs, white blood cells (WBCs), and platelets may be made outside the bone marrow. This is called *extramedullary hematopoiesis* or, if it is part of an unregulated myeloproliferative disorder, *extramedullary myeloid metaplasia.* The most prominent sites of extramedullary hematopoiesis are the spleen and liver, which are sites of fetal erythropoiesis.

KINETICS

The stem cell-progenitor cell population is self-sustaining, since stem cells both undergo self-renewal and differentiate into BFU-E. Although lacking the capacity for prolonged self-renewal, BFU-E function as an amplifying population capable of extensive proliferation, as well as differentiation into CFU-E. CFU-E also proliferate but, as shown by their behavior in culture, have a more limited capacity for amplification.

The morphologically recognizable erythroid precursor population is not self-sustaining. CFU-E must continually differentiate into pronormoblasts to replace pronormoblasts maturing into later forms. Between the pronormoblast and the late polychromatophilic normoblast stage, the maturing erythroid precursor divides three to five times. Division stops as the build-up of hemoglobin within the cell represses further DNA synthesis. The nucleus is then extruded from the cell. The newly formed reticulocyte normally matures further for 1 to 2 days in the marrow. Because it still possesses mRNA, ribosomes, and a few mitochondria, the marrow reticulocyte continues to synthesize hemoglobin.

The time elapsing from the pronormoblast stage to entrance of the reticulocyte into the circulation is normally 5 to 6 days. Each pronormoblast gives rise to 8 to 32 RBCs. For each 100 circulating RBCs, there are two morphologically recognizable nucleated erythroid precursors and two reticulocytes in the marrow.

REGULATION

Hematopoiesis may be viewed as a two-tiered process in which growth factors prepare early progenitor forms for the effect of later, more specific trophic hormones for a particular lineage. Thus, erythropoiesis requires the successive participation of a growth factor (or factors) needed to initiate the process and a factor required to sustain the process to its end result—the effective formation of RBCs. These factors have been named:

1. Burst-promoting activity (BPA), an activity released within the marrow itself.
2. Erythropoietin, a hormone carried to the marrow in the blood from its site of production in the kidney.

Local marrow conditions modulate the release of BPA. These conditions influence the secretion from marrow monocytes and macrophages of a soluble factor (monokine; see Chapter 14) called interleukin 1 that then stimulates endothelial cells, fibroblasts, and T-lymphocytes within the marrow microenvironment to release BPA. One should understand that BPA is an operational name. Growth factors for hematopoiesis were discovered from their effects on formation of colonies of blood cells in in vitro marrow cultures, and they were given names reflecting these effects. Thus, BPA got its name because it was an activity required for primitive erythroid progenitors (BFU-E) to give rise in culture to large colonies of nucleated erythroid precursors. An activity discovered differently—because it must be present for very early progenitor cells to give rise in marrow cultures to colonies of granulocytes and macrophages—was given the name GM-CSF (granulocyte, macrophage-colony stimulating factor). Purified GM-CSF has now been prepared by recombinant DNA technology. It was found to stimulate formation of granulocyte/macrophage colonies and to function as BPA. However, one should not conclude from this that GM-CSF functions as the only physiologic BPA; other materials could exist that are equally important physiologic sources of BPA.

As differentiation progresses, a series of intermediate erythroid progenitor cells are formed that are less and less responsive to burst-promoting activity and increasingly responsive to the specific trophic hormone, erythropoietin. Presumably, this reflects the progressive loss with differentiation of cell surface receptors for burst-promoting activity and the acquisition of cell surface receptors for erythropoietin. Finally, the most differentiated erythroid progenitor is formed, the CFU-E, which is responsive only to erythropoietin.

In certain circumstances bone marrow lymphocytes can suppress erythropoiesis. When a particular type of lymphocyte is added to in vitro marrow cultures, the number of erythroid colonies formed from CFU-E is reduced. The lymphocyte responsible may be a suppressor T-lymphocyte with cytotoxic properties (see Chapter 14) or a closely related lymphocyte called a natural killer (NK) cell. Suppression of erythropoiesis by lymphocytes is thought important in the pathogenesis of some hypoproliferative anemias (see Chapters 11 and 17). Whether suppressor lymphocytes play a role in the physiologic regulation of erythropoiesis is not yet clear.

Erythropoietin

Despite the need for burst-promoting activity for early differentiation, erythropoietin functions as the major, established, physiologic regulator of erythropoiesis. Differentiation of BFU-E into CFU-E in vivo apparently requires erythropoietin, and CFU-E will not form colonies in vitro in cultures lacking added erythropoietin. Erythropoietin also regulates the rate at which morphologically recognizable erythroid precursors mature and are released from the marrow. Increased amounts of erythropoietin shorten the time required for new RBCs to be made, causing cell divisions to be skipped during maturation and reticulocytes to enter the blood as soon as they are formed. As a result, large RBCs, staining a purplish color because of increased amounts of persisting cytoplasmic RNA (polychromatophilic macrocytes), will be found on a peripheral blood smear (see Fig. 2-4). Their discovery provides a clinical clue that RBC production may be stimulated by increased amounts of erythropoietin.

Erythropoietin is secreted from cells in the glomerulus or juxtaglomerular body of the kidney. Tissue hypoxia stimulates increased release of erythropoietin. The tissue hypoxia may result from a decreased blood hemoglobin content (anemia), from impaired oxygenation of hemoglobin in the lungs (due to high altitude, lung diseases, some congenital heart diseases), or from impaired release of oxygen from hemoglobin at normal tissue oxygen tensions (e.g., when blood carbon monoxide levels are elevated; see Chapter 13).

In end-stage renal disease, normal basal production of erythropoietin is decreased and patients become anemic because of impaired erythropoiesis. However, nephrectomized patients maintained by renal dialysis have diminished but not absent erythropoiesis. Another organ, probably the liver, can supply small amounts of erythropoietin that can support a minimal level of erythropoiesis.

Iron Availability

The developing RBC must make a large amount of hemoglobin (33 g/dL of RBCs). The synthesis of a molecule of hemoglobin requires:

1. The production of two pairs of polypeptide chains of globin (see Chapter 5).
2. The production of four molecules of the oxygen-binding compound, heme. A heme molecule is inserted into each of the polypeptide chains of globin. The synthesis of heme requires:
   a. The production of the tetrapyrrole ring compound protoporphyrin.
   b. The binding of an atom of iron to the protoporphyrin molecule.

The developing normoblast intrinsically possesses everything it needs to make hemoglobin except iron. The plasma transport protein, transferrin, must deliver the iron to the normoblast. A 70-kg man normally needs 21 mg of iron daily for hemoglobin synthesis. Its primary source is iron released to transferrin from the breakdown of senescent RBCs in the mononuclear phagocytic system (reticuloendothelial system). If this man had a sudden major hemorrhage, the kidney would rapidly secrete added erythropoietin into the blood to stimulate erythropoiesis to replace the lost RBCs. For the rate of erythropoiesis to increase threefold, the normoblasts would need not 21 mg but 63 mg of iron daily. Although 21 mg of iron are readily available from the normal daily break down of senescent RBCs, the remaining 42 mg must come from body iron stores. If the stores are low, the rate at which iron can be mobilized will be insufficient to supply the full additional 42 mg. Lack of iron for increased hemoglobin synthesis would then limit the increase in erythropoiesis. Thus, in addition to erythropoietin, the availability of iron regulates the rate of RBC production.

Other Regulatory Factors

Testosterone and related androgenic steroids stimulate erythropoiesis. They apparently act in three ways: by stimulating production of erythropoietin, by potentiating the effect of erythropoietin, and by poorly understood mechanisms independent of erythropoietin. Large doses of androgenic steroids are sometimes given to patients with hypoproliferative anemias in an attempt to increase RBC production.

In compensated hemolytic states, hemoglobin levels remain normal despite increased RBC breakdown because increased RBC production keeps pace with destruction. Since the tissues are not anoxic when the hemoglobin level is normal, it is not clear how increased erythropoietin release can be responsible for maintaining the increased RBC production. Consequently, a second mechanism for stimulating RBC production has been postulated but has yet to be identified.

SYNTHESIS OF HEME

The initial and final steps of protoporphyrin synthesis (Fig. 1-2) and the incorporation of iron into protoporphyrin to form heme take place within the mitochrondria. The intermediate steps of protoporphyrin synthesis take place outside the mitochondria in the soluble portion of the cytoplasm (the cytosol). The mitochrondria encircle the nucleus of the erythroid precursor. In certain disorders iron that fails to be incorporated into heme accumulates within the mitochondria as a ring of coarse granules around the nucleus (ring sideroblasts; see Fig. 11-2).

Most of the mitochondria are extruded from the cell with the nucleus, and the few remaining mitochondria are lost within a day or two after the RBC enters the circulation. Thus, the mature RBC, lacking both RNA and mitochondria, can synthesize neither the globin chains nor the heme moiety of hemoglobin. The enzymatic reactions leading to the formation of heme may be summarized as follows:

1. Succinyl CoA, formed in the mitochondria in the Krebs cycle, combines with glycine to form δ-aminolevulinic acid (δ-ALA). The enzyme catalyzing this reaction, δ-ALA synthetase, is rate limiting for heme synthesis. Pyridoxal phosphate is needed as a coenzyme for the reaction.
2. Two δ-ALA molecules combine to form a pyrrole compound, porphobilinogen.
3. Four porphobilinogen molecules are linked together to form a tetrapyrrole ring compound called uroporphyrinogen.
4. Successive decarboxylations of the side chains of uroporphyri-

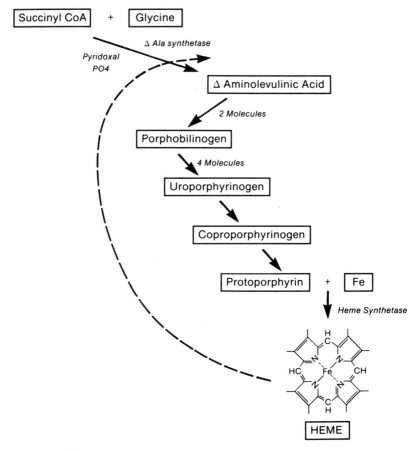

Fig. 1-2. The steps of heme synthesis and a schematic representation of the ring structure of the heme molecule. The dotted line represents feedback inhibition of protoporphyrin synthesis by heme.

nogen lead to the formation first of a compound called coproporphyrinogen and then of protoporphyrin. The enzyme catalyzing the latter reaction is a mitochondrial enzyme.

5. An atom of ferrous iron is added to protoporphyrin to form heme. This reaction is catalyzed by the enzyme ferrochelatase (heme synthetase).

As heme accumulates, it decreases further protoporphyrin synthesis through feedback inhibition of production of the first enzyme of the reaction sequence, δ-ALA synthetase. When the normoblast contains insufficient iron for normal heme synthesis, this feedback inhibition is impaired, and excess protoporphyrin accumulates within the RBC. Measuring RBC protoporphyrin has come into increasing use as a simple screening test for iron-deficient erythropoiesis (see Chapter 3).

SELECTED READING

1. Eaves AC, Eaves CJ: Erythropoiesis in culture. Clin Haematol 13:371, 1984.
2. Finch CA: Erythropoiesis, erythropoietin, and iron. Blood 60:1241, 1982.
3. Mangan KF, Hartnett MF, Matis SA, Winkelstein A, Abo T: Natural killer cells suppress human erythroid stem cell proliferation in vitro. Blood 63: 260, 1984.

2

Diagnosis of Anemia

CRITERIA

Adults

Anemia is not a diagnosis but a sign of disease. Like fever, it means underlying disease is present and demands an explanation, not just treatment. At sea level, anemia should be suspected in an adult when:

	MEN	WOMEN
Red blood cells ($\times 10^6$ per μL)	< 4.5	< 4.0
Hemoglobin (g per deciliter)	<14.0	<12.0
Hematocrit (per cent)	<41	<37

These lower limits were derived from statistical analysis of tests performed on a large group of normal subjects. A person whose values fall below those listed is much more likely to be anemic than not. However, individuals with values higher than those listed are not necessarily normal. For example, an apparently healthy man had always had a hemoglobin level between 16 and 17 g per deciliter (dL) on yearly physical examinations until one year, when he was found to have a hemoglobin level of 14.5 g per dL. Although this value is still within the "normal" range, it was not normal for this patient, and a search disclosed an underlying cause.

Infants and Children

The infant has a mean cord blood hemoglobin concentration of 16.5 g per dL and a mean venous blood hemoglobin concentration a few hours after birth of 19.0 g per dL. The rise results from a loss of plasma volume in the first hours of life. Erythropoiesis almost stops for several weeks after birth, and the hemoglobin level falls to about 11 g per dL by 6 weeks of age. The normal range at 1 year of age is between 11 and 12 g per dL of blood.

The mean hemoglobin concentration persists at 12 g per dL throughout childhood and rises to 13 g per dL in the young teenager. The difference between the values for men and women cited above appear at puberty and disappear in the elderly. They reflect the effect of increased testosterone secretion on erythropoiesis in the male.

PATIENT HISTORY

The history of an anemic patient should provide the physician with an understanding of:

1. *When the anemia began.* Continuous anemia or bouts of anemia for many years suggest a hereditary disorder, for example, hereditary spherocytosis or sickle cell disease. Anemia of recent onset (e.g., when the patient has had normal blood counts on prior examinations or has been accepted as a blood donor in the past) suggests an acquired disorder.
2. *The severity of cerebral and circulatory symptoms relative to the severity of the anemia.* When anemia develops slowly or has been present for a long period of time, a patient with a hemoglobin level in the 6 to 8 g per dL range may be asymptomatic or complain only of feeling "washed out." In contrast, when an anemia of this severity develops rapidly, a patient will complain of symptoms of cerebral and circulatory distress, for example, light-headedness on standing up, palpitations, and breathlessness on slight activity. A patient taking a beta adrenergic blocking agent (e.g., propranolol) may complain of similar symptoms at a relatively high hemoglobin level, for example, 9 to 10 g per dL, because he or she cannot increase cardiac output effectively in response to the anemia.
3. *The possibility of chronic blood loss.* A patient may slowly lose

great amounts of blood from the gastrointestinal tract and be unaware of bleeding. Therefore, an anemic patient must be questioned carefully for symptoms suggestive of lesions that bleed (peptic ulcer, hiatal hernia, carcinoma of the colon) and for a history of black stools. Women may bleed excessively during menstruation without realizing it. A detailed menstrual history must include information about the length of periods, the number of pads or tampons used, their saturation, the use of double pads, and the passage of clots.

4. *The possibility of episodes of hemolysis.* The patient should be asked specifically about episodes of weakness associated with slight icterus, dark urine, and normal to dark stools. Hemolysis does not produce deep jaundice unless there is complicating liver disease. Jaundice with light stools is never the result of hemolysis.

5. *The presence of neurologic symptoms.* An altered mental state, numbness and burning of the hands and feet, and difficulty in walking because of weakness of the legs or loss of balance should alert the physician to the possibility of subacute combined degeneration of the nervous system and, therefore, of pernicious anemia.

6. *Prior therapy for anemia.* A patient with a severe anemia who has received large amounts of a specific agent for many weeks, for example, repeated injections of vitamin B_{12}, obviously does not have an anemia due to deficiency of the factor he or she has received. Conversely, a patient with a specific deficiency of vitamin B_{12} may have received an injection of vitamin B_{12} from another doctor several days earlier. He or she will still be anemic, but the earlier injection will have altered the characteristic features of the untreated disorder. A patient who has taken iron may still present with an iron deficiency anemia if:
   a. The medication was used irregularly or contained inadequate amounts of iron.
   b. The patient has continued to lose large amounts of iron because of continued heavy blood loss.

7. *Use of other drugs and exposure to toxins.* Because many drugs may cause anemia by a variety of mechanisms, the physician must know about *every* drug the patient has been taking. One should also ask specifically about exposure to lead, benzene, and pesticides.

8. *Dietary history.* In the United States the only two common nutritional deficiency anemias are:

    a. Iron deficiency

      (1) In infants fed only milk for many months.

      (2) In adolescent and young women in whom a diet marginal in total calories and heme iron may supply inadequate dietary iron to keep up with normal menstrual iron loss.

    b. Folate deficiency in the alcoholic with chronic liver disease who has been drinking heavily and not eating, or in the neglected elderly patient existing on a marginal diet.

  9. *Family history and racial background.* Anemia, splenomegaly, or both in other family members arouses suspicion of a hereditary cause for anemia, for example, hereditary spherocytosis or a hemoglobinopathy. Genetic causes for anemia differ in frequency in different ethnic groups. In black patients, one thinks particularly of the possibility of a sickle cell syndrome or of glucose-6-phosphate dehydrogenase (G6PD) deficiency. In ethnic groups from the Mediterranean basin, the Middle East, or Southeast Asia, one thinks particularly of the possibility of a thalassemic syndrome.

  10. *Underlying disease.* Three nonhematologic disorders appear frequently enough as an unexplained anemia to require specific questioning for symptoms suggestive of their presence. These are uremia, chronic liver disease, and hypothyroidism.

PHYSICAL EXAMINATION

The anemic patient deserves a thorough physical examination with attention focused on the following aspects of the examination.

Skin

Pallor alone suggests a nonhemolytic anemia (e.g., iron deficiency anemia); pallor plus slight jaundice suggests an anemia with a hemolytic component (e.g., pernicious anemia, hereditary spherocytosis); and pallor plus petechiae or purpura suggest a disorder with an associated thrombocytopenia (e.g., acute leukemia). Spider angiomas and liver palms may imply anemia due to chronic liver disease. Splinter hemorrhages in the nail beds arouse suspicion of anemia secondary to infective endocarditis or systemic lupus erythematosus.

Eye Grounds

Spectacular hemorrhages may be seen in very severe anemia from any cause. Hemorrhages with white centers may be seen in infective endocarditis. The combination of marked venous dilatation with sausage-like indentations of the veins, hemorrhages, exudates, and sometimes papilledema is an important finding of the hyperviscosity syndrome associated with macroglobulinemia of Waldenström (see Fig. 20-7). Extreme tortuosity of the vessels may be seen in sickle cell anemia.

Mouth

A smooth tongue suggests the possibility of pernicious anemia or severe iron deficiency. Marked hypertrophy of the gums raises the suspicion of acute monocytic leukemia.

Heart

Cardiac dilatation, a forceful cardiac impulse, tachycardia, loud systolic and even diastolic murmurs, and peripheral edema may all result from severe anemia alone. The presence of underlying cardiac disease may be difficult to evaluate until the anemia is corrected. The distinction between a hemic murmur and an organic valvular murmur becomes particularly important when other findings raise the possibility of infective endocarditis.

Abdomen

The combination of dilated abdominal veins and moderate splenomegaly suggests the possibility of congestive splenomegaly secondary to chronic liver disease; the liver need not be palpable. Massive splenomegaly filling the whole left abdomen may occur in chronic myelogenous leukemia, in myelofibrosis with extramedullary myeloid metaplasia, and in certain lymphocytic leukemias or lymphomas (e.g., hairy cell leukemia).

Lymph Nodes

Prominent lymphadenopathy in an anemic patient suggests the possibility of a lymphocytic leukemia or lymphoma, or of an infectious disease involving lymph nodes (e.g., AIDS-related complex, tuberculosis).

Nervous System

The findings of subacute combined degeneration mean pernicious anemia until proved otherwise. Slow return of tendon reflexes alerts one to the possibility of hypothyroidism.

INITIAL LABORATORY EVALUATION

One begins the laboratory investigation of an anemia with simple procedures:

1. A blood count that includes determination of the RBC count, the hemoglobin, the hematocrit, and the RBC indices (of which, as discussed below, the MCV is the key value). Electronic blood counters routinely provide these values. Newer counters also measure variation in RBC size (anisocytosis), for example, as an RBC histogram (Fig. 2-1) or as a calculated value for RBC volume distribution width (RDW, see below).
2. Study of the peripheral blood smear by the physician.
3. A reticulocyte count.

    The purposes of these initial examinations are:

1. To classify the anemia on the basis of RBC cell size.
2. To establish the presence or absence of RBC morphologic abnormalities suggestive of disordered RBC production or hemolysis.
3. To search for morphologic clues to the diagnosis from the WBCs and platelets on the peripheral blood smear.
4. To identify the kinetic basis for the anemia as failure of RBC production, rapid RBC loss, or both.

    The history, physical examination, and this initial laboratory evaluation often yield the diagnosis. At the very least, they provide the information necessary for selecting further laboratory tests with discrimination.

RBC INDICES

Mean Corpuscular Volume

When blood counts were performed manually, the mean corpuscular volume (MCV) was a calculated value obtained by dividing the hematocrit by the RBC count. With the most commonly used method of

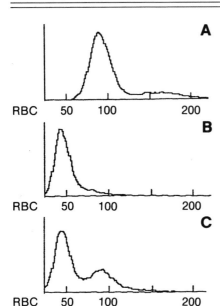

Fig. 2-1. Histograms of red cell volume distribution obtained with an electronic counter (Coulter, Model S Plus IV). The number of red cells is plotted on the y axis and red cell size in fL is plotted on the x axis. (A.) A normal adult. Hgb is 15 g/dL, MCV, 91.5 fL, and RDW 13.5%. (B.) A 15-month-old infant with severe iron deficiency anemia. Hgb is 6.3 g/dL, MCV is markedly reduced to 46.6 fL, and RDW is increased to 25.8%. (C.) The same infant after beginning iron therapy. A second population of normocytic RBCs is now present. Hgb is 10.3 g/dL, MCV 60.5 fL, and because of the second population of cells, the RDW is now markedly increased to 42.4%.

machine blood counting, the MCV is measured directly and very accurately because the intensity of the signal in a counter that an RBC generates varies with its volume. The normal mean value for the MCV is 90 fL (femtoliter or 10^{-15} liter) with a normal range of from 80 to 100 fL. A low MCV means microcytosis, and a high MCV means macrocytosis. Because evaluation of RBC size is key to the diagnosis of an anemia, *the MCV is the most important of the RBC indices.* (Even when the RBC count is normal, one should note the value for the MCV on the blood count report, since an abnormality in mean RBC size may precede the development of overt anemia.)

Mean Corpuscular Hemoglobin

Mean corpuscular hemoglobin (MCH) is the average weight of hemoglobin in the RBC and is calculated by dividing the hemoglobin by the RBC count. The normal range is 27 to 34 pg (picogram, or 10^{-12}

gram). Although the weight of hemoglobin in an RBC depends on both the concentration of hemoglobin within the cell and the volume of the cell, plots of machine-generated values for MCH against machine-generated values for MCV yield a linear correlation over a wide range. Apparently, the concentration of hemoglobin does not change except in conditions with very severely impaired hemoglobin synthesis (see below). Thus, with electronic counting, the MCH has become redundant for the clinician, serving only to confirm the directly measured MCV. It is useful, however, to laboratory personnel as a check of the accuracy of the counter.

Mean Corpuscular Hemoglobin Concentration

Although hemoglobin is present only within the RBC, the RBCs are lysed in measuring the hemoglobin concentration, and the test result is expressed as per dL of whole blood. To convert this value to hemoglobin concentration within the RBCs—the mean *corpuscular* hemoglobin concentration (MCHC)—one divides the hemoglobin by the hematocrit, that is, by the volume of whole blood occupied by the RBCs. The normal range for the MCHC is 32 to 36 g per dL of RBCs (usually written simply as 32%–36%).

Before the advent of electronic counting, a low MCHC was commonly found when the RBCs on a blood smear had an increased area of central pallor, that is, appeared hypochromic. Hypochromia was therefore accepted as visual evidence of a reduced RBC hemoglobin concentration. However, hematocrits obtained manually by centrifuging blood may be falsely high in an anemic patient because of trapping of plasma within the RBC column. When machine hematocrits (calculated from very accurately measured values for the MCV and RBC count) replaced manual hematocrits, normal values for the MCHC were found in patients whose RBCs were moderately but definitely hypochromic on the blood smear. Apparently, moderate hypochromia stems not from a reduced RBC hemoglobin *concentration* but from the presence of RBCs that are smaller and thinner than normal.

Paradoxically, correcting the hematocrit error by converting to machine-generated values for the MCHC has diminished the clinical usefulness of the MCHC, since it is no longer abnormal in early iron deficiency anemia. A low MCHC by machine counting is found only in patients with markedly impaired hemoglobin synthesis, for example, the patient with very severe iron deficiency anemia or the patient with a major thalassemic disorder. Since such patients are readily identified by a markedly reduced MCV and striking hypochromia on the blood smear (see Fig. 2-10), the MCHC has also become a redundant determination.

Red Cell Distribution Width

Newer counters display histograms of RBC volume distribution curves (Fig. 2-1). A determination called the red cell distribution width (RDW) is also included in the printout from the Coulter counter. The RDW, which is the coefficient of variation of the normally gaussian-shaped RBC volume distribution histogram, is determined by dividing the standard deviation of the MCV by the MCV and multiplying by 100 to convert the value to a percentage. Thus, the RDW provides a quantitative measure of variation in size of the circulating RBC (anisocytosis). Its normal value is 13.5 $\pm$ 1.5%.

PERIPHERAL BLOOD SMEAR

One must know how to evaluate a peripheral blood smear to work up an anemic patient optimally. Looking at RBC indices on the blood count report does not replace looking at the blood smear. The morphology of the RBC on the blood smear (Fig. 2-2) often yields important additional information.

RBC Morphology

RBCs are best evaluated on a blood smear made by the slide method. One looks a short distance inside the feather edge of the smear for fields where individual RBCs just touch each other (Fig. 2-3). Fields in the feather edge or in the thick portion of the smear are unsatisfactory. While looking at the RBCs one asks the following questions:

1. How does the appearance of the RBCs on the blood smear amplify the information about RBC size obtained from the MCV and RDW?
2. Are polychromatophilic macrocytes frequently seen? As discussed in Chapter 1, finding polychromatophilic macrocytes on a blood smear (Fig. 2-4) usually means that erythropoiesis has been stimulated by increased amounts of erythropoietin. It also usually means that the rate of RBC production is increased. However, small numbers of polychromatophilic macrocytes, of-

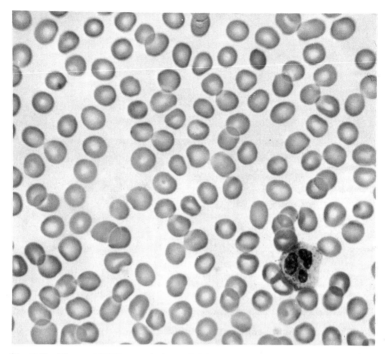

Fig. 2-2. Normal RBC morphology. RBCs are round with little variation in size. A central pale area is seen in most cells because the normal RBC is a biconcave disc.

ten accompanied by proportionately large numbers of nucleated RBCs, may be found on the blood smear in the absence of an increased rate of RBC production in disorders that allow immature hematopoietic cells to escape readily into the circulation (e.g., marrow infiltrative disease with extramedullary myeloid metaplasia).
3. Are there morphologic changes suggestive of disordered RBC production or of a hemoglobinopathy? For example:
   a. *Oval cells and teardrop forms,* which are seen in megaloblastic anemias (Fig. 2-5) and in myelofibrosis with extramedullary myeloid metaplasia.
   b. *Siderocytes,* which are cells containing nonhemoglobin iron as bunched ferritin granules (Fig. 2-6) and which may indicate impaired hemoglobin synthesis not due to iron deficiency.

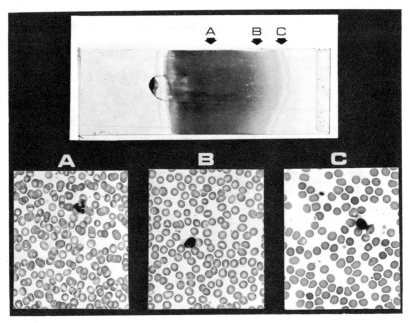

Fig. 2-3. The different appearance of RBCs on different portions of the same blood smear. In the feather edge *(C)*, normal cells lose their central pallor and look like spherocytes. In the thick portion *(A)*, clumping prevents evaluation of individual RBCs. Inside the feather edge, fields are found *(B)* in which individual RBCs just touch. RBC morphology can be evaluated in fields like this.

    c. *Target cells,* which are cells whose membranes are too large for the cells (Fig. 2-7) and which are found in patients with liver disease, in patients with hemoglobins C, E, or S, and in thalassemic syndromes.

    d. *Basophilic stippling,* which results from precipitation of ribosomal RNA. The increased amounts of RNA in polychromatophilic macrocytes occasionally precipitate during staining of a blood smear with Wright's stain. This gives rise to *fine basophilic stippling,* a finding of no significance beyond that of the polychromatophilic macrocyte itself. However, in certain disorders of erythropoiesis, such as lead poisoning and thalassemia, RBCs may contain residual abnormal aggregates of ribosomal material that precipitate during staining as *coarse basophilic stippling* (Fig. 2-8).

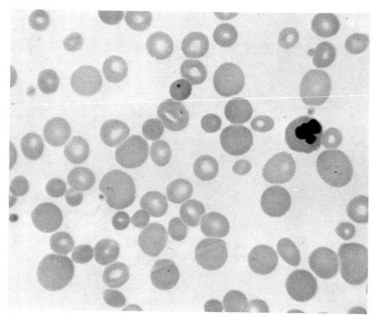

Fig. 2-4. Polychromatophilic macrocytes and spherocytes on a blood smear from a patient with an acute, acquired autoimmune hemolytic anemia. A single nucleated RBC with an atypical cloverleaf nucleus is also seen.

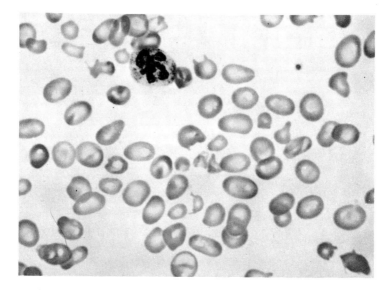

Fig. 2-5. Oval macrocytes plus smaller cells, including teardrop forms, on a blood smear from a patient with pernicious anemia. Also note the hypersegmented polymorphonuclear leukocyte.

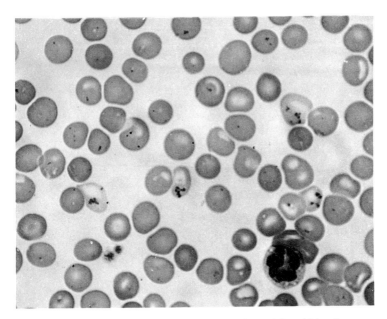

Fig. 2-6. Many siderocytes are present on this peripheral blood smear. The iron is seen as coarse, bunched granules, usually in cells that appear to contain less hemoglobin than other RBCs on the smear.

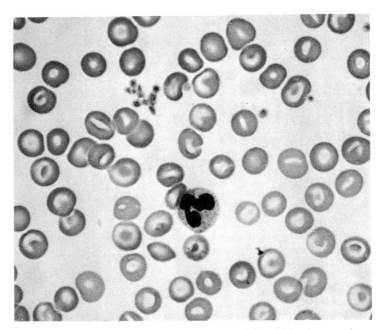

Fig. 2-7. Macrocytes and target cells on a peripheral blood smear from a patient with chronic liver disease.

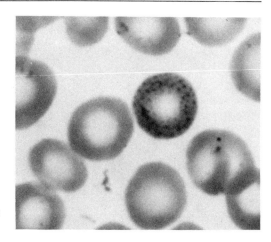

Fig. 2-8. Coarse basophilic stippling in an RBC of a patient with lead poisoning.

Other Findings

Obviously the WBC on the blood smear should also be examined carefully. Immature WBCs raise the possibility of leukemia or other marrow infiltrative disease. Hypersegmented WBCs are a key finding in the megaloblastic anemias (see Fig. 2-5). The number and appearance of the platelets must be evaluated. Large, bizarre platelets are sometimes seen when the marrow is infiltrated by tumor or leukemic cells. Rouleaux (see Fig. 20-5) indicate hyperglobulinemia and raises the possiblity of an immunoproliferative disorder.

CLASSIFICATION OF ANEMIAS BY CELL SIZE

Although overlaps exist, the mean size of the RBCs provides important information about the possible cause for an anemia (Fig. 2-9).

Microcytic Anemias (MCV <80 fL)

Microcytosis represents morphologic evidence of a diminished capacity of maturing RBC precursors to make hemoglobin. This can result from:

1. *Insufficient iron* reaching normoblasts for normal hemoglobin synthesis, as when:
   a. Total body iron content is reduced (iron deficiency anemia).
   b. Release of iron from mononuclear phagocytes is impaired de-

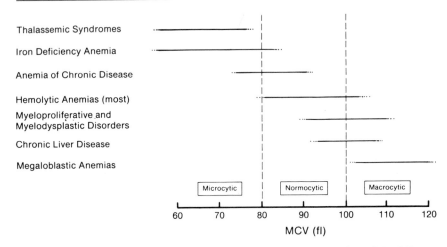

Fig. 2-9. The range of values for the mean corpuscular volume (MCV) in different types of anemia.

spite an adequate total body iron content (anemia of chronic disease).

2. Hereditary genetic defects that diminish synthesis of one of the polypeptide chains of globin (thalassemic syndromes).

3. Uncommon disorders impairing the function of enzymes catalyzing heme synthesis, as in:

   a. Rare types of sideroblastic anemia in which one or more steps in the synthesis of protoporphyrin are impeded (see Chapter 11).

   b. Lead poisoning, because lead impairs the function of the enzyme ferrochelatase, which catalyzes incorporation of iron into protoporphyrin.

A mild to moderate microcytic anemia, with a hemoglobin level in the range of 10 to 12 g per dL, usually results from iron deficiency, from the anemia of chronic disease, or from a mild thalassemic syndrome. The RDW may provide a clue to the cause, since it often is increased in iron deficiency anemia but normal in the anemia of chronic disease and in mild thalassemic syndromes. Definitive evaluation requires examination of iron availability for erythropoiesis and of iron stores (as described in Chapter 3).

A severe microcytic anemia, with an MCV below 70 fL and with microcytosis and hypochromia of the degree seen on the blood smear illustrated in Figure 2-10, has only one common cause in the United

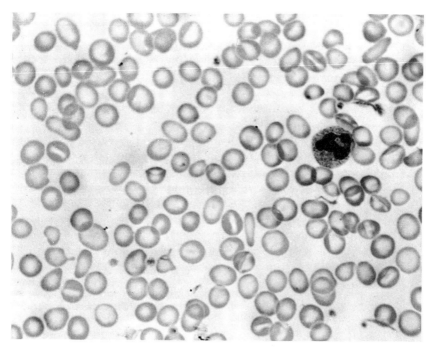

Fig. 2-10. Hypochromic, microcytic RBCs on a peripheral blood smear from a patient with severe iron deficiency anemia secondary to chronic blood loss.

States—*iron deficiency*. Another cause—one of the severe thalassemic syndromes—is rare in the United States except in communities in which large numbers of members of ethnic groups from the Mediterranean basin, Middle East, or Southeast Asia may reside.

Normocytic Anemias (MCV 80–100 fL)

The large group of normocytic anemias may be subdivided as follows:

1. *Normocytic anemias without abnormally shaped RBCs (poikilocytes) or polychromatophilic macrocytes.* The RBCs look normal (see Fig. 2-2) although slight hypochromia or slight microcytosis is sometimes noticed. (This is because the RBCs in the anemia of chronic disease may vary from normocytic to microcytic.) The RDW is normal. The lack of poikilocytosis rules out conditions with disordered erythroid maturation; the lack of polychromatophilic macrocytes means that the marrow is not being stimulated

by erythropoietin to increase RBC production. Disorders producing this type of anemia include:

  a. Chronic infectious and inflammatory states.
  b. Malignancies (unless there has been chronic blood loss or bone marrow invasion).
  c. Chronic renal disease.
  d. Endocrine hypofunction (hypopituitarism, hypothyroidism, hypogonadism).
  e. Marrow suppression by drugs or toxins.

2. *Normocytic anemias with prominent poikilocytosis and occasional polychromatophilic macrocytes.* Disorders that markedly disturb erythrocyte maturation frequently produce this pattern. Sometimes, however, the RBCs are predominantly macrocytic instead of normocytic. Such disorders include:

  a. The leukemias.
  b. Myelofibrosis with extramedullary myeloid metaplasia (see Chapter 16).
  c. Myelodysplastic syndromes with refractory anemia (see Chapter 11).
  d. Carcinoma invading bone marrow.

3. *Normocytic anemias with numerous polychromatophilic macrocytes.* Very large numbers of polychromatophilic macrocytes strongly suggest hemolysis. (Sometimes the polychromatophilic macrocytes will be so numerous that the MCV rises into the macrocytic range.) Often, but by no means always, other alterations in red cell morphology signifying hemolysis are also present (see Fig. 2-4).

Macrocytic Anemias (MCV >100 fL)

Macrocytes result from skipped divisions during RBC maturation and are found in disorders of erythropoiesis with abnormal *nuclear* maturation and also when RBC production is stimulated by erythropoietin (polychromatophilic macrocytes). The macrocytic anemias fall into two morphologic categories:

1. *Macrocytic anemias with oval macrocytes and teardrop cells.* These morphologic findings of markedly disordered erythropoiesis are found in:

  a. Megaloblastic anemias, in which one also finds hypersegmented neutrophils on the blood smear (see Fig. 2-5).
  b. Myelofibrosis with extramedullary myeloid metaplasia, in

which one also finds a scattering of nucleated RBCs, immature WBCs, and large platelets on the blood smear.
2. *Macrocytic anemias with predominantly round macrocytes.* This
type of macrocytic morphology is found in:
   a. Chronic liver disease, in which macrocytes are uniform and
   target cells may be frequent (see Fig. 2-7).
   b. Patients treated with cytotoxic chemotherapeutic agents.
   (Some of these drugs may also induce megaloblastic changes
   with oval macrocytes.)
   c. Aplastic anemia and myelodysplastic refractory anemia (some
   patients).
   d. Myxedema.
   e. Hemolytic anemias with such marked reticulocytosis that the
   MCV is macrocytic (see Fig. 2-4).

The routine measurement of the MCV by means of machine
counting has led to the discovery of patients with an increased MCV
but no or only minimal anemia. Some of these patients will be in an
early stage of a disorder that would progress to a full-blown macrocytic anemia if left untreated, for example, early vitamin B_{12} deficiency. Others are patients who drink excessive amounts of alcohol,
yet may have no evidence of two known alcohol-related causes for
macrocytosis—alcoholic liver disease and folate deficiency. The macrocytosis disappears if such a patient stops drinking.

THE RETICULOCYTE COUNT

One can assess effective RBC production simply because the RBC is
"labeled" for the first 24 to 36 hours of its circulating life. It still
possesses residual RNA, which certain dyes, such as new methylene
blue, will precipitate. The precipitate may form clumps or a fine
reticulin network (Fig. 2-11), hence the name reticulocyte. Since the
new RBC remains a reticulocyte for only 1.0 to 1.5 days and the RBC
circulates normally for 120 days, blood normally contains about one
reticulocyte per 100 RBCs (50,000 to 75,000 per μL).

Reticulocytes are counted by noting the number seen while
counting 1,000 RBCs. Results are usually expressed simply as a percentage (number per 100 RBCs). This may give a false impression of
the number of new RBCs. For example, a patient with an RBC count
of 1 million per μL and an uncorrected reticulocyte count of 5% has
the same number of circulating reticulocytes (50,000 per μL) as a

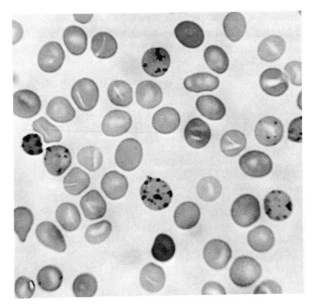

Fig. 2-11. Appearance of reticulocytes in a permanent preparation stained with brilliant cresyl blue.

patient with an RBC count of 5,000,000 per μL and an uncorrected reticulocyte count of 1%.

Therefore, when the laboratory reports the reticulocyte count as an uncorrected value, one should convert the result either into an absolute number or into a corrected reticulocyte percentage. For the former, one multiplies the observed reticulocyte count in percent by the RBC count/100; for the latter, one multiplies the observed reticulocyte count in percent by the patient's hematocrit/45 (normal hematocrit value). Thus, in the example cited above of a patient with an RBC count of 1 million per μL (hematocrit of 9%) and an uncorrected reticulocyte count of 5%, the absolute reticulocyte count would be $5 \times 1,000,000/100$ or 50,000 per μL, and the corrected reticulocyte count would be $5 \times 9/45$ or 1%.

When RBC production is stimulated by increased amounts of erythropoietin, newly made reticulocytes are released into the circulation without first maturing for 1 to 2 days in the marrow. Therefore, they retain precipitable RNA and will stain as reticulocytes for 2 to 3 days, rather than for 1.0 to 1.5 days. Consequently, when polychromatophilic macrocytes are seen on the blood smear, the corrected reticulocyte percentage should be divided by 2. The final value in percent after this further correction, which is called the *reticulocyte index,* provides an estimate of the rate of effective erythropoiesis as a multiple of the normal rate of one. For example, a patient with a reticulocyte index of 3 has an effective erythropoietic rate of three times normal.

Reticulocyte Levels and Anemia

ELEVATED RETICULOCYTE COUNTS

Modestly elevated uncorrected reticulocyte counts may result from the escape of immature RBCs into the circulation in the absence of increased production of RBCs. This occurs primarily in infiltrative marrow disorders associated with prominent extramedullary erythropoiesis. Immature RBCs escape not only from the marrow, but also from sites of production in the sinusoids of the liver and spleen. A reticulocytosis from this cause can be recognized because:

1. The absolute number of reticulocytes after correcting for polychromasia (or the reticulocyte index) is not increased.
2. Scattered RBCs on the Wright-stained smear have a blue cast indicative of disordered maturation with loss of the nucleus in a cell containing very little hemoglobin and much residual RNA.
3. Nucleated RBCs are often present on the smear in numbers greater than expected from the degree of reticulocytosis. (Nucleated RBCs are also found on blood smears from patients with hemolysis and markedly increased RBC production, but these patients will also have very high corrected reticulocyte counts.)

Anemia with a prominent reticulocytosis that gives an elevated absolute reticulocyte count after correcting for polychromasia (or an elevated reticulocyte index) suggests the following possibilities:

1. *Hemolysis.* In severe hemolysis the RBC count may fall despite a very high reticulocyte count. In acute hemolytic states, RBC production can increase to about five times its normal basal rate. In chronic hemolytic states with an expanded active marrow space, RBC production may increase up to about eightfold.
2. *Acute blood loss.* After acute blood loss, the uncorrected reticu-

locyte count doubles within 24 hours owing to a shift of marrow reticulocytes into the peripheral blood. After several days, the reticulocyte count rises further up to a maximum reticulocyte index of about 3, which reflects an increased rate of erythropoietin-stimulated RBC production. The higher reticulocyte counts of hemolytic states are not achieved because the iron made available for RBC production by increased RBC breakdown in hemolytic states is not available for RBC production after acute blood loss (see Chapter 1).

3. *Response of a "starved" marrow to specific replacement therapy.* When anemia stems from the lack of a specific factor needed to make RBCs (e.g., iron, vitamin B_{12}, folic acid), a brief burst of accelerated RBC production occurs when the missing factor is supplied. The resultant reticulocytosis is evidence that the anemia was caused by a deficiency of the specific factor supplied.

DEPRESSED RETICULOCYTE COUNTS

A markedly depressed corrected reticulocyte count (e.g., 0.1% or 0.2%) in an anemic patient arouses suspicion of:

1. Very serious marrow disease, for example, marrow aplasia or replacement of erythroid precursors by leukemic cells.
2. Marked temporary depression of erythropoiesis by an infectious agent, toxin, or drug (e.g., chloramphenicol, an alkylating agent).

NORMAL RETICULOCYTE COUNTS

A "normal" corrected reticulocyte count is not normal in an anemic patient, because the marrow should respond to anemia by increasing effective RBC production. Thus, a normal corrected reticulocyte count means that the anemia stems at least partly from a failure of the marrow to respond to the anemia. Causes include:

1. Lack of a specific factor needed to make RBCs, as in iron deficiency.
2. Failure to increase erythropoietin production, as occurs in chronic renal disease.
3. Both of the above, as may occur in the anemia of chronic disease.

EVALUATION OF RBC DESTRUCTION

RBC Morphology

Hemolysis is frequently associated with evidence of damaged or otherwise abnormal RBC on the peripheral blood smear. One looks for the following:

1. *Spherocytes.* These are RBCs that are round instead of biconcave because they have lost pieces of their cell membrane. On the smear they appear smaller in diameter than normal RBCs and denser, without the normal central area of pallor (see Fig. 2-4). Discovery of spherocytes is presumptive evidence of hemolysis but two notes of caution apply:
   a. Normal RBCs may look like spherocytes in the feather edge of the smear (see Fig. 2-3). RBC morphology must be evaluated in an area of the smear where the RBCs just touch each other.
   b. Small numbers of spherocytes may be noted on the blood smear after transfusions.
   Sometimes it is difficult to be sure if significant spherocytosis is present. *Osmotic fragility* studies are then helpful. Spherocytes cannot swell as much as normal cells because the cell membrane is too tight. Thus, they lyse at concentrations of hypotonic saline solution that fail to lyse normal cells, that is, they exhibit increased osmotic fragility.
   Spherocytosis indicates increased RBC destruction because:
   a. The process leading to spherocytosis in some cells may often directly destroy other cells.
   b. Spherocytes are sequestered and destroyed by mononuclear phagocytes in the spleen, liver, and other organs.
   Finding spherocytes does not pinpoint the cause for hemolysis. Spherocytes may be found in hereditary spherocytosis, which is a group of genetic disorders affecting the RBC membrane skeleton protein, spectrin; in acquired autoimmume hemolytic anemia, a disorder in which macrophages attack RBC membranes coated with antibody; and in clostridial septicemia, a condition in which a bacterial toxin damages the RBC membrane.
2. *Fragmented RBCs.* Mechanical damage to RBCs leads to hemolysis characterized by fragmented, irregularly contracted cells (helmet cells, triangular cells, twisted cells) plus a scattering of

spherocytes (Fig. 2-12). Such mechanically damaged cells are produced:

a. In disorders in which fibrin is deposited in small blood vessels (e.g., thrombotic thrombocytopenic purpura, hemolytic-uremia syndrome); as the RBCs move through such vessels they stick to the fibrin and pieces of the RBCs break off.

b. In an occasional patient after insertion of a prosthetic heart valve.

3. *Ghost cells.* With marked intravascular hemolysis, broken cells that have lost their hemoglobin may be found on the blood smear.

4. *Agglutinated cells.* When hemolysis is caused by an RBC antibody (e.g., a cold agglutinin), clumps of agglutinated cells are sometimes noted on the smear. These clumps are different from rouleaux, in which the red cells line up and look like stacks of coins.

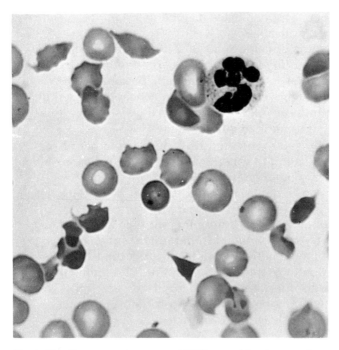

Fig. 2-12. Numerous fragmented RBCs on a blood smear from a patient with thrombotic thrombocytopenic purpura.

5. *Sickled cells.* In sickle cell disorders some RBCs may become irreversibly sickled. Since such cells cannot revert to a normal shape when blood is exposed to the oxygen of room air, they will be found on the blood smear (Fig. 2-13).
6. *"Bite cells."* Oxidative damage to hemoglobin causes aggregates of precipitated hemoglobin to form in cells (Heinz bodies, see below). As cells containing such precipitates pass through the red pulp of the spleen, mononuclear phagocytes may remove these aggregates, leaving RBCs that look as if a bite has been taken out of them (Fig. 2-14).

Although the discovery of one of the above abnormalities on the blood smear indicates that hemolysis is contributing to the pathogenesis of an anemia, the failure to find abnormal RBCs on the smear does not rule out hemolysis.

Since hemolysis usually calls forth a vigorous marrow response,

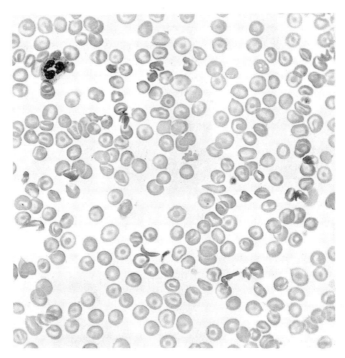

Fig. 2-13. Sickled cells and target cells on the peripheral blood smear of a patient with Hgb SC disease.

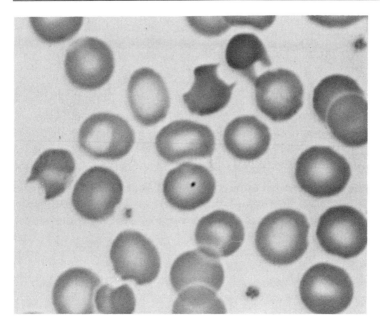

Fig. 2-14. Bite cells on the peripheral blood smear of a patient who developed hemolysis while receiving the oxidant drug dapsone for treatment of leprosy.

one also expects to find many polychromatophilic macrocytes on the blood smear (see Fig. 2-4). In a severe hemolytic crisis, many nucleated RBCs may also be found on the blood smear.

Reticulocyte Count

As already mentioned, the corrected reticulocyte count is usually high. Occasionally, however, the marrow fails to respond, and the reticulocyte count is low. In this situation, the hematocrit falls extremely rapidly, and the patient is often desperately ill.

The stain used for the reticulocyte count will also stain Heinz bodies, which, because they are aggregates of precipitated hemoglobin, stain red with Wright's stain like the rest of the hemoglobin in the cell and, therefore, are not usually visible on the blood smear. Heinz bodies are characteristically located at the RBC membrane (Fig. 2-15). The discovery of large numbers of Heinz bodies while doing the reticulocyte count arouses suspicion of hemolysis secondary

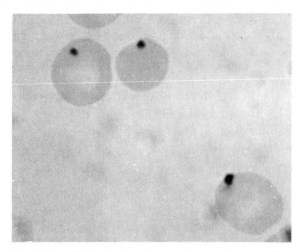

Fig. 2-15. Heinz bodies in a wet mount preparation stained with methyl violet.

to glucose-6-phosphate dehydrogenase (G6PD) deficiency or to an unstable hemoglobin.

Plasma and Urine Pigments

Hemolysis produces serum and urinary pigment patterns that vary, depending on whether the hemolysis is primarily extravascular or intravascular.

EXTRAVASCULAR HEMOLYSIS

Extravascular hemolysis means hemolysis resulting from an increased phagocytosis of RBCs by mononuclear phagocytes in the spleen, liver, and bone marrow. Since senescent RBCs are normally removed by this mechanism, the pigment changes of extravascular hemolysis represent an exaggeration of the normal pigment pattern.

When hemoglobin is catabolized in a macrophage, the globin is broken down to amino acids that are reused; the iron is split from the heme and reused; but the protoporphyrin molecule is broken down and excreted. The ring structure of the protoporphyrin molecule opens, and a straight-chain tetrapyrrole called biliverdin is formed.

Biliverdin is reduced in the macrophage to bilirubin. The bilirubin then enters the plasma, where it binds to albumin and, therefore, is measured as indirect-reacting bilirubin. The liver removes the bilirubin and converts it to bilirubin glucuronide, which is measured as direct-reacting bilirubin. The bilirubin glucuronide is excreted in the bile. Intestinal bacteria convert the bilirubin to urobilinogen, which is excreted in the feces; however, a small amount of urobilinogen is reabsorbed. Most of this is reexcreted by the liver into the gut, but a small fraction is excreted in the urine.

Each gram of hemoglobin gives rise to 35 mg of bilirubin. Since about 6 g of hemoglobin are normally broken down daily, about 200 mg of bilirubin must be excreted daily. The normal liver can handle this load without difficulty; consequently, serum normally contains less than 0.2 mg of direct-reacting bilirubin and less than 0.8 mg of total bilirubin per dL. About 150 mg of urobilinogen are excreted daily in the stools. Normal urinary excretion does not exceed 4 mg per 24 hours. In extravascular hemolysis, the normal removal mechanism may be operating at as high as 10 times the normal rate. The resultant markedly increased bilirubin load produces the following:

1. *In the plasma,* an elevation of the indirect bilirubin. Levels may reach 3 to 4 mg per dL but do not rise higher unless there is associated impaired liver function.
2. *In the urine,* an increased excretion of urobilinogen, which makes the urine turn darker on standing. The urine does not contain bilirubin, because bilirubin bound to albumin (indirect bilirubin) is not normally excreted into the urine.

In addition, since hemolysis that is primarily extravascular often has a small associated intravascular component, plasma haptoglobin levels may fall (see below).

INTRAVASCULAR HEMOLYSIS

About 10% of the normal daily breakdown of RBCs occurs intravascularly. Therefore, about 0.6 g of hemoglobin is liberated each day into the plasma. The hemoglobin molecule, made up of two pairs of polypeptide chains ($\alpha_2 \beta_2$), breaks down in plasma into $\alpha\beta$ dimers. The dimers bind immediately to a globulin with a high affinity for hemoglobin dimers called *haptoglobin*. Hepatic parenchymal cells remove the haptoglobin–hemoglobin dimer complex from the circulation. Consequently, normal plasma hemoglobin levels are very low, less than 5 mg per dL. Binding to haptoglobin prevents excretion of dimers into the urine, and, therefore, conserves the 1.5 mg of iron that would otherwise be lost into the urine each day from the intravascular breakdown of 0.6 g of hemoglobin.

Normal plasma haptoglobin concentration, measured as the amount of added hemoglobin that a serum sample can bind, is about 150 mg per dL. Massive intravascular hemolysis overwhelms this hemoglobin-binding capacity. As a result the following occurs:

1. *In the plasma*
    a. Haptoglobin disappears owing to its conversion to haptoglobin–hemoglobin dimer complexes and the hepatic removal of such complexes faster than new haptoglobin can be produced.
    b. Free dimers of hemoglobin and methemoglobin (hemoglobin whose iron is oxidized to the ferric state) are found and give the plasma a pink to purple color. The free dimers may:
       (1) Be excreted in the urine.
       (2) Be taken up by hepatic parenchymal cells and by mononuclear phagocytes.
       (3) Dissociate within the plasma to form ferriheme (oxidized heme) and globin.
    c. *Methemalbumin* is formed. Ferriheme in plasma binds to a globulin having a high affinity for free heme called *hemopexin*. However, the heme-binding capacity of hemopexin is soon exceeded, and the ferriheme then binds to albumin, giving rise to methemalbumin.

       Methemalbumin appears within about 5 hours after the onset of intravascular hemolysis and persists for 24 to 48 hours. During this interval, methemalbumin gradually gives up its heme to new hemopexin synthesized by the liver. The slow disappearance of methemalbumin contrasts with the rapid disappearance of hemoglobin and methemoglobin, which are cleared from the plasma within about 6 to 12 hours after an episode of acute intravascular hemolysis. Therefore, methemalbumin, rather than free plasma hemoglobin, is the plasma pigment one looks for when seeking evidence that an episode of intravascular hemolysis, for example, a transfusion reaction, may have occurred 12 or more hours earlier. (Methemalbumin, which gives plasma a muddy brown look, can be readily quantitated spectroscopically.)
2. *In the urine*
    a. *Hemoglobinuria.* The hemoglobin and methemoglobin dimers that are filtered into the urine are excreted when the amount filtered exceeds the limited capacity of the tubule cells to

reabsorb dimers. The resultant hemoglobinuria causes the
urine to turn reddish-purple to black in color.

b. *Hemosiderinuria.* Reabsorbed dimers are broken down within
the renal tubule cells. Therefore, when intravascular hemolysis is chronic, iron accumulates within the tubule cells as
hemosiderin granules. The tubule cells are shed into the
urine, producing hemosiderinuria, which can be demonstrated by staining the urinary sediment for iron. Consequently, whereas hemoglobinuria is found in acute, massive
intravascular hemolysis, hemosiderinuria is the hallmark of
chronic intravascular hemolysis.

Lactic Acid Dehydrogenase

RBCs contain lactic acid dehydrogenase (LDH). When circulating
RBCs undergo hemolysis or when RBC precursors undergo intramedullary hemolysis (ineffective erythropoiesis; see Chapter 6),
plasma LDH levels rise. Therefore, plasma LDH is often measured
to confirm suspected hemolysis and occasionally is used to monitor
changing rates of hemolysis.

SELECTED READING

1. Bessman JD, Gilmer PR Jr, and Gardner FH: Improved classification of
   anemias by MCV and RDW. Am J Clin Pathol 80:322, 1983.
2. Gartner LM, and Arias IM: Formation, transport, metabolism and excretion of bilirubin. N Engl J Med 280:1339, 1969.
3. Hillman RS, and Finch CA: Red Cell Manual, 5th ed. Philadelphia, FA
   Davis, 1985.

3

Iron Deficiency Anemia

IRON METABOLISM

Distribution Of Body Iron

A normal man weighing 70 kg has about 3.5 g (50 mg per kg) of iron in his body, and a normal woman weighing 60 kg has about 2.1 g (35 mg per kg) of iron in her body. The vast majority of this iron is present within cells as:

1. Heme iron, which is iron chelated to the porphyrin ring prosthetic group of proteins involved in oxygen transport (hemoglobin), oxygen storage (myoglobin), and oxygen activation in biologic oxidations (heme tissue enzymes).
2. Storage iron in the form of ferritin and hemosiderin.

At any moment a few mg of iron are present in the plasma and extracellular fluid, bound to the iron transport protein, transferrin. This iron is primarily en route to normoblasts in the bone marrow for incorporation into heme.

IRON IN HEME

Iron in hemoglobin makes up the great bulk of heme iron. Each gram of hemoglobin contains 3.4 mg of iron. Thus, a 70-kg man with 15 g of Hgb per 100 mL of blood and a blood volume of 5000 mL will have:

3.4 mg/g × 15g/100 mL × 5000 mL = 2550 mg of hemoglobin iron

In addition, he will have about 150 mg of heme iron in muscle myoglobin and about 15 mg in trace heme tissue enzymes (cytochromes, catalases).

IRON IN STORES

Iron stores in normal men are 500 to 2000 mg; the amount gradually rises with age. Average iron stores for normal young American women are estimated as 250 mg, but about 25% of young American women have no iron stores. After menstruation ceases, iron stores in women rise.

Iron is stored as:

1. *Ferritin,* which is made up of subunits of a protein, apoferritin, arranged as a shell around a central storage cavity. Variable amounts of iron are present in the storage cavity as microcrystals of ferric hydroxyphosphate. Iron moves freely into and out of the storage cavity through channels in the protein shell and, thus, is readily available for metabolic use. Individual ferritin particles are too small to be seen by light microscopy.

2. *Hemosiderin,* which is made up of precipitated aggregates of ferritin whose protein component has been partially degraded. The aggregates are visible as granules that stain golden-brown with hematoxylin-eosin and stain blue with a specific iron stain (Prussian blue reaction). Iron is more slowly released from hemosiderin for metabolic use.

Iron is stored normally in two types of cells: in macrophages of the liver, spleen, and bone marrow, and in hepatic parenchymal cells. When a normal individual is in positive iron balance, the stores increase in both macrophages and hepatic parenchymal cells.

In disease states with abnormally increased iron stores, different tissue storage patterns have been observed:

1. Accumulation of iron within hepatic parenchymal cells (and later within the parenchymal cells of other organs such as the pancreas and heart) but not within macrophages. This pattern is found in hemochromatosis, a disorder of failure of mucosal regulation of absorption (see below) in which many grams of excess iron may accumulate within the body.

2. Accumulation of iron within macrophages but not within hepatic parenchymal cells. This pattern is found in patients receiving multiple transfusions for aplastic anemia, a disorder in which erythropoiesis ceases because hematopoietic stem cells have been destroyed or suppressed. Iron is liberated within the macrophages during the breakdown of transfused RBCs and stays within the macrophages because its release to support production of new RBCs is not needed.

3. Accumulation of iron both within macrophages and within hepatic parenchymal cells. This pattern is found in patients with anemias characterized by chronic ineffective erythropoiesis (e.g., thalassemic syndromes). Iron accumulates from multiple transfusions and, to a lesser extent, from increased dietary absorption (see below). Iron flow through the plasma is increased because macrophages release large amounts of iron to support an augmented but defective RBC production. As a consequence, the excess iron is distributed both within macrophages and hepatic (and later other) parenchymal cells.

Iron Loss

The body conserves iron; loss is negligible, amounting in a normal man to about 0.9 mg per day from cells shed into the gut and urinary tract and from the skin. *Only when blood is lost* are significant amounts of iron lost from the body. One dL of blood contains about 50 mg of iron in hemoglobin (15 g Hgb per dL × 3.4 mg iron per g Hgb). Therefore, a simple way to estimate changes in body iron content from loss or gain of blood is to assume that 2 mL of blood contain 1 mg of iron.

Women normally lose 30 to 90 mL of blood during a menstrual period (mean loss, 45 mL). A woman's daily iron loss from other sources is estimated as 0.6 mg. If one adds to this an increment to compensate for monthly menstrual iron loss, a woman's daily iron loss may be considered to be 1.1 to 2.1 mg (average, 1.3 mg).

Iron Absorption

AVAILABILITY FOR ABSORPTION OF DIETARY IRON

The American diet contains about 7 mg of iron per 1000 calories. Dietary iron varies in its availability for absorption. Iron in meat, which is iron in the heme of myoglobin and hemoglobin, is readily available for absorption, apparently as the intact heme molecule. However, most dietary iron is non-heme iron, for example, iron in wheat and eggs. Non-heme iron is of limited availability for absorption because it may form insoluble complexes in the stomach with phosphates, tannates, and oxalates from food and insoluble polymers of ferric hydroxide in the alkaline medium of the duodenum. Therefore, both the total caloric intake and the content of the diet determine the adequacy of dietary iron supply.

In health, only enough iron is absorbed from the diet to balance daily iron loss (0.6–2.1 mg) and to allow the accumulation of up to 2000 mg of iron stores over the course of a lifetime. In women, most of this storage iron accumulates after menstruation ceases. Indeed, the diet of a substantial fraction of American women contains insufficient absorbable iron to allow them to accumulate any iron stores during their menstrual years. When the body absorbs iron from a good diet as avidly as possible (as occurs in iron deficiency anemia), the amount absorbed increases to only between 3 and 4 mg per day.

Iron is absorbed primarily in the duodenum and upper jejunum. Gastric surgical procedures in which the stomach is connected to the jejunum (gastroenterostomy), with resultant bypass of the absorptive surface of the duodenum, impair the absorption of dietary iron. Injury to the mucosa of the upper small intestine, as occurs in celiac disease, also impairs absorption of dietary iron.

REGULATION OF ABSORPTION BY THE INTESTINAL MUCOSA

Transferrin, the iron transport protein, and *ferritin*, the iron storage protein, are both present in intestinal mucosal cells, and their balance within the cell is thought to regulate iron absorption. Mucosal cell transferrin moves iron from the gut lumen into the mucosal cell and from the cell into the blood. Mucosal cell ferritin binds iron within the cell. Such bound iron is passed back into the intestinal lumen when the mucosal cell dies and is shed.

Mucosal cell transferrin increases in conditions in which plasma transferrin levels rise—namely, iron deficiency anemia and pregnancy—and supports increased absorption of iron in these states. This is "appropriate," since added body iron is needed in these conditions for increased erythropoiesis and for the growing fetus. However, iron absorption is also increased in certain chronic anemic disorders in which the marrow uses increased amounts of iron for increased ineffective erythropoiesis (see Chapter 6). In this circumstance, increased intestinal absorption is "inappropriate," since the body contains adequate iron from the break down of the ineffectively made RBCs to support the increased erythroid activity. Presumably, increased absorption in this circumstance also stems from an increased concentration or function of mucosal cell transferrin, but the signal mechanism for this is not clear.

Mucosal regulation limits iron absorption to the amount needed to replace daily iron loss—0.6 to 2.1 mg instead of the 3 to 4 mg that might otherwise be absorbed from a normal diet. Failure of mucosal regulation to prevent maximal iron absorption from the diet, as in hemochromatosis, can lead over years to the accumulation of many grams of excess body iron.

Even with a normal mucosal regulatory mechanism, excess iron may accumulate in the body from increased absorption in two circumstances:

1. If large amounts of iron are ingested over a long time, for example, if a patient takes unnecessary medicinal iron for many years as a "tonic".
2. In lifelong anemic disorders with marked ineffective erythropoiesis in which, as mentioned above, the mucosa receives a continuous signal to absorb iron maximally.

Internal Iron Circuit

The RBC's life span is 120 days. Therefore, each day the mononuclear phagocytic system of an adult with a blood volume of 5000 mL removes the RBCs of 42 mL of blood (1/120 of 5000 mL equals 42 mL). Since 2 mL of blood contain 1 mg of iron, 21 mg of iron are transferred daily from RBCs to macrophages (Fig. 3-1).

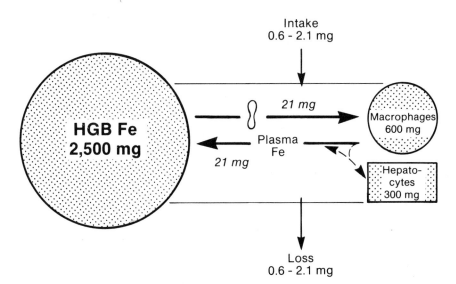

Fig. 3-1. Closed circulation of iron within the body.

At equilibrium, an equal number of new RBCs are made, which means that at least 21 mg of iron must return each day from macrophages into maturing RBCs. This iron is carried back to the marrow in the plasma, bound to transferrin. Receptors on the developing RBC bind transferrin, which is then taken into the cell, releases its iron, and moves back out of the cell to reenter the plasma.

The amount of iron that passes through the plasma in 24 hours, which is called the *plasma iron turnover*, can be calculated from the plasma iron concentration, the plasma volume, and the plasma iron clearance (the rate of disappearance of a trace amount of radioactive iron that has been complexed in vitro to transferrin and then injected intravenously). The plasma iron turnover for a 70-kg man is not 21 mg—the expected value if all iron moving through the plasma were incorporated into circulating RBCs—but 30 mg.

About 2 mg of the excess can be accounted for by iron incorporated into hemoglobin of faulty red cells that are destroyed before they circulate (ineffective erythropoiesis). An additional, variable portion of the excess may reflect flow of iron to non-erythroid tissues, particularly the liver. Hepatocytes possess high-affinity receptors for transferrin, and when the plasma iron concentration is high, a significant fraction of plasma iron turnover may reflect movement of iron from plasma transferrin into hepatocytes. Finally, a portion of the excess may reflect error due to diurnal variation in the plasma iron level. The plasma iron level affects the ratio in the plasma of diferric transferrin (transferrin containing two iron atoms per molecule) to monoferric transferrin (transferrin containing one iron atom per molecule). The two forms of transferrin differ in their efficiency of delivery of iron to tissues and, therefore, in their effect upon the measurement of plasma iron clearance.

EVALUATION OF IRON DEFICIENCY

Body iron deficiency may be divided into three stages that represent arbitrarily selected points on a continuum of manifestations of increasing iron depletion. These are:

1. *Depletion of iron stores*, which may be recognized by:
   a. The absence of stainable iron in macrophages in the bone marrow.
   b. A low serum ferritin level.

   c. An elevated total iron binding capacity (TIBC) of the plasma
     (see below).
2. *Iron deficient erythropoiesis.* At this stage, insufficient iron is
  supplied to developing red cell precursors for normal hemoglobin synthesis, but the patient is not yet frankly anemic. In addition to the abnormalities listed above, one finds:
    a. A substantially reduced percent saturation of transferrin with
      iron (see below).
    b. An elevated free erythrocyte protoporphyrin (FEP).
    c. Beginning microcytosis (MCV approaching or already slightly
      below 80 fL).
3. *Iron deficiency anemia.* At this stage, all of the above findings
  are present, and the hemoglobin level has fallen below the normal range. As the anemia worsens, microcytosis increases, anisocytosis becomes increasingly apparent, and abnormally shaped
  cells indicative of disordered erythropoiesis, for example, elon-
  gated cells, called "pencil cells", are found on the blood smear
  (see Fig. 2-10).

    The interpretation of the tests used to evaluate body iron status
are discussed further in the following sections.

Bone Marrow Iron

On low-power microscopic examination of a histologic section of a
bone marrow particle or a needle biopsy specimen of normal marrow
stained for iron (Prussian blue stain), one will see dark blue granular
material scattered throughout the marrow. This is storage iron (hemosiderin) within macrophages (Fig. 3-2). It diminishes and then
disappears as a patient becomes iron deficient. With rare exception,
the presence of storage iron within macrophages rules out body iron
deficiency as a cause for an anemia.

    If one looks with an oil-immersion objective at aspirate smears
of normal marrow stained for iron, one can also see tiny blue-staining
dots, which are aggregates of ferritin, in the cytoplasm of many normoblasts. This is not storage iron, but iron awaiting incorporation into
hemoglobin. Normoblasts containing such stainable iron are called
sideroblasts. Abnormal sideroblasts containing coarse iron granules
(see Fig. 11-2) are found in several disorders of erythropoiesis in
which hemoglobin synthesis is impaired for reasons other than iron
deficiency.

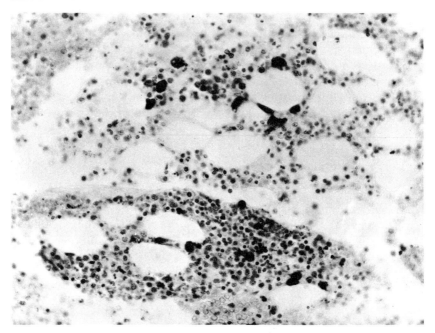

Fig. 3-2. Iron stain of bone marrow particle showing increased amount of iron. Iron, which stains dark blue, appears here as black granules. The patient, an elderly woman with diabetes, episodes of vomiting, and a history of tarry stools, was admitted to the hospital in ketoacidosis. Hematocrit was 31%, RBCs were microcytic, stools contained occult blood, and serum iron was 36 µg per dL (6.6 µmol per L) with a total iron-binding capacity of 170 µg per dL (31 µmol per L). The increased iron in her bone marrow established that iron deficiency was not contributing to the cause for her anemia and confirmed that her low serum iron level was secondary to chronic infection or inflammation.

Serum Ferritin

Minute amounts of ferritin, measured in µg per liter (L), are present in plasma and can be quantitated by immunologic techniques. This ferritin, which either is secreted from or leaks out of macrophages, has an intravascular half-time of only 5 to 10 minutes and is cleared from plasma primarily by hepatic parenchymal cells. Its physiologic function, if any, is unknown. However, its presence in plasma provides a convenient method for assessing iron stores, since the amount of ferritin present in plasma mirrors the amount of ferritin present in macrophages.

Mean values for serum ferritin in *normal subjects* are about 35 μg per L in women and about 100 μg per L in men. Mean values rise to about 160 μg per L in older people of both sexes. When the serum ferritin level is less than 12 μg per L, iron will not be seen in the macrophages of the bone marrow, that is, iron stores are depleted. In healthy persons whose serum ferritin level is above 12 μg per L, one may estimate tissue iron stores in mg by multiplying the number for the serum ferritin level by ten. For example, a healthy man with a serum ferritin of 100 μg per L would have 1000 mg of tissue iron stores.

In *sick patients*, a serum ferritin level of less than 12 μg per L also means depleted iron stores, but a value above 12 μg per L does not rule out depleted stores because:

1. Chronic inflammatory disease serves as a stimulus for macrophages to synthesize ferritin independent of tissue iron stores.
2. In patients with hepatocellular disease, for example, alcoholic liver disease or viral hepatitis, ferritin from injured liver cells escapes into the plasma.

Studies relating serum ferritin levels to bone marrow iron content in various chronic disorders suggest that serum ferritin levels in sick patients without liver disease (for example, a patient with rheumatoid arthritis or a patient on chronic hemodialysis in whom blood loss during hemodialysis requires periodic assessment of iron stores) may be interpreted as follows:

1. Less than 30 μg per L—iron stores depleted.
2. Between 30 and 50 μg per L—iron stores probably depleted.
3. Between 50 and 150 μg per L—iron stores uncertain.
4. Above 150 μg per L—iron stores present.

Plasma Iron and Total Iron Binding Capacity

Plasma iron circulates bound to transferrin. A diurnal variation exists; plasma iron levels in the morning may be one third higher than levels in the evening. For diagnostic purposes, the serum iron level is measured in blood drawn in the morning from a fasting patient. Its normal range is 75 to 150 μg per dL.

Transferrin is not measured in the clinical laboratory as mg of protein but indirectly as the amount of iron that a serum sample can bind. This value, called the total iron binding capacity (TIBC), is the sum of the value for the serum iron determination plus the amount of additional iron that the transferrin in the serum sample can bind. A normal TIBC of 300 μg per dL corresponds to a transferrin protein concentration of approximately 250 mg per dL. Transferrin is normally about one-third saturated with iron (Fe/TIBC × 100 = 33%).

In an otherwise healthy person, the TIBC rises as iron stores fall; an *elevated TIBC*, like a *low* serum ferritin, represents evidence of storage iron depletion. Unfortunately, just as for serum ferritin, the presence of chronic disease complicates interpretation of the TIBC. Chronic disease depresses transferrin levels, and so the TIBC usually fails to rise in a patient with both iron deficiency and chronic disease.

The serum iron level reflects a balance between iron release from macrophages and iron uptake by normoblasts. The serum iron level falls:

1. In iron deficiency, because the macrophages are depleted of iron.
2. In chronic infections and inflammatory states, because although the macrophages contain plenty of iron, its release is impaired.
3. Transiently, when there is a sudden burst of erythropoiesis (for example, immediately after a patient with vitamin B_{12} deficiency megaloblastic anemia is treated with vitamin B_{12}), because the large number of erythroid precursors starting to mature at once remove iron at a rate temporarily exceeding its release from macrophages.

In iron deficiency, the TIBC level rises as the plasma iron level falls and, therefore, the saturation of transferrin falls below 15%. In chronic disease, the plasma iron level and the TIBC both fall; consequently, the saturation of transferrin usually does not fall below 15%. However, it does fall below 15% often enough to prevent one from using this value as a reliable cutoff point that distinguishes iron deficiency anemia from the anemia of chronic disease.

Free Erythrocyte Protoporphyrin

In the last step of heme synthesis, iron is incorporated into protoporphyrin to form heme. Protoporphyrin in the RBC (usually referred to as free erythrocyte protoporphyrin, or FEP, even though it is measured in the RBC as zinc protoporphyrin) can now be quantitated simply and rapidly on a drop of blood by a fluorescent technique with an instrument called a hematofluorometer. Normal levels are less than about 35 μg per dL of whole blood. Protoporphyrin accumulates in the RBC when:

1. Iron supply to the RBC for incorporation into heme cannot keep up with the rate of protoporphyrin synthesis. This occurs in both iron deficiency anemia and the anemia of chronic disease.
2. The activity of ferrochelatase, the enzyme catalyzing incorporation of iron into protoporphyrin, is impaired, as occurs in lead poisoning. (The FEP is widely used as a screening test for exposure to lead.)

Measuring FEP is simpler and cheaper than determining transferrin saturation and serves as an equally valid indicator of iron deficient erythropoiesis. Because the test can be performed rapidly on the same sample of blood taken for a blood count, it has proved particularly useful as a presumptive test for iron deficiency in small children.

CAUSES OF IRON DEFICIENCY

Infants

A newborn infant weighing 3.4 kg (7.5 lb) will possess 250 mg of iron, of which about about 185 mg will be iron in hemoglobin, about 25 mg (7 mg per kg) will be tissue iron in myoglobin and heme tissue enzymes, and about 35 mg will be iron in stores. At 1 year of age, an infant weighs about 10.5 kg. If the infant absorbed no iron at all from the diet during the first year, he or she would have 250 mg of iron minus 74 mg (7 mg per kg of persisting tissue iron × 10.5 kg) or 176 mg of iron available for hemoglobin synthesis. The total hemoglobin would be 51 g; the blood volume would be 840 mL (8% of body weight); and the hemoglobin level would be approximately 6 g per dL.

The mean hemoglobin level of normal infants at 1 year of age is 11.5 g per dL. Thus, the normal infant absorbs enough iron to synthesize the difference between 6 and 11.5 g of hemoglobin per dL or a total of 46 g of hemoglobin (5.5 g per dL × 8.4 dL). This requires the absorption of 156 mg of iron during the first year of life.

Milk is a poor source of iron, containing only 0.5 mg per L of which only about 10%, or 0.05 mg per L, is absorbed. At large metropolitan hospitals, many infants between the ages of 9 and 24 months have been seen with severe iron deficiency anemia. Usually these infants have been fed almost entirely on milk. Often such babies have also been born with a low total body iron content for one or more of the following reasons:

1. Prematurity. The fetus receives most of its iron during the last trimester of pregnancy, and each day of prematurity robs the fetus of 3 to 4 mg of iron.
2. Severe iron deficiency in the mother. This causes the mother's plasma iron level to fall and so hinders transfer of iron across the placenta.
3. Twin births, with resultant competition for maternal iron.
4. Fetal blood loss at delivery.

Moreover, some infants fed large quantities of whole cow's milk develop a hypersensitivity to proteins in cow's milk that lasts for several months. Continuing exposure to cow's milk during this period causes RBCs and plasma proteins to be lost into the gut from a friable gastrointestinal mucosa. Thus, RBC loss may contribute to the severity of the iron deficiency anemia of infants fed primarily upon cow's milk.

Erythropoiesis decreases sharply in the first few days after birth, and the hemoglobin level falls from 18 g per dL at birth to 11 g per dL by 6 weeks of age. Consequently, the normal infant has plenty of iron from the breakdown of senescent RBCs for hemoglobin synthesis during the first 4 to 6 months. Thereafter, however, the normal infant must absorb 0.8 to 1.0 mg of iron daily to provide for optimal hemoglobin synthesis. Dietary iron is best supplied by commercial, iron-fortified cereals. Feeding such cereals to age 18 months has been suggested to assure optimal iron intake.

Adolescents

The growth spurt of adolescence creates an increased need for iron for erythropoiesis. In boys, increased postpubertal testosterone synthesis further stimulates erythropoiesis and adds to the need for iron. In girls, menstrual iron loss adds to the need for iron. The "junk food" diet of many youngsters provides insufficient dietary iron to meet these physiologic needs and a mild iron deficiency anemia results. The anemia may persist into adult life in some women because of the combination of a continuing iron-poor diet and menstrual blood loss.

Adults

Because the normal daily requirement is so small, it would take years for an adult with normal iron stores to develop an iron deficiency anemia from insufficient iron intake alone. Therefore, discovery of iron deficiency in an adult requires evaluation of the patient for abnormal blood loss.

The patient may or may not be aware of excessive blood loss. In a man, the gastrointestinal tract is the only site from which enough blood may be lost to produce iron deficiency anemia without the patient realizing that he is losing blood. Because of lower or absent iron stores, a woman develops iron deficiency anemia after less blood loss than does a man. One must decide whether iron loss from menstrual bleeding and pregnancies (500 mg per pregnancy) can account for the iron deficiency—and so make a search for a gastrointestinal cause for blood loss unnecessary. Occasionally, a woman may lose as much as 200 mL of blood during a menstrual period and be unaware that she is bleeding unusually heavily.

DIAGNOSIS OF IRON DEFICIENCY ANEMIA

Mild Anemia

A microcytic (MCV <80 fL) anemia with a hemoglobin value in the 9 to 12 g per dL range may represent

1. Iron deficiency anemia.
2. The anemia of chronic disease.
3. A mild form of thalassemia.

Mild thalassemia is readily recognized: the microcytosis (decrease in MCV) exceeds that expected from the value for the RBC count, which frequently is normal despite a reduced hemoglobin concentration; the red cell distribution width (RDW) is not increased; and the FEP is not elevated. In beta thalassemia, the diagnosis can be confirmed by demonstrating an elevated Hgb A_2 level (see Chapter 5).

The diagnosis of iron deficiency anemia can often be made simply by demonstrating that

1. The FEP is elevated (>35 µg per L), which indicates that erythropoiesis is iron deficient.

2. The serum ferritin is low (<12 μg per L), which indicates that iron stores are depleted.

In the anemia of chronic disease, the FEP will also be elevated; erythropoiesis is iron deficient, but for a different reason—impaired iron release from macrophages. However, the serum ferritin level should be greater than 150 μg per L. Diagnostic difficulty arises when serum ferritin values in the 35 to 150 μg per L range are found. Then, one may not be sure whether body iron deficiency is contributing to the anemia of a patient with chronic disease. Two approaches are possible:

1. If the presence or absence of iron deficiency needs to be established without delay, a bone marrow specimen may be examined for stainable iron in macrophages (see Fig. 3-2).
2. If the diagnosis is not urgent, the patient may be given a therapeutic trial of oral iron therapy. A rise in hemoglobin level of 2 g per dL within 4 weeks represents reliable evidence of iron deficiency; a rise in hemoglobin level of 1 g per dL is suggestive but not definitive evidence of iron deficiency.

Severe Anemia

A microcytic anemia with markedly hypochromic and microcytic cells on the peripheral blood smear (see Fig. 2-10) means either iron deficiency or a thalassemic syndrome. In the United States, the latter needs to be considered only in ethnic groups from the Mediterranean basin or from Southeast Asia. Iron deficiency can usually be established without difficulty by demonstrating either a low serum ferritin level or a low percent transferrin saturation. Further diagnostic effort in an adult is then directed toward determining the cause for chronic blood loss.

TREATMENT OF IRON DEFICIENCY ANEMIA

For the adult, the cardinal therapeutic rule is to *correct the cause of the chronic blood loss*. Treating the anemia with iron without discovering the reason for the blood loss could harm a patient, for example, by delaying the discovery of a resectable carcinoma of the ascending colon.

Oral Iron Therapy

The selection of an oral iron preparation and its dosage is based upon the following:

1. Only ferrous iron should be used because it is absorbed much better than ferric iron.
2. About 180 mg of iron should be given daily. (If 20% of the iron is absorbed, this would supply 36 mg, or enough iron to synthesize about 10 g of new hemoglobin daily. In a patient with a 5000-mL blood volume, this would raise the hemoglobin level by 0.2 g per dL daily.)
3. Any ferrous iron salt will be satisfactory; the dosage needed to provide 180 mg of iron will vary with the weight of the non-iron portion of the preparation. No agent is better or cheaper than ferrous sulfate for routine use. A 320-mg ferrous sulfate tablet contains 60 mg iron. Therefore, one tablet is given three times daily, preferably on an empty stomach to avoid binding of iron to complexes in food.

RESPONSE

A rise in hemoglobin level of 2 g per dL in 4 weeks is an acceptable response to oral ferrous sulfate therapy. Treatment should continue, not only until the hemoglobin level has returned to normal, but until iron stores, as measured by the serum ferritin level, have been replaced.

Occasionally, the hemoglobin level fails to return to normal despite seemingly adequate doses of oral iron. Usually the patient has not been taking the iron as instructed. Less frequent causes include:

1. Persistent bleeding that results in the patient continuing to lose substantial amounts of iron.
2. Some reason for impaired gastrointestinal absorption of iron, e.g., concurrent administration of large amounts of an antacid (which will bind iron) as treatment for a peptic ulcer.
3. An additional reason for impaired erythropoiesis, for example, chronic infection.

Parenteral Iron Therapy

Parenteral iron is not often indicated but may be helpful in the following situations:

1. When a patient needs to receive 100 to 250 mg of iron daily, for example, a severely iron-depleted patient with hereditary telangiectasia in whom continued frequent bleeding episodes are expected during the period of iron replacement.
2. When the patient has serious gastrointestinal disease limiting oral replacement therapy, for example, ulcerative colitis or regional ileitis.
3. When the patient has demonstrated that he or she cannot be relied upon to take daily oral iron.

SELECTED READING

1. Bothwell TH, Charlton RW, Cook JD, Finch CA: Iron Metabolism in Man. Oxford, Blackwell Scientific Publications, 1979.
2. Cook JD: Clinical evaluation of iron deficiency. Semin Hematol 19:6, 1982.
3. Finch CA, and Huebers H: Perspectives in iron metabolism. N Engl J Med 306:1520, 1982.
4. Marsh WL, Jr, Nelson DP, and Koenig HM: Free erythrocyte protoporphyrin (FEP) II. The FEP test is clinically useful in classifying microcytic RBC disorders in adults. Am J Clin Pathol 79:661, 1983.

4

Megaloblastic Anemias

Understanding the megaloblastic anemias requires knowledge of two vitamins essential for normal DNA synthesis in rapidly proliferating cells. These vitamins are the cobalamins and folate.

PROPERTIES OF COBALAMINS AND FOLATE

Nomenclature and Structure of Cobalamins

The *cobalamins* are a group of molecules of similar structure, ability to bind to specific binding proteins, and biologic properties. Their structure consists of a nucleotide (5, 6-dimethylbenzimidazole) connected to a porphyrin-like corrin ring, which contains a central cobalt atom. A ligand is attached to this central cobalt atom, and the various cobalamins differ only in this ligand. Although *vitamin* B_{12} is often loosely used as a name for all cobalamins, vitamin B_{12} is the name of a specific cobalamin in which cyanide is the ligand attached to the cobalt (cyanocobalamin). Because vitamin B_{12} is stable, it is the cobalamin available for pharmaceutical use; however, vitamin B_{12} is not found naturally in the human body. The two cobalamins found in humans are:

1. Methylcobalamin, in which a methyl group is the ligand attached to the cobalt.
2. Adenosylcobalamin, in which 5'-deoxyadenosyl is the ligand attached to the cobalt.

Cobalamins participate in two known human metabolic reactions:

1. The conversion of homocysteine to methionine, in which methionine synthase is the enzyme and methylcobalamin is a coenzyme.
2. The conversion of methyl malonyl-coenzyme A to succinyl-coenzyme A, in which methyl malonyl CoA mutase is the enzyme and adenosylcobalamin is a coenzyme.

Microorganisms contain molecules called *cobalamin analogues*, which, although only slightly modified in structure from true cobalamins, cannot replace cobalamin in the above reactions. As discussed later, cobalamin analogues have been identified in human plasma.

Nomenclature and Structure of Folates

Folate is an inclusive term for folic acid and its derivatives. *Folic acid* is a molecule made up of a pteridine double ring attached to para-aminobenzoic acid, which, in turn, is attached to from one to nine molecules of glutamic acid (Fig. 4-1A). An enzyme called *dihydrofolate reductase* reduces folic acid, causing double bonds to be broken and hydride ions to be added at the fifth, sixth, seventh, and eighth positions of the molecule (Fig. 4-1B). The reduced molecule, called tetrahydrofolate, functions as a carrier of single carbon atom units—methyl, methylene, formyl, or forminino groups—which can bind to the N^5, to the N^{10}, or to both positions of the reduced molecule. Different folate coenzymes are thus formed. These coenzymes participate in a number of metabolic reactions involving the transfer of single carbon atom units: the formation of inosinic acid in purine biosynthesis, the catabolism of histidine to glutamic acid, the conversion of serine to glycine, the methylation of homocysteine to form methionine, and the methylation of deoxyuridilate to form thymidylate. As discussed in the next section, these last two reactions are essential for normal DNA synthesis.

COBALAMIN AND FOLATE IN DNA SYNTHESIS

Pathways of Synthesis of Thymidylate

DNA and RNA consist of chains of *nucleotides*. Nucleotides are compounds made up of a nitrogenous base—either a purine (adenine or guanine) or a pyrimidine (cytosine, uracil, or thymine)—joined to a

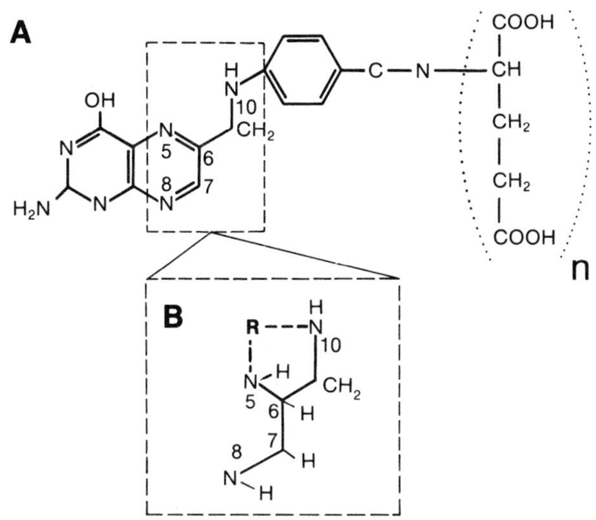

Fig. 4-1. The upper portion of the figure *(A)* is a representation of the folic acid molecule. The pteridine double ring is shown on the left; the para-aminobenzoic acid is positioned horizontally in the center; the glutamic acid molecule is shown on the right. Additional glutamic acid molecules are attached by peptide bonds between successive glutamic acid molecules to form polyglutamates. The key 5, 6, 7, 8, and 10 positions of the molecule have been numbered. In the lower portion of the figure *(B)*, the 5, 6, 7, 8, and 10 positions of the molecule have been enlarged. The reduced, tetrahydrofolate form of the molecule is shown; the double bonds between the 5 and 6 positions and the 7 and 8 positions have been replaced by hydride ions. This then allows different one-carbon fragments, labeled R, to bind to the N^5, the N^{10}, or to both sites of the molecule.

sugar molecule (ribose in RNA, deoxyribose in DNA) and to one or more phosphate groups attached as an ester to the sugar molecule. An intermediate compound, a *nucleoside*, is made up of a base plus a sugar molecule but lacks a phosphate group.

One of the pyrimidine bases of RNA, uracil, is replaced in DNA by *thymine*, which is methylated uracil. Two pathways exist for generating the nucleotide *thymidylate* (the base thymine plus deoxyribose plus a phosphate group) in DNA synthesis:

1. A *salvage pathway* in which the nucleoside thymidine formed during the breakdown of old DNA is phosphorylated to form thymidylate.
2. A pathway involving *synthesis of new thymine*. Uracil present in the nucleotide deoxyuridilate is methylated to yield thymi-

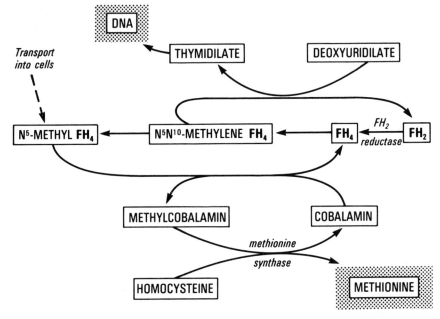

Fig. 4-2. The pathways whereby folate participates in the synthesis of DNA and the synthesis of methionine. Note that N^5-methyl folate must give its methyl group to cobalamin in the synthesis of methionine. Note also that N^5,N^{10}-methylene tetrahydrofolate may be utilized either for DNA synthesis or, by its conversion to N^5-methyl folate, for methionine synthesis. (See text for discussion.) Abbreviations: FH_2, dihydrofolate; FH_4, tetrahydrofolate.

dylate. N^5,N^{10}-Methylene tetrahydrofolate supplies the methyl group for the reaction (Fig. 4-2).

The salvage pathway cannot generate enough thymidylate for DNA synthesis in tissues, such as bone marrow or gastrointestinal epithelium, that rapidly produce new cells; therefore, the proliferating cells must maintain intracellular concentrations of N^5,N^{10}-methylene tetrahydrofolate adequate for methylating deoxyuridilate to thymidylate at rates needed to make the new DNA for normal cell turnover in these tissue.

CAUSES OF INTRACELLULAR N^5,N^{10}-METHYLENE TETRAHYDROFOLATE DEFICIENCY

Intracellular N^5,N^{10}-methylene tetrahydrofolate deficiency can result from:

1. A reduced intracellular folate concentration. This, in turn, can stem from:
   a. Impaired delivery of folate to the cells because of inadequate body folate stores.
   b. Loss of folate from cells because of impaired synthesis of folate polyglutamates, a reaction required to prevent folate from leaking out of cells.
2. Impaired intracellular recycling of N^5,N^{10}-methylene tetrahydrofolate. As can be seen from Figure 4-2, N^5,N^{10}-methylene tetrahydrofolate stands at a metabolic crossroads in that:
   a. N^5,N^{10}-methylene tetrahydrofolate can be utilized as the coenzyme supplying the methyl group to convert deoxyuridilate to thymidylate for DNA synthesis. In so doing, it is oxidized to dihydrofolate. The enzyme dihydrofolate reductase must be available to reduce dihydrofolate to tetrahydrofolate, which can then be converted back into N^5,N^{10}-methylene tetrahydrofolate. Materials that compete with dihydrofolate for dihydrofolate reductase will therefore prevent the recycling of N^5,N^{10}-methylene tetrahydrofolate that has taken this pathway. (The important antimetabolite used in cancer chemotherapy, methotrexate, acts by this mechanism.)
   b. N^5,N^{10}-methylene tetrahydrofolate can be converted to N^5-methyl tetrahydrofolate and so enter a pathway that results in synthesis of methionine. In so doing, N^5-methyl tetrahydrofolate is converted to tetrahydrofolate, which can then be recycled to N^5,N^{10}-methylene tetrahydrofolate. Any process blocking the synthesis of methionine prevents the recycling of N^5,N^{10}-methylene tetrahydrofolate entering this pathway by causing accumulation of N^5-methyl tetrahydrofolate.

LINKAGE OF IMPAIRED METHIONINE SYNTHESIS TO THE AVAILABILITY OF N^5,N^{10}-METHYLENE TETRAHYDROFOLATE FOR THYMIDYLATE SYNTHESIS

As seen in Figure 4-2, inhibition of conversion of homocysteine to methioine can result from:

1. Decreased availability of the coenzyme for the reaction, cobalamin, which accepts the methyl group from N^5-methyl tetrahydrofolate and transfers it to homocysteine. This is a major cause of megaloblastic anemia in man.
2. Inhibition of the enzyme catalyzing the reaction, methionine

synthase. This is the cause for a megaloblastic anemia induced by excessive exposure to the anesthetic gas NO_2.

Impaired synthesis of methionine depletes the cell of N^5,N^{10}-methylene tetrahydrofolate by two mechanisms:

1. *Trapping of folate as N^5-methyl folate.* The cell attempts to compensate for impaired synthesis of methionine by diverting N^5,N^{10}-methylene tetrahydrofolate from the thymidylate synthesis pathway to the methionine synthesis pathway. Folate therefore accumulates in the cell as N^5-methyl folate. Moreover, new folate, which enters cells as N^5-methyl folate, cannot be converted to tetrahydrofolate and then to N^5,N^{10}-methylene tetrahydrofolate. Intracellular folate becomes "trapped" as N^5-methyl tetrahydrofolate useless for thymidylate synthesis.

2. *Diminished synthesis of folate polyglutamates.* The methyl group of methionine serves as a major source of intracellular formate for the formation of N^5,N^{10}-methylene tetrahydrofolate and of two other folate cofactors not shown in Figure 4-2— N^5-formyl tetrahydrofolate (folinic acid or leucovorin) and N^{10}-formyl tetrahydrofolate. These three folate cofactors are the principal substrates for the enzyme converting folate from its monoglutamate form—the form in which it enters the cell —to folate polyglutamates—the form in which the cell can retain folate.

COBALAMIN METABOLISM

Certain bacteria and molds found in water, soil, and the rumen of animals synthesize cobalamin. Man obtains cobalamin from eating animal protein: meat, poultry, fish, and dairy products. An average American daily diet contains 5 to 30 μg. The recommended daily allowance for an adult is 5 μg. Daily body loss, primarily in the feces through biliary excretion, is 1 to 3 μg.

Absorption of Cobalamin

Cobalamin binds to two types of proteins in gastric juice:

1. *Intrinsic factor,* a glycoprotein secreted by the parietal cell of the gastric mucosa. *Binding to intrinsic factor is essential for the absorption of cobalamin.*

2. *R proteins*, which are members of a family of structurally similar cobalamin-binding proteins present in many tissues and body fluids, including saliva, gastric juice, and intestinal fluid. (The first R protein was discovered as an additional cobalamin-binding protein of gastric juice that moved more rapidly on electrophoresis than intrinsic factor; hence, the name R (for rapid) protein.) *Cobalamin bound to R protein cannot be absorbed.*

In the stomach, intrinsic factor and R proteins compete for cobalamin liberated from food. In the small intestine, trypsin in pancreatic juice breaks down R proteins but does not attack intrinsic factor, thus liberating additional cobalamin to bind to intrinsic factor. (Although this process is impaired in patients with severe pancreatic deficiency, the resultant decrease in cobalamin available for binding to intrinsic factor is insufficient to produce clinically significant cobalamin deficiency.) Cobalamin bound to intrinsic factor is absorbed in the presence of calcium ions by attachment of intrinsic factor to specific receptors in the brush border of mucosal cells of the terminal ileum.

From 1 to 10 μg of cobalamin are excreted daily into the bile. Most of this cobalamin is reabsorbed by the same mechanism as for cobalamin from food.

Plasma Cobalamin

Two proteins that bind cobalamin, transcobalamin (TC) I and TC II, were initially identified in plasma. Later, a small amount of a binding protein with an electrophoretic mobility different from either TC I or TC II was also recognized. Called TC III, it was subsequently found to differ from TC I only in its carbohydrate content.

TC II, which is synthesized by the liver, is a key transport protein that carries cobalamin from the plasma and extracellular fluids into cells. It has an intravascular half-life measured in minutes. Cells take up the TC II-cobalamin complex by pinocytosis; proteolysis of the TC II by lysosomal enzymes then frees the cobalamin. Rare infants have been discovered with a severe megaloblastic anemia due to a hereditary deficiency of TC II. This experiment of nature establishes that TC II is essential for normal cobalamin metabolism.

TC I, a member of the family of R proteins, is synthesized within granulocyte precursors and released into plasma from the specific granules of granulocytes. TC I has an intravascular half-life measured in days. The liver slowly catabolizes TC I, with resultant partial excretion of its bound cobalamin into the bile. The role of TC I in cobalamin metabolism is unknown but not essential, since individuals with a hereditary deficiency of TC I have no recognized manifestations of cobalamin deficiency.

Normal plasma cobalamin (vitamin B_{12}) levels are 150 to 800 picograms (pg) per mL. Levels fall below 100 pg per mL in severe cobalamin deficiency. Very high plasma cobalamin levels may result from:

1. Increased production of TC I in conditions with increased granulopoiesis, for example, chronic myelogenous leukemia or polycythemia vera.
2. Liver disease with release of cobalamin from damaged hepatocytes.

Plasma Cobalamin Analogues

Cobalamin analogues have recently been identified in human plasma; their plasma concentration in some individuals approaches that of cobalamin. Their binding properties differ from those of cobalamin. Cobalamin binds equally well to intrinsic factor (its intestinal transport protein), to TC II (its plasma transport protein), and to R proteins. Cobalamin analogues do not bind to intrinsic factor, bind poorly to TC II, but bind readily to R proteins, including the R protein in plasma, TC I.

Cobalamin analogues cannot replace cobalamin in metabolic reactions. Thus, despite their presence in the plasma of patients with pernicious anemia within the range found in normal subjects, they cannot prevent the severe clinical manifestations of cobalamin deficiency of that disease. Moreover, cobalamin analogues may possibly exert deleterious effects, for example, by acting as a cobalamin inhibitor.

The sources of human plasma cobalamin analogues are not fully identified, but include vitamin B_{12} that degrades to cobalamin analogues in stored multivitamin tablets that contain mineral supplements. Habitual use of such tablets may result in significant body uptake of cobalamin analogues despite their inability to bind to intrinsic factor.

One measures "serum vitamin B_{12}" clinically as a substance in serum competing with radiolabeled vitamin B_{12} for a binder. Since cobalamin analogues can bind to R proteins, falsely elevated values for "serum vitamin B_{12}" will be obtained if the binder contains free R proteins. This has caused diagnostic confusion, for example, reports of "vitamin B_{12} levels" within normal limits in patients with pernicious anemia. To prevent this error, a laboratory must use an assay kit in which the binder is either free of R proteins or contains added cobalamin analogue to saturate the binding sites of contaminating R proteins.

Tissue Cobalamin

Tissue cobalamins are found as methylcobalamin and adenosylcobalamin tightly bound to the enzymes required for their coenzyme activities. A storage form of cobalamin does not exist. The total body content of cobalamin varies between 2 and 5 mg (2000 to 5000 μg), of which about 1 mg is found in the liver. Since only 1 to 3 μg of cobalamin is lost daily, it takes 3 to 5 years of failure to absorb cobalamin to induce cobalamin deficiency in a previously normal individual.

FOLATE METABOLISM

Folates are found in fresh green vegetables, many fruits, beans, nuts, liver, and kidney. Folate is lost rapidly during cooking. Heating during canning may also destroy folate. Dietary folate intake varies widely in different socioeconomic groups, reflecting both the content of the diet and its manner of preparation. The normal daily requirement is 50 to 100 μg. Need increases in pregnancy to 400 μg, an amount the diet can provide only if it contains uncooked fruit, fruit juice, or fresh or lightly cooked vegetables.

Absorption of Folate

Folates in food are polyglutamates that must be broken down to monoglutamates before absorption. Enzymes called conjugases, which are present in the brush border of jejunal mucosal cells, catalyze the reaction. No cofactor is needed for absorption of folate, which occurs preferentially in the upper small intestine. As folate is transported through the intestinal mucosal cell, it is converted to N^5-methyl tetrahydrofolate. Sulfasalazine, a compound used to treat inflammatory bowel disease, phenytoin (Dilantin), and oral contraceptives may impair folate absorption with resultant depressed levels of serum and red cell folate in many individuals and megaloblastic anemia in a rare individual.

Plasma Folate

Folate circulates in plasma as N^5-methyl tetrahydrofolate monoglutamate, which is free or only loosely bound to albumin. (This is why a uremic patient receiving hemodialysis treatments loses enough folate into the dialysis fluid to become folate deficient unless given supplemental folic acid therapy.)

Plasma folate is taken up by all tissues but with particular avidity by the liver, where it both participates in metabolic reactions and is stored. The liver releases stored folate for use by other tissues, but only by a circuitous route that involves its excretion into the bile and reabsorption from the small intestine into the plasma. This enterohepatic circulation of folate appears to be necessary to maintain normal plasma folate levels. Thus, when normal subjects are given alcohol, release of folate from liver cells into the bile is impaired, the enterohepatic circulation of folate is interrupted, and plasma folate levels begin to fall within hours.

The normal serum folate level is 6 to 20 nanograms (ng) per mL. When a person stops ingesting folate, the serum folate level falls below 3 ng per mL within 3 weeks. However, tissue stores are not exhausted until several weeks later. Conversely, when a folate-deficient patient begins to eat normally, the serum folate level rises before tissue stores are repleted. The rapidity with which serum folate levels change with diet diminishes the value of serum folate measurements as a test for clinically significant folate deficiency.

Tissue Folate

As already mentioned, folate is present in tissues in the polyglutamate form, the additional glutamyl residues being required for cells to retain folate. RBC folate levels can be measured as a convenient indicator of tissue folate stores. However, RBC folate levels have limited usefulness in the differential diagnosis of a megaloblastic anemia because, as discussed earlier, depletion of either body folate or cobalamin can reduce intracellular folate levels.

Normal tissue stores of folate are estimated as 5 to 10 mg (5000 to 10,000 µg). Since the daily requirement is 50 to 100 µg, tissue stores of folate, unlike tissue stores of cobalamin, are limited in relation to the daily requirement. If a previously normal subject stops ingesting folic acid, he or she will develop a megaloblastic anemia within about 5 months.

MANIFESTATIONS OF COBALAMIN OR FOLATE DEFICIENCY

As already mentioned, the block to normal DNA synthesis imposed by cobalamin or folate deficiency most affects tissues that make new cells rapidly: the bone marrow and the mucosal lining of the gastrointestinal tract. Impaired DNA synthesis can account for the cytologic changes observed in these tissues, namely:

1. The nucleus of the cells has a fine, lacy chromatin pattern with prominent parachromatin spaces. Nuclear maturation appears to lag behind cytoplasmic maturation.
2. The cells are larger than normal, which implies a reduced number of cell divisions during maturation.

Megaloblastic Anemia

The defect in DNA synthesis in hemopoietic cells gives rise to an anemia with characteristic peripheral blood and bone marrow morphology, which is referred to as a megaloblastic anemia. In its early stages, the hemoglobin level may be only minimally reduced and the disorder is recognized by the altered morphology of developing and mature RBCs and granulocytes. As the deficiency state worsens, the anemia becomes progressively more severe. In a patient with advanced megaloblastic anemia, the hemoglobin level may fall to 3 to 4 g per dL.

The *peripheral blood findings* of a megaloblastic anemia are:

1. *RBC.* An *oval macrocyte* well filled with hemoglobin is the characteristic cell. Poikilocytosis is prominent, as is expected in disordered RBC production. Although macrocytes predominate on the blood smear, small teardrop cells are also frequently noted (see Fig. 2-5). The macrocytosis usually results in an MCV in the 110 to 125 fL range. However, in an occasional patient who has both a megaloblastic anemia and iron deficiency, the MCV may be within the normal range (<100 fL). The reticulocyte count is not elevated.
2. *WBC.* A moderate leukopenia is usually found. Large granulo-

cytes (macropolycytes) with hypersegmented nuclei (greater than five lobes) are an early, distinctive feature of the peripheral blood morphology (Fig. 4-3). Regardless of the appearance of the RBCs, one must consider the possibility of a megaloblastic anemia whenever hypersegmented macropolycytes are discovered on a blood smear. Conversely, their absence raises doubts as to the diagnosis despite compatible RBC morphology.

3. *Platelets.* Mild thrombocytopenia is frequent. Rarely, severe thrombocytopenia with bleeding may be encountered.

The characteristic *bone marrow findings* are:

1. *Megaloblastic erythropoiesis* with marked erythroid hyperplasia. The characteristic feature of a megaloblast (Fig. 4-4) is that at each stage of development its nucleus has finer chromatin and more prominent parachromatin spaces than the nucleus of a normoblast of comparable cytoplasmic maturity. Evidence of aberrant nuclear division is also found, for example, erythroid precursors with a cloverleaf nucleus instead of a round nucleus and cells containing a main nuclear mass plus satellite pieces of nuclear material.

The erythroid hyperplasia results from stimulation by erythropoietin. It is associated with increased plasma iron turnover but not with an increased reticulocyte count. Thus, despite the evidence that the marrow is making erythroid precursors more rapidly than normal, new RBCs are not found in increased numbers in the peripheral blood. Erythropoiesis is ineffective, that is, most of the developing RBCs are destroyed

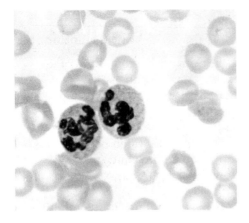

Fig. 4-3. Hypersegmented neutrophils on a blood smear from a patient with pernicious anemia.

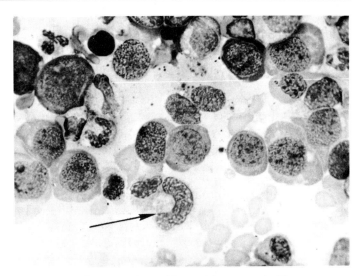

Fig. 4-4. Bone marrow smear from a patient with pernicious anemia. The numerous megaloblasts are readily recognized by their fine nuclear chromatin and prominent parachromatin spaces. The arrow points to a giant metamyelocyte.

within the bone marrow before they mature. (It is believed that enough deoxyuridilate accumulates within the developing RBC that this abnormal nucleotide is incorporated into DNA. This then activates excision and repair mechanisms of DNA to remove the faulty nucleotide—with resultant irreversible damage to the developing RBC.)

2. *Giant metamyelocytes*, the forerunners of the hypersegmented macropolycytes, are always found in truly megaloblastic marrows (see Fig. 4-4) and should be looked for as an important confirmatory finding.

3. *Large megakaryocytes* with more than the usual number of nuclei are frequently noted and, if the patient is thrombocytopenic, imply ineffective thrombocytopoiesis (see Chapter 25).

4. *Iron stores are increased* with prominent coarse hemosiderin granules in macrophages.

The megaloblastic anemia of cobalamin deficiency and of folate deficiency are morphologically indistinguishable in the untreated patient; however, the megaloblastic anemia of folate deficiency is most often seen in the United States in an alcoholic patient whose diet has been deficient in folate and in whom alcohol has imposed a block in folate metabolism. Hospitalization removes the patient from alcohol and provides the patient with a diet containing folate. Consequently, the megaloblastic changes in the bone marrow begin to regress without other therapy. Unless the bone marrow is examined promptly after admission, the marrow of such a patient may appear "dimorphic" with erythroid precursors that appear intermediate between megaloblasts and normoblasts.

Giving appropriate therapeutic doses of cobalamin or folate causes megaloblastic erythroid precursors to disappear from the bone marrow within 3 to 6 days of beginning therapy. Giant metamyelocytes and hypersegmented granulocytes may persist in the bone marrow, and hypersegmented granulocytes may persist in the peripheral blood for about 2 weeks, which is the time required to exhaust the postmitotic marrow pool of these cells (see Chapter 14).

Gastrointestinal Tract Alterations

The impaired DNA synthesis of cobalamin or folate deficiency leads to atrophy of the mucosa of the gastrointestinal tract. Intestinal malabsorption can result, including a secondary malabsorption of cobalamin and folate that can intensify the primary deficiency state.

The adult patient with cobalamin deficiency due to pernicious anemia will invariably have marked *gastric atrophy.* This gastric atrophy, which leads to a failure of secretion of intrinsic factor, is the cause, rather than the result, of cobalamin deficiency. Giving vitamin B_{12} does not reverse the gastric atrophy. In contrast, vitamin B_{12} corrects the secondary mucosal atrophy responsible for the smooth tongue often seen in the patient with pernicious anemia and also responsible for a secondary intestinal malabsorption of cobalamin that may complicate the interpretation of the Schilling test (see below).

In gluten enteropathy (celiac disease, non-tropical sprue) or in tropical sprue, folate deficiency developing as a consequence of malabsorption increases the severity of the malabsorption. Jejunal biopsies show changes of increasing severity reflecting the primary disease process: blunting of intestinal villi, fusion of villi, and finally total villous atrophy. Folate deficiency contributes an additional morphologic abnormality; individual mucosal epithelial cells become enlarged with an empty-looking nucleus ("megaloblastic" changes). Giving folic acid may partially improve clinical manifestations of malabsorption. However, definitive treatment requires management of the primary disorder, which consists of the removal of gluten from the diet in gluten enteropathy or the long-term administration of tetracycline in tropical sprue.

When the folic acid antagonist methotrexate is given to toxicity, DNA synthesis may be so severely impaired that the gastrointestinal epithelium desquamates. A patient may develop multiple, painful ulcers in the mouth and esophagus.

Subacute Combined Degeneration of the Nervous System

As a general rule, *cobalamin deficiency but not folate deficiency* can cause subacute combined degeneration of the nervous system. Since nerve cells do not divide, they do not synthesize DNA. Thus, cobalamin deficiency must damage the central nervous system by a mechanism unrelated to DNA synthesis. Methionine supplies a methyl group for the methylation of myelin basic protein, and blocked methionine synthesis induced by cobalamin deficiency is now thought to cause subacute combined degeneration of the nervous system by impairing the formation of myelin.

This mechanism would explain why subacute combined degeneration occurs only on the rarest occasion in folate deficiency. As mentioned earlier, diminished methionine synthesis diverts N^5,N^{10}-methylene tetrahydrofolate from the thymidylate synthesis pathway to the methionine synthesis pathway (see Fig. 4-2). This would protect against developing subacute combined degeneration in all but most extreme folate deficiency but at the expense of enhancing the development of megaloblastic anemia.

The full-blown neurologic pattern of subacute combined degeneration consists of the following:

1. *Peripheral neuritis*: numbness, burning, tingling of the fingers and toes.
2. *Posterior column damage*: impaired sense of position and vibration, positive Romberg's sign.
3. *Lateral column damage*: spasticity, hyperactive deep reflexes, positive toe signs.
4. *Disturbances of cerebration*.

CLASSIFICATION OF MEGALOBLASTIC ANEMIAS

A classification of megaloblastic anemias based upon the mechanism responsible for cobalamin or folate deficiency is outlined in Table 4-1. In the United States, pernicious anemia is the common cause of megaloblastic anemia due to cobalamin deficiency. Occasionally, me-

Table 4-1. Classification of Megaloblastic Anemias

MECHANISM	DISEASE
MEGALOBLASTIC ANEMIAS DUE TO COBALAMIN DEFICIENCY	
Insufficient dietary intake of cobalamin	
Lack of animal protein in the diet for many years	Tropical macrocytic anemia (rare)
Lack of intrinsic factor	
Failure to secrete intrinsic factor by otherwise normal gastric mucosa	One form of juvenile pernicious anemia (rare)
Failure to secrete intrinsic factor secondary to marked gastric atrophy	Adult pernicious anemia (common)
Surgical removal of cells secreting intrinsic factor	Postgastrectomy megaloblastic anemia
Abnormalities of the ileum	
Disease damaging ileal mucosa	Regional enteritis, tropical sprue*
Surgical removal of cells absorbing cobalamin	Ileal resection
Specific inability to absorb cobalamin in absence of other abnormalities of the ileum	Second form of juvenile pernicious anemia (rare)
Failure of plasma transport	Megaloblastic anemia secondary to hereditary transcobalamin II deficiency (rare)
Inhibition of methionine synthase plus oxidation of cobalamin to cobalamin analogues	Megaloblastic anemia secondary to exposure to nitrous oxide

galoblastic anemia is also seen in patients who have diseases that interfere with absorption of cobalamin in the terminal ileum (for example, regional enteritis). Other causes of megaloblastic anemia due to cobalamin deficiency, for example, an intestinal lesion resulting in bacterial overgrowth or excessive exposure to the anesthetic gas NO_2, are rare. Since even poor diets in the United States contain some animal protein, a megaloblastic anemia due to inadequate dietary intake of cobalamin is virtually unheard of.

In contrast, megaloblastic anemia in the United States due to folate deficiency usually results from poor dietary intake, often combined with the heavy use of alcohol. It also occasionally results from the combination of an increased folate requirement and a suboptimal dietary folate intake. This may be seen in patients with chronic hemolytic disease (for example, sickle cell anemia), in pregnancy, and

Table 4-1. Continued

MECHANISM	DISEASE
MEGALOBLASTIC ANEMIAS DUE TO FOLATE DEFICIENCY	
Reduced intake of folate	
Diet lacking folate often coupled with alcohol-induced block in folate metabolism	Nutritional megaloblastic anemia
Markedly increased requirement for folate	
Chronic hemolysis exhausting folate stores because of increased utilization for RBC synthesis	Megaloblastic anemia complicating thalassemia major, sickle cell disease, other chronic hemolytic states
Increased demand of fetus, sometimes coupled with increased demand of a chronic hemolytic state	Megaloblastic anemia of pregnancy
Abnormal absorption of folate	
Induced by drugs	Megaloblastic anemia induced by phenytoin (Dilantin^R)
Mucosal disease affecting the jejunum	Gluten enteropathy, tropical sprue*
Interference with folate metabolism by drugs competing for dihydrofolate reductase	Megaloblastic anemia induced by methotrexate or by antimicrobial agents (pyrimethamine)

* In tropical sprue, the whole small intestine may be involved. Although the megaloblastic anemia is usually corrected by administration of folic acid and although subacute combined degeneration does not occur, serum vitamin B_{12} levels are frequently low and the Schilling test may reveal evidence of impaired absorption of vitamin B_{12}.

particularly in the patient who is both pregnant and has a hemolytic disorder. Diseases interfering with absorption in the upper small intestine (for example, gluten enteropathy) represent another cause for a clinically significant incidence of megaloblastic anemia due to folate deficiency.

TESTS TO DETERMINE THE CAUSE OF A MEGALOBLASTIC ANEMIA

Although the clinical setting often provides a strong clue to the cause of a megaloblastic anemia, laboratory tests are required to establish whether the anemia stems from cobalamin deficiency or folate deficiency.

Serum Vitamin B$_{12}$ and Folate Levels

Routinely ordering serum vitamin B$_{12}$ and folate levels on every anemic patient, regardless of the morphology of the anemia, wastes money and may yield misleading results. For example, a patient may have an anemia from some other cause yet have a low serum folate level due to a recent poor diet. In contrast, *if examination of the peripheral blood or bone marrow reveals morphologic evidence of a megaloblastic anemia*, then serum vitamin B$_{12}$ and folate levels often help to establish the cause for the anemia. The following patterns of test values may be found:

1. A serum vitamin B$_{12}$ level below 100 pg per mL and a normal or elevated serum folate level, which indicates that cobalamin deficiency is the cause for the megaloblastic anemia.
2. A serum folate level below 3 ng per mL and a normal serum vitamin B$_{12}$ level, which strongly suggests that folate deficiency is the cause of the megaloblastic anemia.
3. A serum folate level below 3 ng per mL and a serum vitamin B$_{12}$ level below 150 pg per mL. This pattern may be found:
   a. When the megaloblastic anemia stems from true combined folate and cobalamin deficiency.
   b. When the megaloblastic anemia stems from pure folate deficiency. For an unknown reason, an occasional patient with folate deficiency may have a reduced serum vitamin B$_{12}$ level.
   c. When the megaloblastic anemia stems from cobalamin deficiency but the patient's recent diet has been deficient in folate.
4. Normal serum vitamin B$_{12}$ and folate levels. This pattern may be found:
   a. In an occasional patient with megaloblastic RBC precursors due, not to cobalamin or folate deficiency, but to a myelodysplastic syndrome (see Chapter 11). The absence of giant metamyelocytes and hypersegmented granulocytes usually provides a morphologic clue to this circumstance.
   b. Due to error if:
      (1) The binder used in the vitamin B$_{12}$ assay binds cobalamin analogues.
      (2) The deficient factor has been given to the patient before blood for the assays is drawn.

Because subacute combined degeneration of the nervous system and megaloblastic anemia are independent manifestations of cobalamin deficiency, the serum vitamin B_{12} level should also be measured in patients with neurologic findings suggestive of subacute combined degeneration, regardless of whether anemia or morphologic evidence suggestive of megaloblastic changes (elevated MCV, hypersegmented granulocytes) is present.

Response to Physiologic Replacement Doses of Cobalamin or Folate

Ten μg of parenteral vitamin B_{12} given to a patient with megaloblastic anemia due to cobalamin deficiency or 100 to 200 μg of folic acid given parenterally to a patient with a megaloblastic anemia due to folate deficiency will cause a brisk reticulocytosis 5 to 7 days after beginning treatment. A reticulocyte response to such doses in the physiologic range establishes that a megaloblastic anemia is due to lack of the replacement material that has been given. Large replacement doses must not be used. A megaloblastic anemia due to vitamin B_{12} deficiency will respond to large doses of folic acid (for example, 10 mg daily) and, conversely, a megaloblastic anemia due to folic acid deficiency may respond to large doses of vitamin B_{12} (for example, 100 μg daily).

This approach to diagnosis was particularly useful before serum vitamin B_{12} and folate levels became generally available; however, it delays diagnosis and optimal replacement therapy and is not used often today. It should never be used in the critically ill patient.

The Deoxyuridine Suppression Test

In this test, either lymphocytes from peripheral blood or bone marrow cells are incubated with *radioactive thymidine* in the presence and in the absence of *nonradioactive deoxyuridine*. The incorporation of radioactivity into DNA is measured. In normal subjects, the added deoxyuridine is converted into nonradioactive thymidylate and this suppresses the salvage pathway conversion of radioactive thymidine to radioactive thymidylate. In the patient with either cobalamin or folate deficiency, adding deoxyuridine does not suppress incorporation of radioactivity into DNA. One then repeats the test in the presence of added folate or vitamin B_{12} to determine which one corrects the abnormal test result. The deoxyuridine suppression test has yet to come into general use.

Schilling Test

The Schilling test provides indirect evidence for the cause of a megaloblastic anemia by testing the ability of a patient to absorb oral cobalamin given first without and then with an exogenous source of intrinsic factor. The test is particularly useful:

1. In a patient with a megaloblastic anemia and a known low serum vitamin B_{12} level to determine the mechanism for the impaired absorption of cobalamin.
2. In a patient with a questionable diagnosis of pernicious anemia who is first seen after being treated elsewhere with vitamin B_{12}. Although the prior treatment will have caused morphologic evidence of a megaloblastic anemia to disappear, the Schilling test will detect a persistent defect in cobalamin absorption.
3. In a nonanemic patient with neurologic disease compatible with subacute degeneration of the nervous system and a low to borderline low serum vitamin B_{12} level to strengthen the evidence for cobalamin deficiency as a cause for the nervous system damage.

The Schilling test is performed by giving a patient an oral tracer dose of radioactive vitamin B_{12} followed by a large parenteral dose of nonradioactive vitamin B_{12}. The urine is collected for 24 to 48 hours. The parenteral dose of cold vitamin B_{12} saturates the plasma vitamin B_{12} binding proteins and "flushes" vitamin B_{12} into the urine. If the radioactive oral dose has been absorbed normally, more than 7% of the administered radioactivity will be excreted into a 24-hour urine collection. If absorption is impaired, usually less than 3% of the administered dose will be recovered in the urine. Falsely low values may result from an incomplete collection of urine or from impaired urinary excretion due to renal insufficiency.

When the test result is abnormal, the test is repeated, giving oral radioactive vitamin B_{12} together with hog intrinsic factor. Adding exogenous intrinsic factor will correct abnormal absorption due to lack of endogenous intrinsic factor (pernicious anemia) but not abnormal absorption due to intestinal disease. Test results may be misleading if the second test is performed in a patient with pernicious anemia who is not first treated with vitamin B_{12} for several weeks to correct complicating intestinal malabsorption stemming from the effect of cobalamin deficiency upon gastrointestinal mucosal function.

Recently, test kits have become available in which both parts of the Schilling test are performed simultaneously by giving oral vitamin B_{12} labeled with two cobalt isotopes. One isotope is used to label free vitamin B_{12} and the other isotope is used to label vitamin B_{12} complexed with intrinsic factor. For the reason just cited and also because the patient who turns out to absorb cobalamin normally receives an unnecessarily increased radiation exposure, the author avoids the use of the simultaneous Schilling test technique. An exception would be a patient in whom one anticipates difficulty in obtaining a complete 24-hour urine collection. Then, determining the ratio between excretion of the two forms of radioactive cobalamin helps to compensate for error due to inadequate urine collection.

PERNICIOUS ANEMIA

Pathogenesis

The pathogenetic lesion of pernicious anemia is severe gastric atrophy with consequent failure to secrete intrinsic factor. Autoimmune injury is strongly suspected to cause the gastric atrophy. A cell-mediated immune process is the likely mechanism, since pernicious anemia has developed in a small number of patients with agammaglobulinemia. Nevertheless, most patients with pernicious anemia have antibodies to gastric parietal cell antigens and many patients also have antibodies to intrinsic factor in their serum. These antibodies are thought to result from the gastric mucosal injury rather than to cause it.

History and Physical Findings

Pernicious anemia is rare before age 35 years. Weakness and fatigability secondary to marked anemia are the usual complaints. Gastrointestinal symptoms, for example, a sore tongue or diarrhea, may be prominent. Numbness and tingling of the hands and feet is a common complaint. Rarely, difficulty in walking due to loss of balance or spasticity of the legs causes the patient to seek medical care.

The patient often looks well nourished but pale and slightly icteric. He or she is usually afebrile (although fever may develop after treatment in association with a marked reticulocytosis). The tongue is usually smooth. Sometimes the tip of the spleen is palpable. Evidence of subacute combined degeneration may be found on examination of the nervous system.

Laboratory Findings

1. *Peripheral blood and bone marrow.* Macrocytic anemia is present with RBC morphology as already described, leukopenia with hypersegmented neutrophils, sometimes a mild thrombocytopenia, and rarely a severe thrombocytopenia. The marrow is megaloblastic (see earlier description). The reticulocyte count is not elevated before treatment but rises several days after the first injection of vitamin B_{12}, with a peak at 5 to 7 days.

2. *Serum vitamin B_{12} and folate levels.* If measured accurately, the serum vitamin B_{12} level is almost always below 100 pg per mL. The serum folate level is normal or elevated unless the patient's recent diet has been folate deficient.

3. *Schilling test.* Less than 3% of an oral dose of radioactive vitamin B_{12} is recovered in a 24-hour urine specimen. When the patient is treated for 2 months with vitamin B_{12} and the test is then repeated with the addition of intrinsic factor, at least 7% of the administered dose of radioactivity is recovered in a 24-hour specimen.

4. *Other blood chemistries.* A high serum iron level, a markedly elevated serum lactic acid dehydrogenase level, and a slightly elevated indirect bilirubin are usually found as manifestations of ineffective erythropoiesis with hemolysis of defective RBCs within the marrow.

5. *Gastric analysis.* A low volume of gastric juice and absent free acid after stimulation is found. This was formerly used as the major presumptive evidence for lack of secretion of intrinsic factor. The availability of the serum vitamin B_{12} assay and of the Schilling test has reduced the frequency with which gastric analysis is performed today.

6. *Antibodies.* About 90% of patients will have serum antibodies to parietal cell antigens and about 50% will have serum antibodies to intrinsic factor. The latter is strong indirect evidence for the diagnosis of pernicious anemia. Many patients with pernicious anemia also have antithyroid antibodies, which suggests that these patients may have an underlying generalized immunologic abnormality.

Management

In the patient who is not critically ill, one may approach diagnosis and treatment as follows:

1. Draw blood for serum vitamin B_{12} and folate levels.
2. Perform the first part of the Schilling test without delay.
3. Begin replacement therapy with 200 μg of vitamin B_{12} intramuscularly daily for 1 week, then 1000 μg weekly for 7 weeks.
4. Check the reticulocyte response 7 days after the first parenteral injection of vitamin B_{12}.
5. Ascertain that the hemoglobin level has returned to normal 2 months after beginning therapy.
6. Perform the second part of the Schilling test 2 months after beginning therapy.
7. Maintain replacement therapy indefinitely with 200 μg of vitamin B_{12} intramuscularly every month.
8. Perform an upper gastrointestinal radiographic series early in the course of therapy because of the increased risk of gastric carcinoma in the patient with pernicious anemia. Check stools for occult blood at 3- to 6-month intervals. Initiate further investigation if the stool becomes positive for occult blood.

Complications

1. *Fever.* The patient with severe anemia may develop fever after beginning vitamin B_{12} therapy because of an increased metabolic production of heat associated with a burst of effective erythropoiesis. However, intercurrent pulmonary or urinary tract infection must not be overlooked as possible causes of fever. If the patient is infected, the initial reticulocyte response to therapy may be blunted.
2. *Hypokalemia.* The serum potassium level may fall after beginning vitamin B_{12} therapy because of an increased need for intracellular potassium to support new RBC production. An occasional patient requires supplemental potassium therapy.
3. *Failure of the hemoglobin level to rise to normal.* Despite an initial good reticulocyte response to vitamin B_{12}, the hemoglobin may fail to rise to a normal level within 2 months. One must then search for a second cause for anemia, particularly:
   a. Iron deficiency, which can be masked initially by the changed

distribution of iron resulting from intramedullary hemolysis in the untreated patient.
b. An underlying chronic inflammatory state.
c. Coexistent myxedema.

FOLIC ACID DEFICIENCY ANEMIAS

Megaloblastic anemia due to folate deficiency is frequently suspected from the clinical setting, for example, an alcoholic patient who has been drinking heavily and eating poorly, an elderly person on a "tea and toast" diet, a pregnant woman. Serum folate and vitamin B_{12} levels confirm the diagnosis. The usual patient will respond with a prompt reticulocytosis to the daily oral administration of 1 mg of folic acid. Therapy should be continued for a period determined by the cause of the deficiency. Two points deserve emphasis:

1. In megaloblastic anemia of pregnancy, one should be alert to the possibility of an underlying chronic hemolytic disorder adding to the demand for folic acid, particularly an unsuspected hereditary spherocytosis.
2. In a patient from the Caribbean area or from Southeast Asia with a history of poor diet and possibly also of alcoholism, one should not attribute folate deficiency solely to these causes until the possibility of underlying tropical sprue has been eliminated. A D-xylose excretion test should be carried out as a screening test after treatment with folic acid to look for persisting malabsorption. If positive, small-bowel radiographs and a jejunal biopsy may be indicated.

THE CRITICALLY ILL PATIENT WITH MEGALOBLASTIC ANEMIA

An elderly patient may be seen who is critically ill with a severe megaloblastic anemia, for example, a hemoglobin level below 5 g per dL. It may then be wisest to proceed as follows:

1. Draw blood for serum vitamin B_{12} and folate levels.
2. Delay all other diagnostic procedures.
3. Begin immediate combined parenteral therapy with 200 μg of vitamin B_{12} and 5 mg of folic acid daily.

The patient will usually also require a transfusion. A single unit of packed RBCs should be given cautiously because of the danger of precipitating left heart failure. Over the next several days, one or more additional units of packed RBCs may be needed before the patient's own new RBCs begin to enter the circulation in large numbers. After the patient's condition has stabilized, further diagnostic procedures, for example, the first part of the Schilling test, can be carried out.

FOLIC ACID ANTAGONISTS

As mentioned earlier, certain drugs can interfere with DNA synthesis by competing with dihydrofolate for the enzyme dihydrofolate reductase. One such folic acid antagonist, methotrexate, is used to treat certain hematologic and other malignancies. When pushed to toxicity, methotrexate may cause serious pancytopenia and gastrointestinal ulcerations. Administering a source of tetrahydrofolate in the form of N^{10}-formyl tetrahydrofolate (Leukovorin[R]) can ameliorate the toxic effects of methotrexate by bypassing the steps of folate metabolism catalyzed by dihydrofolate reductase (see Fig. 4-2). Certain folic acid antagonists have a higher affinity for microbial dihydrofolate reductase than for human dihydrofolate reductase. Such compounds are used clinically as antibacterial (trimethoprim) and antiprotozoal (pyrimethamine) agents either alone or in combination with a sulfa drug.

SELECTED READING

1. Chanarin I: The Megaloblastic Anemias, 2nd Ed. Oxford, Blackwell Scientific Publication, 1979.
2. Herbert V: The nutritional anemias. Hosp. Practice 15:65, 1980.
3. Hillman RS, and Steinberg SE: The effects of alcohol on folate metabolism. Ann Rev Med 33:345, 1982.
4. Lindenbaum J: Aspects of vitamin B_{12} and folate metabolism in malabsorption syndromes. Am J Med 67:1037, 1979.
5. Schilling RF: Vitamin B_{12}: assay and absorption testing. Lab Management 20:31, 1982.
6. Weir DG, and Scott JM: Interrelationships of folates and cobalamins. In Lindenbaum J (ed.): Nutrition in Hematology, New York, Churchill Livingston, 1983.

5

Hemoglobinopathies and Thalassemia Syndromes

In 1949, the hemoglobin of patients with sickle cell anemia was discovered to differ in electrophoretic mobility from normal hemoglobin. This landmark observation, which related sickle cell anemia to a molecular abnormality of a polypeptide chain of globin, initiated an era of investigation into the structure of the hemoglobin molecule. The accomplishments of the ensuing years have been remarkable. The sequence of amino acids and their steric relationship to each other has been worked out for each of the globin polypeptide chains of the normal hemoglobins. How the different segments of each polypeptide chain are folded to give rise to a three-dimensional structure is also known. Moreover, the changing spatial relationship with degree of oxygenation between the different globin chains of a hemoglobin molecule has been delineated. During this period, more than 400 variant hemoglobin molecules have been characterized, and the list continues to grow. Only a very few occur with sufficient frequency to cause a significant incidence of disease. Nevertheless, the discovery of rare variants has been important for the clues they have yielded to the relation between the structure and properties of a polypeptide globin chain. Finally, the powerful tools of modern molecular genetics have been applied to the study of genetic mutations that impair the synthesis of the polypeptide chains of globin. Such studies have strikingly enhanced our knowledge of the structure and organization of human globin genes.

NORMAL HUMAN HEMOGLOBINS

Adult Hemoglobin: Hgb A $(\alpha_2\beta_2)$

Normal adult hemoglobin consists of identical half molecules, each containing two unlike polypeptide chains. These chains are called α and β chains. Normal adult hemoglobin may be pictured as shown in Figure 5-1. Over 90% of the hemoglobin of the normal adult is Hgb A (Table 5-1). An additional approximate 5% of hemoglobin is glucosylated Hgb A, which is hemoglobin A to which sugar molecules have become slowly but irreversibly bound during the 120-day life span of the circulating RBC. (The percent of Hgb A present as the major form of glucosylated hemoglobin, Hgb A_{Ic}, in a blood sample varies with the blood glucose concentration to which the RBCs have been exposed during their circulating lifetime. Therefore, Hgb A_{Ic} levels are used to evaluate overall adequacy of control of the blood sugar level in diabetic patients during the preceding 120 days.)

Fetal Hemoglobin: Hgb F $(\alpha_2\gamma_2)$

Hgb F resembles Hgb A in possessing two α chains but differs in possessing two γ chains instead of two β chains. The production of α chains begins during early fetal life and continues unabated thereafter. The production of γ chains begins to taper off shortly before birth and is replaced by increasing production of β chains. At birth,

Fig. 5-1. A schematic diagram of a molecule of Hgb A to illustrate that each molecule is made up of identical half-molecules, each containing an α chain and a β chain. A molecule of heme, containing an atom of iron (Fe), is associated with each chain.

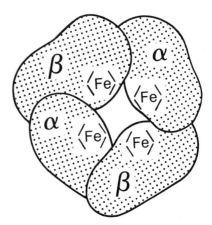

Table 5-1. Hemoglobins Found in the Normal Adult

NAME	GLOBIN CHAINS	OF TOTAL Hgb (%)
Hgb A	$\alpha_2\beta_2$	95
Hgb A$_{1c}$	$\alpha_2\beta_2$	<3.5
Hgb A$_2$	$\alpha_2\delta_2$	<3.5
Hgb F	$\alpha_2\gamma_2$	<1

Hgb F still makes up about 75% of the total hemoglobin, but the level of Hgb F drops to below 5% by age 6 months. The normal adult synthesizes only traces of Hgb F ($<1\%$).

Hgb F levels are measured clinically in evaluating genetic mechanisms for certain sickle cell disorders and thalassemic syndromes. Since Hgb F may not separate completely from Hgb A on routine hemoglobin electrophoresis, electrophoretic techniques are not usually used for its measurement. However, Hgb F, unlike Hgb A, does not decolorize rapidly in an alkaline solution. This forms the basis of a simple clinical test for quantitating Hgb F—the alkali-denaturation test. Moreover, pink-staining cells containing residual Hgb F (F cells) can be readily distinguished from ghost cells that contained only Hgb A by examining stained blood smears that have been first incubated in an acid buffer that elutes Hgb A but not Hgb F from the RBC. This technique permits evaluation of the evenness of distribution of Hgb F in the RBCs in patients with elevated Hgb F levels, an important variable influencing the severity of anemia in patients with certain unusual forms of sickle cell disease or thalassemia. This technique has also been used to detect fetal cells in the maternal circulation during pregnancy or after delivery.

Hemoglobin A$_2$ ($\alpha_2\delta_2$)

When hemoglobin from a normal adult is subjected to electrophoresis, a small portion fails to migrate with the main component and remains close to the origin. This minor fraction has been named Hgb A$_2$ ($\alpha_2\delta_2$). It contains α chains, but the β chains have been replaced by δ chains. Quantitation of Hgb A$_2$, which is required for precise diagnosis of β-thalassemia syndromes (see later), involves either elution of Hgb A$_2$ after electrophoresis on cellulose acetate or microcolumn chromatography. Hemoglobin A$_2$ makes up less than 3.5% of the hemoglobin of a normal adult.

Embryonic Hemoglobins

During early gestation, when erythropoiesis takes place in the yolk sac, an early α-like chain, called a ζ chain, and a polypeptide chain, called an ε chain, are made. Embryonic hemoglobins consisting of a combination of two ζ or two true α chains with two ε chains are formed, as well as an embryonic hemoglobin composed of a tetramer of ε chains. These embryonic hemoglobins disappear after the first 3 months of intrauterine life.

HEMOGLOBIN NOMENCLATURE

Normal adult hemoglobin was named Hgb A and normal fetal hemoglobin was named Hgb F. The first of the abnormal hemoglobins to be discovered, sickle cell hemoglobin, was named Hgb S. Later variants were assigned successive letters of the alphabet, beginning with Hgb C. (B was left out to avoid confusion with ABO blood typing.) An abnormal hemoglobin causing methemoglobinemia was named Hgb M. By the time Hgb Q was reached, it was clear that another nomenclature was needed. Investigators agreed to give new hemoglobins names indicating their place of discovery, for example, Hgb Zurich, Hgb Kansas.

Occasional variants were discovered with electrophoretic properties identical to an earlier hemoglobin with an established letter name but with a different amino acid substitution responsible for the altered electrophoretic properties. For example, several different hemoglobins with the electrophoretic properties of Hgb D were identified. Moreover, five different amino acid substitutions were found to give rise to hemoglobins associated with methemoglobinemia—that is, five Hgbs M have been identified. In these situations, different hemoglobins are identified by a letter plus a place name, for example, Hgb D-Punjab, Hgb M-Saskatoon.

An individual with an α-chain variant of Hgb A will also make a variant Hgb F and a variant Hgb A_2 because these hemoglobins also contain α chains. However, an individual who makes a variant Hgb F with an abnormal γ chain or a variant Hgb A_2 with an abnormal δ chain will not make an abnormal Hgb A. Variants of Hgb F or A_2 are named with the letter F or A_2 followed by a place name. (An exception is a γ chain tetramer found in thalassemia, called Hgb Bart's.)

Today, the amino acid substitutions responsible for the majority of the variant hemoglobins are known. This information is now added as a superscript in the complete name of a variant hemoglobin. For example, the complete name for Hgb S is Hgb $S\alpha_2\beta_2^{6Glu \rightarrow Val}$, which informs one at a glance that the structural abnormality of Hgb S stems from replacement of a glutamic acid by a valine in the sixth position from the amino terminus of the β polypeptide chain of globin.

HUMAN GLOBIN GENES

The human α globin genes are found on chromosome 16 as part of a cluster consisting of the following (as one moves downstream from the 5' to the 3' end of DNA): the gene for the α-like embryonic globin chain, ζ; two pseudogenes, that is, DNA segments which have sequence homology to functional genes but which have become functionally inactive during evolution; and *two* α chain genes. Thus, the α gene has undergone duplication during evolution, and each normal diploid cell contains 4 functional α genes, two on the paternal chromosome 16 and two on the maternal chromosome 16. The duplicated genes produce identical 141 amino acid residue polypeptide chains.

The γ, δ, and β genes are found in a cluster on chromosome 11 (Fig. 5-2), and their polypeptide chain products are strongly analogous to each other. Each has 146 amino acid residues, of which the γ chain differs by 39 amino acids from the β chain, and the δ chain differs in only 16 amino acids from the β chain; however, the δ gene has undergone additional mutations in its regulatory region that has converted it into a "thalassemic gene" (see below), capable of supporting only very limited polypeptide chain synthesis.

Like the α gene, the γ gene has been duplicated during evolution. The duplicated γ genes give rise to polypeptide chains that differ only at a single residue, which is glycine for one gene, the $^G\gamma$ gene, and alanine for the other, the $^A\gamma$ gene. In contrast to α- and γ-chain production, β-chain production is dependent upon only a single gene transmitted from each parent. Since all known variants affecting a given polypeptide chain are controlled by genes which are alleles

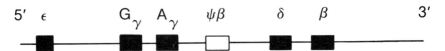

Fig. 5-2. A schematic representation of the related gene cluster on chromosome 11. The open box, identified by the symbol, $\psi\beta$, represents a pseudogene.

(present at the same locus) of a normal gene for that chain, an individual can, at the most, make only two different kinds of β chains.

ABNORMAL GLOBIN CHAIN SYNTHESIS

Genetic Mechanisms

Genetic abnormalities may give rise to a structural hemoglobin variant, may impair the production of a polypeptide chain, or may cause both. The great majority of structural abnormalities result from single amino acid substitutions as a consequence of single nucleotide substitutions in a codon (the triplet of nucleotides that code for an amino acid). Rare structural variants stem from deletion of a nucleotide from a codon, which results in a shift in the reading frame of downstream codons with consequent deletion of one or more amino acid residues or, conversely, extension of the polypeptide chain because the termination codon is altered. Rarely, a mutation of the terminal codon itself causes elongation of a polypeptide chain.

Depending on its site and type, an amino acid substitution in a globin chain may or may not alter the behavior of the hemoglobin molecule. If the structural abnormality produces clinical manifestations, the patient is said to have a *hemoglobinopathy.* In order of their worldwide prevalence, the important structural variants are three β chain variants: Hgb S (α_2 $\beta_2^{6 \ Glu \rightarrow Val}$), Hgb E ($\alpha_2$ $\beta_2^{26 \ Glu \rightarrow Lys}$), and Hgb C ($\alpha_2$ $\beta_2^{6Glu \rightarrow Lys}$). In the United States, Hgb S and Hgb C are found with rare exceptions only in blacks, and Hgb E is encountered primarily in the recent immigrant population from southeast Asia.

Mutations markedly impairing or preventing synthesis of one of the chains of globin give rise to the *thalassemia syndromes.* These mutations may be of two general types:

1. Mutations that either suppress or markedly reduce chain synthesis without altering the amino acid sequence of the chain. The small amounts of polypeptide chain that may be made are of normal structure. Such mutations may result from:
   a. Gene deletion, which accounts for most but not all instances of α chain suppression (α-thalassemia).
   b. Single base substitutions or deletions of one or more bases in an otherwise intact gene, which accounts for most types of β-thalassemia. These mutations occur at sites important for the transcription, processing, stability, or nuclear to cytoplasmic

transport of RNA. Since they do not affect the nucleotide sequence of whatever mature RNA is translated, they do not affect the structure of the polypeptide chain.

2. Mutations that both reduce chain synthesis and give rise to a structurally abnormal polypeptide chain. Examples are:

a. Hgb E, in which the mutation is at a site that affects both structure and splicing of RNA during processing.

b. Hgb Lepore, a fusion gene made up of the amino terminal portion of the δ gene and the carboxy terminal portion of the β gene. (During meiosis, the reduction division in which ova and sperm are formed containing only one pair of chromosomes, the paired chromosomes line up side by side before division. Genes may cross over from one chromosome to its partner. Abnormal crossing over of a portion of a gene may give rise to a fusion gene.) Since the δ gene can support only limited polypeptide chain synthesis, the Hgb Lepore gene gives rise to a reduced amount of an abnormal, part δ and part β polypeptide.

Mechanisms Responsible for Clinical Disease

When a genetic abnormality of globin synthesis gives rise to clinical disease, one of the following mechanisms is involved:

1. *Intracellular polymerization and gelation of hemoglobin molecules.* In RBCs containing large amounts of Hgb S, this phenomenon, which increases with increasing deoxygenation of the hemoglobin molecule, initiates the formation of rigid, deformed cells. Such cells, called sickled cells, have markedly shortened survival and are unable to make their way normally through the microcirculation. A chronic hemolytic anemia and painful vascular occlusive crises result. To a lesser extent, Hgb C also tends to aggregate and give rise to cells more rigid than normal.

2. *Suppression of globin chain synthesis.* As already mentioned, this gives rise to the thalassemic syndromes. Anemia stems not only from an overall reduction in Hgb A synthesis but, just as importantly, from *unbalanced globin chain synthesis.* In the β-thalassemias, excess α chains accumulate in the developing RBC. These form precipitates of aggregated α chains, resembling Heinz bodies, that become attached to the cell membrane. Developing erythroid precursors containing such precipitates may be destroyed within the bone marrow, giving rise to

the markedly ineffective erythropoiesis characteristic of the severe β-thalassemias. RBCs that manage to enter the circulation are rapidly removed by mononuclear phagocytes in the spleen. Under marrow stress, some erythroid precursors revert to a more primitive pathway of differentiation with resultant formation of RBCs containing varying amounts of Hgb F. Because this reduces the excess of free α chains, such RBCs are able to survive longer.

In α-thalassemia, excess β chains in the cell form tetramers (β₄) that can remain in solution for a period of time as an abnormal hemoglobin in circulating cells. This hemoglobin was first identified because of its abnormally fast electrophoretic mobility (Fig. 5-10) and was given the name Hgb H. Patients with limited α-chain synthesis will also form an abnormal Hgb F, containing γ-chain tetramers (Hgb Bart's).

3. *Denaturation of unstable hemoglobins.* A variety of structural abnormalities, for example, amino acid substitutions that destabilize the binding pocket in a globin polypeptide chain for heme, increase the susceptibility of the hemoglobin molecule to denaturation. Either spontaneously or after exposure of RBCs to oxidant stress (for example, exposure to a sulfa drug), denatured hemoglobin precipitates and attaches to the cell membrane, forming Heinz bodies that cause the RBCs to be ingested by mononuclear phagocytes with resultant development of a hemolytic anemia.

4. *Accumulation of methemoglobin.* In the rare Hgbs M, an amino acid substitution in a chain of globin enhances the tendency for the iron of heme to oxidize to form methemoglobin. Since methemoglobin cannot bind oxygen, the homozygous state is incompatible with life. The heterozygote has about 40% hemoglobin M and persistent cyanosis as his or her primary clinical manifestation.

5. *Abnormal oxygen affinity.* A number of instances of familial erythrocytosis have been described in which the erythrocytosis stems from an abnormal hemoglobin with an amino acid substitution in globin that has increased the affinity of heme for oxygen (for example, Hgb Chesapeake, Hgb Yakima). The abnormal hemoglobin binds oxygen so tightly that it fails to be released normally to the tissues as the partial pressure of oxygen in the capillaries falls. The tetramers Hgb H (β₄) and Hgb Bart's (γ₄) also bind oxygen so tightly that they cannot function as oxygen transport proteins.

SICKLE CELL STATES

About 8% of American blacks carry a gene for Hgb S, which means that the statistical chance of carriers marrying and giving birth to an infant homozygous for the Hgb S gene is about 1:650. Since homozygosity produces severe disease with a decreased likelihood of having children, the gene frequency could not have built up unless heterozygosity conferred an offsetting advantage. Epidemiologic studies have related the frequency of Hgb S in a population to the exposure of the population to malaria. Apparently, heterozygosity for Hgb S increases an individual's chance for survival in a malarious region. (The same explanation has been proposed for the high prevalence of the gene for G6PD deficiency in blacks and for the high frequency of thalassemic genes in ethnic groups from the Mediterranean basin and from southeast Asia.)

The principal sickle cell states encountered in the United States are summarized in Table 5-2. Note that the term *sickle cell anemia* refers only to the homozygous state for the Hgb S gene. Disorders resulting from double heterozygosity, that is, an interaction of one gene for Hgb S with a second, different abnormal β chain gene, are included along with sickle cell anemia in the definition of the more general term, *sickle cell diseases.*

Sickle Cell Trait

PATTERN OF MANIFESTATION

The individual with sickle cell trait has one β^S gene and one β^A gene and essentially no resultant clinical disease. Although extensive deoxygenation will cause the RBCs to sickle in vitro, the degree of deoxygenation resulting from passage of blood through the microcirculation does not lead to significant sickling in vivo. The one exception is in the renal medulla. Rare individuals with sickle cell trait have developed gross hematuria due to ischemic ulceration of the renal papillary mucosa. Older individuals also usually develop a fixed urinary specific gravity of 1.010 as a probable consequence of a reduction of renal medullary capillaries (vasa recta) due to occlusion by sickled cells. In every other aspect the individual is completely normal, should be told so, and should be viewed so by others for purposes of employment or life insurance. However, prudence dictates that extreme conditions leading to tissue hypoxia be avoided, for example, strenuous exercise at a high altitude. There is no con-

Table 5-2. The Principal Sickle Cell States

DIAGNOSIS	β GENOTYPE	HEMOGLOBIN PATTERN	MANIFESTATIONS	
			Hgb Level (g/dL)	Sickle Cell Crises
Sickle cell trait	$\beta^A\beta^S$	Hgb A > Hgb S	> 12	None
Sickle cell anemia	$\beta^S\beta^S$	Hgb S, no Hgb A	6–9	4+
SC disease	$\beta^S\beta^C$	Hgb S = Hgb C	10–12	2 to 4+
Sickle-thalassemia	$\beta^S\beta^0$	Hgb S, no Hgb A	7–10	4+
	$\beta^S\beta^+$	Hgb S > Hgb A	9–11	2 to 3+

The symbol β^0 indicates a thalassemic gene that completely blocks β-chain synthesis; the symbol β^+ indicates a thalassemic gene that limits but does not completely block β-chain synthesis.

traindication to flying in a pressurized aircraft. The physical examination is normal.

LABORATORY FINDINGS

The peripheral blood count is normal, and sickled cells are not seen on a routine blood smear. Screening tests for sickling will be positive, for example, one will find:

1. Increased turbidity of an RBC lysate treated with sodium dithionite due to the decreased solubility of deoxygenated Hgb S (dithionite tube test).
2. Sickled RBCs on microscopic examination of the patient's RBCs after incubation with sodium metabisulfite in a coverslipped preparation (Fig. 5-3).

Hemoglobin electrophoresis (see strip 2 of Fig. 5-4) reveals about 60% to 70% Hgb A and about 30% to 40% Hgb S. The increased proportion of Hgb A is thought to reflect the greater affinity of α chains for β^A chains than for β^S chains. Hgb F levels are not elevated.

Sickle Cell Anemia

PATTERN OF DISEASE

The RBCs of the patient homozygous for the gene for Hgb S undergo continuous sickling in vivo. Therefore, the patient has an unrelenting, severe hemolytic anemia that begins within weeks of

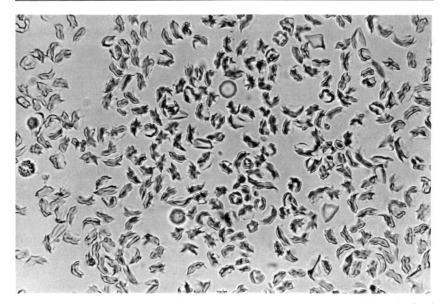

Fig. 5-3. Sickled cells from a patient with sickle cell anemia. A drop of blood mixed with sodium metabisulfite was placed on a glass slide, covered with a coverslip, and allowed to stand for a few minutes. A similar picture would be obtained with blood from a patient with sickle cell trait or with Hgb SC disease.

birth (as Hgb S replaces Hgb F) and lasts throughout life. Masses of sickled RBC repeatedly plug vessels in the microcirculation, leading to painful vascular occlusive crises. In children, these frequently follow an acute, presumably viral, febrile illness, whereas in young adults, crises often occur without an identifiable precipitating cause. For an unknown reason, severe, painful crises are uncommon in older patients. Repeated episodes of ischemic necrosis lead to progressive organ damage, beginning with the spleen, whose function may be impaired even in infancy and which, as a result of repeated infarcts, shrivels into a small remnant later in childhood. Infections are frequent in infants and children; one watches particularly for pneumococcal infection, which can be overwhelming and a cause of sudden death in the infant or small child with absent splenic function. From 5% to 10% of children or young adults experience major cerebral vascular accidents: stroke or hemorrhage resulting from stenosis or aneurysmal dilatation of major cerebral arteries. (The pathogenesis of the arterial wall injury, whether it results from endothelial cell damage by adherent sickled cells or from occlusion by sickled cells of

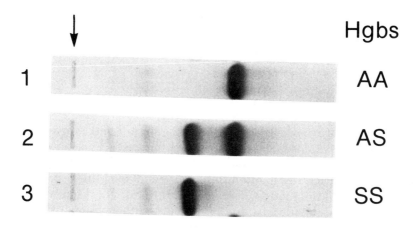

Fig. 5-4. The mobility on cellulose acetate electrophoresis at alkaline pH of Hgb A and Hgb S as demonstrated by hemoglobin electrophoresis strips from a normal person, a person with sickle cell trait, and a person with sickle cell anemia. The arrow denotes the point of application of the hemoglobin. An artifactual band of stained material persists at the point of application. Next in order is a faint band that is not hemoglobin but the enzyme carbonic anhydrase, and then a faint band that is Hgb A_2. The heavy band that migrates in an intermediate position is Hgb S, and the heavy band migrating furthest from the point of application is Hgb A.

nutrient vessels in the arterial wall, is not clear.) Patients are also prone to attacks of an acute chest syndrome characterized by fever, pleural pain, cough, and, often, an infiltrate on chest radiographs. Although usually resulting from pulmonary infarction due to occlusion of pulmonary arterial vessels by sickled cells, the chest findings may be indistinguishable from those of acute bacterial pneumonia.

As patients progress through early adult life, organ damage becomes increasingly evident. The organ or tissue most severely affected varies. For example, right heart failure from pulmonary hypertension due to repeated pulmonary vascular insults may incapacitate one patient; the kidneys may fail in a second patient; aseptic necrosis of the femoral heads may disable a third patient; and repeated ulcers of the lower legs, which take months to heal, may make life miserable for yet a fourth patient. In an occasional patient, an area of ischemic necrosis of bone or bone marrow may serve as a nidus for osteomyelitis due to *Salmonella* or another bacterial organism.

Despite these problems, the majority of adult patients are able to avoid repeated hospitalizations and some do manage to lead productive lives. Present longitudinal studies of large groups of patients should yield reliable statistics on life expectancy and causes of death. A number of patients live beyond 40 years of age, but elderly patients with sickle cell anemia are rarely seen.

PHYSICAL EXAMINATION

Some, but by no means all, patients are tall and thin with long, slender limbs and digits (which reflects increased long bone growth due to delayed closure of epiphyses and hyperemia of the growth plate). Scleral icterus is often detectable and sometimes prominent. Funduscopic examination may reveal tortuous, "corkscrew" retinal vessels. (More detailed evaluation by an ophthalmologist should be sought to evaluate early proliferative retinopathy that will regress with photocoagulation therapy.) The heart is dilated with a hyperdynamic cardiac impulse and murmurs that are usually systolic but rarely also diastolic. The liver is often enlarged and occasionally is massive. Because of atrophy secondary to repeated infarcts, the spleen is not palpable except in childhood. Ulcers or scars of past ulcers may be noted on the shins.

LABORATORY FINDINGS

1. *Peripheral blood count.*
   a. A severe anemia with a hemoglobin level in the range of 6 to 9 g per dL is usually found. Most patients have an MCV in the 90 fL range, but a small subset of patients with concomitant α-thalassemia-2 (see below) have a reduced MCV in the 70 fL range.
   b. An elevated WBC count in the 12,000 to 15,000 per μL range is occasionally found, probably reflecting the effect of splenic atrophy. Platelet counts are often elevated. The sedimentation rate is usually but not invariably very low.
   c. Sickle cells are frequently seen on a routine blood smear and occasionally may be present in large numbers. These represent *irreversibly sickled cells* in which incompletely understood oxidant damage to the RBC membrane, related somehow to formation of Hgb S, has so altered the RBC membrane that the cell can no longer return to a normal shape after it is exposed to the oxygen of room air. Polychromatophilic cells and normoblasts are also found on the smear. RBCs contain-

ing small nuclear remnants (Howell-Jolly bodies) and sidero-cytes are noted and reflect the failure of an atrophic spleen to remove inclusion bodies from circulating RBCs.

2. *Types of hemoglobin.* Hemoglobin electrophoresis reveals a single band of Hgb S (see strip 3 of Fig. 5-4), which makes up from 75% to 95% of the total hemoglobin. Except for a normal, small amount of Hgb A_2, the remainder of the hemoglobin (about 5%–25%) consists of Hgb F. The Hgb F is distributed unevenly in the RBCs; the cells with the highest Hgb F content survive the longest.

3. *Serum bilirubin.* Bilirubin levels may be normal but are usually slightly elevated as a consequence of the increased excretory load resulting from hemolysis. Occasionally, higher bilirubin levels, with elevation of the direct-acting fraction, are found. This usually reflects cholestatic hepatic dysfunction secondary to the effects of sickling within hepatic sinusoids, although the possibility of obstruction of the common bile duct by a bilirubin gallstone must also be kept in mind.

4. *Bone radiographs.* Bone films reflect the effects of two processes:

   a. *Marked erythroid hyperplasia of the marrow*, which causes widening of the medullary spaces, thinning of the cortices, coarsening of the trabeculae, and such lesions as a "fish-mouth" appearance of vertebral bodies.

   b. *Ischemic necrosis of bone*, which produces periosteal thickening and irregular areas of bone lucency and sclerosis. Striking deformity of the femoral heads due to aseptic necrosis is occasionally seen.

TYPES OF CRISES

Three types of crises are seen:

1. *Vascular occlusive crises*, which are by far the most common and which, as mentioned, may plague the patient throughout childhood and young adult life. Infants may develop dactylitis—painful swollen hands and feet due to ischemic infarcts in the small bones of the hands and feet, which have not yet acquired their full vascular supply and are particularly susceptible to necrosis from vascular occlusion. In older children and young adults, bone or bone marrow infarctions tend to develop in the long bones of the extremities, frequently with resultant

painful swelling of the overlying soft tissues. Young adults may also experience attacks of diffuse, severe musculoskeletal pain without associated fever or other objective evidence of organ or tissue damage. As mentioned earlier, vascular occlusion of pulmonary arterial vessels produces an acute chest syndrome. Ischemic necrosis in the renal medulla, with formation of a papillary ulcer, may cause persistent, gross hematuria. Priapism may occur. Rarely, infarcts of the bone marrow may be followed by sudden coma and death from widespread pulmonary and cerebral fat emboli.

2. *Splenic sequestration crises*, which are an uncommon complication seen in small children who still have an enlarged spleen. The spleen suddenly begins to enlarge further and the hemoglobin drops alarmingly as circulating RBCs are trapped within the red pulp of spleen. This emergent situation must be recognized without delay because the child, who is essentially bleeding into the spleen, requires immediate transfusion to prevent hypovolemic shock and even death.

3. *Aplastic crises.* The patient with sickle cell anemia maintains his or her hemoglobin at a certain level (for example, 7 g per dL) for long periods of time because, at that level, increased destruction and increased production of RBCs are balanced. Occasionally, RBC production may suddenly turn off. The reticulocyte count drops, which is the important clue to the presence of an aplastic crisis, and the hemoglobin level falls. An aplastic crisis may result from:

1. Parvovirus and possibly other types of viral infections.

2. Exposure to toxins or drugs that suppress erythropoiesis.

3. Development of a secondary folic acid deficiency.

TREATMENT

No treatment has been discovered that prevents sickling; however, simple measures may reduce the number of crises—keeping the arms and legs from becoming cold at night; drinking large amounts of fluids to prevent dehydration, which develops readily because of a renal concentrating defect secondary to sickling in capillaries of the renal medulla. The patient adjusts to the chronic anemia and, despite a hemoglobin level that may be only 6 or 7 g per dL, may complain only of easy fatigability. Folic acid is often prescribed because of its increased requirement in chronic hemolytic states.

Vascular occlusive crises are treated with intravenous fluids to maintain hydration, oxygen (which is probably of limited value), and analgesics, which may be needed in large amounts to control severe pain. Transfusions are avoided. The patient's "normal" hemoglobin level of 6 to 9 g per dL does not become an indication for transfusion when he or she is hospitalized for a vascular occlusive crisis. Indeed, raising the RBC concentration, which increases blood viscosity, could worsen a vascular occlusive episode. One remains alert to possible other causes for the patient's findings. For example, the author remembers a patient in whom acute gonococcal tenosynovitis was not recognized initially because pain and swelling around a joint was attributed to a periarticular bone infarct.

In contrast to the management of a vascular occlusive crisis, transfusions are usually needed in the patient with an aplastic crisis whose reticulocyte count remains low despite a steadily falling hemoglobin level. As mentioned, the small child with a splenic sequestration crisis urgently requires transfusions.

The availability of automated pheresis equipment makes exchanging a patient's RBCs for normal RBCs feasible, and this has opened a new approach to transfusion therapy in sickle cell anemia. Although transfusions are still avoided whenever possible to reduce the risks of hepatitis, transfusion hemosiderosis, and the development of RBC alloantibodies, partial exchange transfusion—in which 50% to 70% of a patient's RBCs are replaced with normal RBCs—appears to have value in the following circumstances:

1. In pregnancy to reduce maternal morbidity and infant mortality. It is initiated at 28 weeks of gestation and repeated as needed to keep the Hgb A level above 50% through term.
2. In preparing a patient for general anesthesia.
3. In healing recalcitrant leg ulcers.
4. In relieving priapism.
5. In breaking a cycle of recurring vascular occlusive crises.
6. After a stroke to prevent further cerebrovascular episodes.

PRENATAL DIAGNOSIS

A diagnosis of sickle cell anemia can now be made prenatally by analysis of the size of a β-gene DNA fragment obtained from uncultured amniotic fluid cells. Restriction endonucleases are enzymes that cleave DNA into multiple fragments. A particular restriction enzyme called M*st*II cleaves a fragment from the globin gene, beginning in the 5' flanking sequence and normally ending in a position corresponding to amino acids 5, 6, and 7 of the globin chain. The change in DNA nucleotide sequence giving rise to the glutamic acid to valine substitution at residue 6 in Hgb S prevents M*st*II from recognizing this cleavage site, and it does not cleave the β gene until it sees a second site further along the β gene. Thus, M*st*II, which produces a 1.2-kilobase fragment from the normal β gene, produces a larger, 1.4-kilobase fragment from the β^S gene.

In performing the analysis, DNA fragments after digestion of amniotic fluid cell DNA with M*st*II are separated according to size by agarose gel electrophoresis, transferred to nitrocellulose paper, and allowed to react with a ^{32}P radiolabeled probe for the 5' segment of the β- chain gene prepared from a cloned human β-globin gene. The probe will bind (anneal) only to the one DNA fragment on the nitrocellulose paper with complementary base sites, that is, only to the M*st*II fragment from the 5' flanking region of the β gene from the amniotic fluid cells. The position of the bound radioactive probe, visualized by radioautography, permits one to distinguish the 1.2-kilobase fragment from the normal β gene from the 1.4-kilobase fragment from a β^S-gene (Fig. 5-5). The ability to make a prenatal diagnosis of sickle cell anemia early in gestation makes therapeutic abortion an option for prevention of this lifelong, disabling disease.

Hgb SC Disease

The gene frequency of Hgb C is about 2% in American blacks; thus, the statistical chance of an American black possessing one gene for Hgb S and one gene for Hgb C is about 1:2600. Unlike the person with one gene for Hgb S and one gene for Hgb A who has asymptomatic sickle cell trait, the double heterozygote for Hgb S and Hgb C has clinical disease. There are two reasons for this:

1. Whereas the RBCs in sickle cell trait contain more Hgb A than Hgb S, the RBCs in Hgb SC disease contain approximately equal amounts of Hgb S and Hgb C and, therefore, will have a greater propensity to sickle.
2. Red cells containing Hgb C, for unexplained reasons, lose water and develop an abnormally high intracellular hemoglobin concentration (MCHC). The elevated intracellular hemoglobin concentration increases the tendency for Hgb S to polymerize.

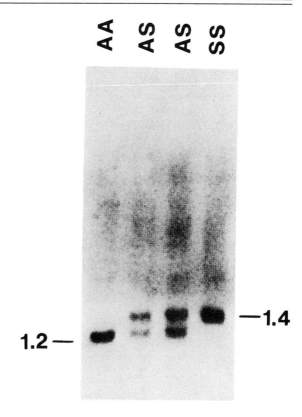

Fig. 5-5. Autoradiograph of a restriction endonuclease digest (Ms*t*II) of amniocyte DNA to illustrate the different migration of the fragment from the β^Agene and the fragment from the β^Sgene. Finding only the latter establishes the prenatal diagnosis of sickle cell anemia. (Reprinted by permission from Warth JA, Rucknagel DL: The increasing complexity of sickle cell anemia. In Brown EB [ed]: Progress in Hematology, vol XIII. New York, Grune & Stratton, 1983).

CLINICAL FINDINGS

Although the patient with Hgb SC disease does not develop severe anemia, he or she may experience severe vascular occlusive crises. Indeed, the increased blood viscosity resulting from a higher RBC concentration appears to increase the risk of ischemic tissue necrosis following vascular occlusion. Thus, aseptic necrosis of the femoral heads and severe proliferative retinopathy are more frequently found in patients with Hgb SC disease than in patients with sickle cell anemia. Moreover, sudden death from fat embolism after bone marrow infarction occurs more frequently in SC disease than in sickle cell anemia, possibly bceause of less erythroid hyperplasia and consequently more fat in the marrow. Jaundice is neither common nor prominent. The spleen is palpable in most but not all patients.

LABORATORY FINDINGS

The hemoglobin level is usually between about 10 and 12 g per dL. Sickle cells may or may not be found on the blood smear. Because of the Hgb C, target cells are prominent (see Fig. 2-13). As already mentioned, approximately equal amounts of Hgb S and Hgb C are seen on hemoglobin electrophoresis (see strip 2 of Fig. 5-6). Hgb F levels are not elevated.

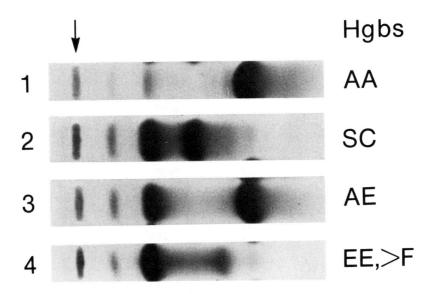

Fig. 5-6. The hemoglobin electrophoresis strips obtained from a patient with SC disease (strip 2), a heterozygote for Hgb E (strip 3), and a double heterozygote for Hgb E and β^0 thalassemia (strip 4). Hgb C and Hgb E migrate only a short distance from the origin, with identical mobilities that prevent their distinction from each other on electrophoresis at an alkaline pH. The double heterozygote for Hgb E and β^0 thalassemia has a single band of Hgb E and an increase in Hgb F, which migrates just behind Hgb A (compare strips 4 and 3). Note also that Hgbs C and E prevent the recognition of Hgb A_2 on electrophoresis at alkaline pH.

Sickle Cell and Thalassemia Interactions

CONCURRENT α-THALASSEMIA

About 15% of blacks have only a single α gene on chromosome 16 (a gene deletion referred to as α-thalassemia-2). Therefore, patients with sickle cell anemia will be seen who are also heterozygotes or homozygotes for α-thalassemia-2. Such concurrence is suspected when one finds a patient with sickle cell anemia and a low MCV in the 70 fL range (since decreased hemoglobin synthesis during erythroid maturation leads to microcytosis). Because reducing intracellular hemoglobin concentration decreases the tendency for Hgb S to gel, patients with sickle cell anemia and concurrent α-thalassemia-2 are usually somewhat less anemic than patients with sickle cell anemia alone. Recent evidence suggests that concurrent α-thalassemia-2 increases survival in sickle cell anemia.

Because limited α-chain synthesis accentuates the effect of the greater affinity of α chains for β^A chains than for β^S chains, the combination of sickle cell *trait* and α-thalassemia-2 widens the difference between the percent of Hgb A and of Hgb S in the RBCs found in sickle cell trait. For example, the usual person with sickle cell trait might have 60% Hgb A and 40% Hgb S, whereas a person with sickle cell trait who is also homozygous for α-thalassemia-2 might have 70% Hgb A and 30% Hgb S.

SICKLE CELL β-THALASSEMIA

Whereas an α-thalassemia gene lessens the expression of a β^S gene, a β-thalassemia gene increases the expression of a β^S gene. Double heterozygosity for a β^S-gene and a β-thalassemia gene increases the proportion of Hgb S in the RBCs and results in clinical disease. If the β-thalassemic gene totally suppresses β^A production (β^0 gene), then the RBCs contain no Hgb A and the severity of the patient's clinical disease approaches that of the homozygous state for Hgb S, that is, sickle cell anemia. If the β-thalassemia gene impairs rather than totally suppresses β^A production (β^+ gene), then the RBCs contain about 15 to 30% Hgb A and disease manifestations are milder than in sickle cell anemia.

Laboratory findings indicative of double heterozygosity for Hgb S and a β-thalassemia gene are:

1. A hemoglobin electrophoretic pattern showing primarily Hgb S but some Hgb A (in a patient who has not been transfused). This

is the reverse of the pattern expected in sickle cell trait and indicates the presence of a β^+ gene.

2. The combination of:
   a. Hgb S without Hgb A.
   b. A reduced MCV in the 70 fL range.
   c. An elevated Hgb A$_2$ (range, 4%–6%).

As mentioned earlier, the first two findings without the third is usually evidence for concurrence of sickle cell anemia and α-thalassemia-2, which is much more common than sickle cell/β-thalassemia°. One recognizes the latter because of the third finding. As will become more apparent later, an elevated Hgb A$_2$ level is characteristic of many β-thalassemic states but never occurs in α-thalassemia.

HETEROZYGOSITY FOR HGB S AND THE HEREDITARY PERSISTENCE OF FETAL HGB (HgbS/HPHF)

The β and δ genes may be deleted by an unusual thalassemic mutation that also somehow prevents the normal switching from γ chain production to β-chain production. Heterozygotes for this HPHF gene mutation make RBCs that contain about 70% Hgb A and 30% Hgb F; homozygotes make RBCs that contain only Hgb F. Rare patients are encountered who are double heterozygotes for Hgb S and for the HPHF gene. Hemoglobin electrophoresis reveals about 70% Hgb S and 30% Hgb F, which is not too different from what is found in occasional patients with sickle cell anemia who may have up to 25% Hgb F. In the patient with Hgb S/HPFH, the Hgb F is *evenly* distributed throughout the RBCs. Consequently, all RBCs have a reduced tendency for sickling and the patient has a much milder disease than sickle cell anemia.

HEMOGLOBIN C

The *heterozygote* for the Hgb C gene does not have clinical disease. Target cells are seen on a peripheral blood smear and Hgbs A and C on hemoglobin electrophoresis.

The *homozygote* for the Hgb C gene has a mild, chronic hemolytic disease with arthralgia, splenomegaly, and slight anemia. Episodes of increased anemia with jaundice may occur. RBC morphology is strikingly disturbed, with a combination of target cells and a population of small, distorted, folded-appearing cells. If blood smears are dried slowly, Hgb C may crystallize and produce occasional rectangular RBCs (Fig. 5-7). Crystals of Hgb C are readily demonstrated on smears made from blood that has been incubated briefly in hypertonic sodium chloride.

HEMOGLOBIN E

Physicians in regions of the United States in which immigrants from southeast Asia have settled need to know the hematologic manifestations of Hgb E, which has an estimated prevalence of 5% to 30% in population groups from Thailand, Cambodia, and Laos. Hgb E, like α-thalassemia trait which is also common in these population groups, produces microcytic RBCs and target cells (Fig. 5-8). The microcytosis stems from diminished β-globin chain synthesis, presumably because the Hgb E mutation, which involves a nucleotide near a splicing site, interferes with normal RNA processing. The microcytosis makes iron deficiency more difficult to recognize when it is also present.

The heterozygote for Hgb E has a normal hemoglobin level; the

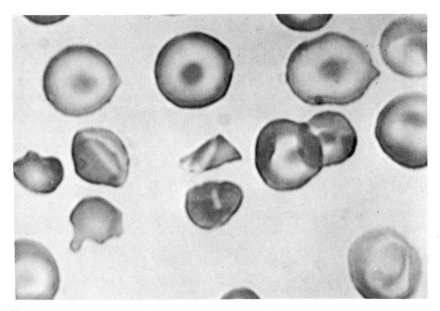

Fig. 5-7. RBC morphology in homozygous Hgb C disease showing target cells and a rectangular cell.

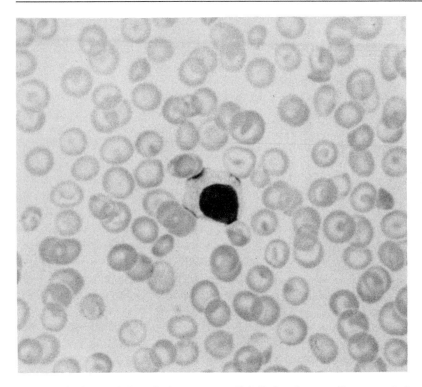

Fig. 5-8. RBC morphology in homozygous Hgb E showing a uniform population of microcytic, hypochromic target cells.

homozygote usually has a mild anemia. As in thalassemia minor and in contrast to uncomplicated iron deficiency, the MCV is much lower than one expects for the level of the RBC count, which is usually normal or even slightly higher than normal (so-called hypochromic polycythemia). Typical findings are as follows:

1. For the heterozygote
   a. A hemoglobin level >12 g per dL.
   b. An MCV in the 70 to 80 fL range, although a few heterozygotes may have a low normal MCV.
   c. About 70% Hgb A and 30% Hgb E on hemoglobin electrophoresis (see strip 3 of Fig. 5-6).
   d. Moderate numbers of hypochromic cells and target cells on a blood smear.
2. For the homozygote
   a. A hemoglobin level between 11 and 13 g per dL.

b. An MCV in the 60 to 70 fL range.

c. Hgb E but no Hgb A on hemoglobin electrophoresis (see strip 4 of Fig. 5-6).

d. A normal Hgb F level (< 5%).

e. Many target cells, microcytes, and hypochromic cells on a blood smear (see Fig. 5-8).

The concurrence of α-thalassemia trait with either heterozygosity or homozygosity for Hgb E does not affect the clinical manifestations of Hgb E. Indeed, recognition of their coexistence requires sophisticated test methods, for example, the measurement of rates of globin polypeptide chain synthesis or restriction endonuclease mapping of the α gene loci.

However, the gene for β° thalassemia is also found in population groups from southeast Asia, and individuals who are double heterozygotes—with one gene for Hgb E and one gene for β° thalassemia—will occasionally be seen. Such individuals will resemble homozygotes for Hgb E in that they will have only Hgb E and no Hgb A on hemoglobin electrophoresis, an MCV in the 60 to 70 fL range, and similar RBC morphology. They will differ, however, in having:

1. A significant anemia, such as, a hemoglobin level in the 8 to 10 g per dL range.

2. An *elevated level of Hgb F* >10% (see strip 4 of Fig. 5-6).

UNSTABLE HEMOGLOBINS

Over 60 different hereditary structural abnormalities of globin have now been described that enhance the propensity of hemoglobin to denature and to form precipitates within the RBC (Heinz bodies). The decreased deformability of such cells causes their enhanced removal from the circulation and a hemolytic anemia. Oxidant stress, as may occur during infection or after administration of oxidant drugs such as certain sulfa preparations, increases the precipitation of hemoglobin within the RBC and worsens the hemolytic anemia. When a patient is discovered with a hemolytic anemia that is worsened by oxidant stress and RBCs that contain Heinz bodies, two diagnoses should be considered:

1. *An unstable hemoglobin.* One can screen for this by incubating a lysate of the patient's RBCs in 17% isopropanol, which causes an unstable hemoglobin to precipitate.

2. *Glucose 6 phosphate dehydrogenase deficiency* (see Chaper 7), for which a simple screening fluorescent spot test is available.

Some of the unstable hemoglobins give rise to a chronic, nonspherocytic hemolytic anemia, which is often recognized in infancy or early childhood. The spleen is palpably enlarged due to hyperplasia resulting from the phagocytosis of large numbers of abnormally rigid RBCs by mononuclear phagocytes in the red pulp. The patient may excrete dark urine containing an unusual dipyrolle pigment thought to arise from the aberrant catabolism of heme within precipitates of aggregated hemoglobin. RBC morphology may appear normal on the blood smear except for polychromatophilic macrocytes reflecting increased erythropoietin-stimulated RBC production. Sometimes "bite cells" (see Fig. 2-14) are found on the blood smear, a result of the pitting of Heinz bodies from RBCs as they traverse the red pulp of the spleen. Hemoglobin electrophoresis may or may not reveal a hemoglobin with abnormal mobility; this depends upon whether the amino acid substitution causing the hemoglobin instability also changes the overall charge of the globin molecule. As already mentioned, precipitation of hemoglobin after incubation in isopropanol establishes that an unstable hemoglobin is present.

In some variants producing a lesser degree of instability, the patient's findings may be normal until he or she is exposed to an oxidant stress. Then, an episode of hemolysis—with the sudden onset of weakness, a falling hemoglobin level, and jaundice—is induced.

THALASSEMIA SYNDROMES

Clinically significant thalassemic syndromes are seen in the United States primarily in ethnic groups from the Mediterranean basin or from southeast Asia and, to a lesser extent, in blacks. As already mentioned, the thalassemic syndromes result from varying degrees of impairment of synthesis of a polypeptide chain of globin. Common to all thalassemic syndromes are:

1. *Impaired overall hemoglobin synthesis*, which results in microcytic, hypochromic RBCs plus added morphologic evidence of disordered RBC production in the form of target cells, ovalocytes, and basophilic stippling.
2. *Unbalanced production of globin chains*. This leads to:
   a. Formation of tetramers of single chains, either in solution (γ_4 or Hgb Bart's, β_4 or Hgb H) or as α_4 precipitates causing rapid cell destruction.

b. Elevated levels of Hgb A_2, Hgb F, or both in the β-thalassemia syndromes.

In the severe β-thalassemia syndromes, the bone marrow shows striking erythroid hyperplasia, but the developing cells containing α_4 precipitates are so defective that the majority are destroyed in the marrow before release or in the spleen promptly after release (ineffective erythropoiesis, see Chapter 6).

α-Thalassemias

Most α-thalassemia results from α-gene deletions. Normal diploid cells contain four genes; possible patterns of deletions are shown in Figure 5-9. Deletion of a single α gene produces no clinical manifestations. Deletion of all 4 α genes causes stillbirth with a hydrops fetalis syndrome. The hemoglobin consists almost entirely of tetramers of γ_4 (Hgb Bart's), which, because it binds oxygen avidly, cannot function effectively as an oxygen-transport protein.

The two forms of α-thalassemia recognized in living patients are:

1. *α-thalassemia trait*, which results from deletion of two genes. Deletions in *cis* (both deletions on the same gene) or in *trans* (one deletion on the paternal gene and one deletion on the maternal gene) produce the same findings. These are:
   a. A minimally reduced hemoglobin level and a normal to slightly elevated RBC count.
   b. Microcytosis out of proportion to the RBC count, with an MCV in the 60 to 75 fL range.

Fig. 5-9. The relation between the number of α-gene deletions and the manifestations of α-thalassemia.

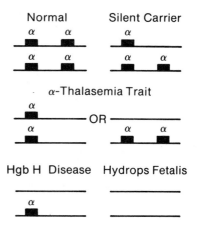

c. No other abnormality measurable by usual clinical test, that is, no elevation of Hgb A_2 or Hgb F and no Hgb E. Small amounts of Hgb H are made but they are insufficient to be recognized on hemoglobin electrophoresis or as inclusion bodies in RBCs incubated with a supravital dye, such as new methylene blue (see below).
Thus, the clinical diagnosis of α-thalassemia trait is largely a diagnosis of exclusion.

2. *Hemoglobin H disease*, which results from deletion of 3 genes. The patient with Hgb H disease has a lifelong, moderately severe microcytic anemia (hemoglobin of 8 to 10 g per dL, MCV 60 to 70 fL), splenomegaly, slight bilirubinemia, and an elevated reticulocyte count. The blood smear shows striking hypochromia, target cells, ovalocytes, and cells with basophilic stippling. On hemoglobin electrophoresis, about 5 to 40% of the hemoglobin moves faster than Hgb A (Fig. 5-10); it is Hgb H. Numerous RBCs containing multiple inclusion bodies of precipitated Hgb H will be noted after incubating blood in vitro with new methylene blue (Fig. 5-11). Hgb H, although soluble in young RBCs, is less stable than Hgb A and begins to precipitate as the circulating RBC ages. RBC containing precipitates lose their deformabil-

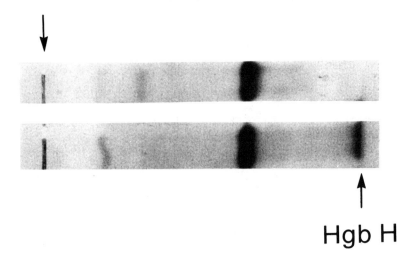

Hgb H

Fig. 5-10. The electrophoretic demonstration of Hgb H as a band moving faster than Hgb A on electrophoresis on cellulose acetate at an alkaline pH.

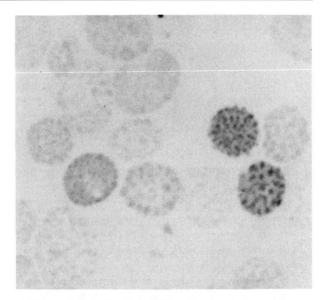

Fig. 5-11. Multiple precipitates of Hgb H within RBCs after incubation with new methylene blue of blood from a patient with Hgb H. The precipitates give the RBCs a diffusely speckled appearance.

ity, with resultant damage in the microcirculation and accelerated removal by mononuclear phagocytes. Like Hgb Bart's, the increased oxygen affinity of Hgb H prevents its functioning as an efficient oxygen transport protein.

In the United States, Hgb H disease is seen in ethnic groups from southeast Asia but not in blacks. Although blacks have a high prevalence of a single α gene deletion from chromosome 16 (known as α-thalassemia-2), deletion of both α genes from chromosome 16 (known as α-thalassemia-1), which is a requisite for the three gene deletions of Hgb H disease, is apparently very rare.

β-Thalassemia

β-thalassemia may result from different types of mutations. A few involve gene deletion: the β gene alone, the β gene plus the δ gene (δβ thalassemia), or the β gene, the δ gene and the $^A\gamma$ gene ($^A\gamma\delta\beta$ thalassemia). Most β-thalassemia, however, results from point mutations—single nucleotide substitutions or deletions in the β gene that cause defective transcription, processing, or transport of β chain mRNA. As discussed earlier, a mutation may either completely suppress β-chain synthesis (β° thalassemia) or may impair but not totally prevent β-chain synthesis (β⁺ thalassemia). The development of synthetic oligonucleotide DNA probes specific for the abnormal nucleotide sequences of various β-thalassemia point mutations now makes possible the prenatal diagnosis of a number of forms of β-thalassemia variants.

The most common type of β-thalassemia seen in the Unites States has the following manifestations:

1. The *heterozygote* is asymptomatic. The spleen tip is frequently palpable. The peripheral blood count reveals a Hgb level of 10 to 13 g per dL, an RBC count which is normal or slightly elevated (for example, 6,000,000 per μL), and an MCV in the 60 to 70 fL range. One notes microcytosis, hypochromia, target and elliptical cells, and RBC with basophilic stippling on the blood smear. The excess production of α over β chains is associated with an increase in Hgb A₂ from normal levels of less than 3.5% to levels of 4 to 6%. Hgb F levels may be normal or slightly elevated.

2. The *homozygote* has a very severe anemia, first detected in early childhood and characterized by increasing hepatosplenomegaly, slight jaundice, and marked bone changes due to an expanded marrow cavity from massive erythroid hyperplasia. A typical facies results, with prominence of the forehead, cheek bones, and upper jaw. Physical growth and development may be impaired. Thinning of the bony cortex may result in pathologic fractures. The hemoglobin level falls to very low levels in the patient who has not been given transfusions, for example, to 3 g per dL. RBCs are markedly hypochromic with bizarre morphology: stippled cells, target cells, elliptical cells, hypochromic cells with polychromatophilic rims, and nucleated RBCs are seen on the blood smear (Fig. 5-12). In patients with a β⁺ variant hemoglobin electrophoresis may reveal a small amount of hemoglobin A. Hgb A₂ levels may be slightly increased. Otherwise all hemoglobin in the nontransfused patient is Hgb F.

Repeated transfusions are necessary to maintain life; some children are "hypertransfused" to maintain the hemoglobin level above 10 g per dL. This will allow normal physical growth and development and prevent bony changes due to an expanded marrow cavity but at a cost of increasing the rate of development of transfusion hemosiderosis. Splenectomy is sometimes performed in an attempt to reduce

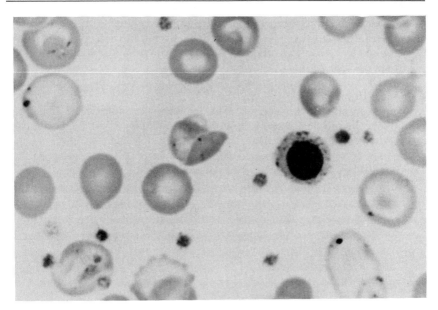

Fig. 5-12. Appearance of the RBCs on a blood smear from a 20-year-old man with homozygous β-thalassemia who was splenectomized in childhood and who receives transfusions at about monthly intervals. The marked hypochromia of the patient's RBCs contrasts strikingly with the normal appearance of the transfused RBCs. Although the patient's RBCs are microcytic, with a low MCV, they appear large on the blood smear because they are thin and spread out more than normal cells do as the blood smear is made. The black granules in the patient's RBCs are siderotic granules (aggregated ferritin), a reflection of the failure of the developing RBC to incorporate iron into hemoglobin, the patient's massive iron overload, and the inability after splenectomy for the mononuclear phagocytic system to "pit" RBCs effectively. A normoblast containing coarse basophilic stippling is also seen.

transfusion requirements. Patients often die in their teens or early adult life from cardiac failure secondary to heavy deposits of iron in the myocardium. Iron chelation therapy with subcutaneous 8 to 12-hour infusions of desferrioxamine 5 or 6 nights a week is now instituted in childhood in an attempt to forestall myocardial damage from iron overload.

SELECTED READING

1. Bunn HF, Forget BG: Hemoglobin: Molecular, Genetic, and Clinical Aspects. Philadelphia, WB Saunders, 1986.
2. Fabry ME, Kaul DK, Raventos-Suarez C, Chang H, Nagel RL. SC eryth-

rocytes have an abnormally high intracellular hemoglobin concentration. Pathophysiological consequences. J Clin Invest 70:1315, 1982.

3. Nienhus AW, Anagnou, NP, and Ley TJ: Advances in thalassemia research. Blood 63:738, 1984.

4. Powars DR: Natural history of sickle cell disease—the first ten years. Semin Hematol 12:267, 1975.

5. Warth JA, and Rucknagel DL: The increasing complexity of sickle cell anemia. In Brown EB (ed.): Progress in Hematology, Vol. 13, p. 25, New York, Grune & Stratton, 1983.

6

Hemolytic Anemias: General Remarks

ERYTHROKINETICS

Marrow Response to Hemolysis

When RBCs are destroyed rapidly, erythropoietin and unknown factors stimulate the marrow to increase RBC production. Erythropoiesis may increase about fivefold over basal levels within 1 week. Increased numbers of erythroid precursors are seen on marrow smears (*erythroid hyperplasia*), and the normal myeloid: erythroid (M:E) ratio of 3:1 is reduced. *Marrow hypercellularity*, with the fat content reduced, is seen on histologic sections of marrow particles or biopsy specimens. When hemolysis is chronic and severe, extreme marrow hypercellularity expands the marrow cavity with resultant thinning of cortical bone and widening of the space between the inner and outer tables of flat bones. Also, islands of erythropoiesis may be found outside the marrow (*extramedullary hematopoiesis*), for example, in periaortic nodes. When hematopoietic marrow expands to this extent, erythropoiesis may increase to about eight times basal levels.

Thus, if the marrow can respond, RBCs may be destroyed at several times the normal rate without a patient becoming anemic. A patient with evidence of brisk hemolysis (for example, spherocytes, reticulocytosis, and elevated indirect bilirubin) but with a normal hematocrit is said to have a *compensated hemolytic anemia*. He or she may become anemic rapidly if:

1. RBC destruction suddenly increases beyond the ability of the marrow to make new RBCs (*hemolytic crisis*).
2. The marrow suddenly stops making RBCs (*aplastic crisis*).

Failure of Marrow Response to Hemolysis

RBC survival is shortened in patients with chronic disease, for example, a chronic infection or rheumatoid arthritis. Hemolysis is not marked enough to alter plasma or urine pigments but is demonstrable as a shortened survival of RBCs labeled with ^{51}Cr (from a normal ^{51}Cr half-life of 28 days to a half-life of 20 days); however, the bone marrow continues to make RBCs at a "normal" rate, failing to speed production to keep pace with destruction. Consequently, the patient becomes mildly to moderately anemic. Although the anemia is associated with an increased rate of RBC destruction, it should not be called a hemolytic anemia. The real fault lies with the inability of the marrow to increase erythropoiesis to compensate for a modest increase in rate of RBC destruction (see further discussion in Chapter 12).

Ineffective Erythropoiesis

Total erythropoiesis may be viewed as consisting of two components:

1. *Effective erythropoiesis*, resulting in the formation of circulating RBCs.
2. *Ineffective erythropoiesis*, resulting in the formation of RBCs so defective that they are either destroyed within the marrow (*intramedullary hemolysis*) or immediately upon entering the circulation.

Total erythropoiesis can be estimated from the following:

1. The number of erythroid precursors seen in a bone marrow aspirate.
2. The plasma iron turnover (see Chapter 3). This primarily reflects total marrow hemoglobin synthesis but also reflects removal of iron from the plasma by liver cells. (The latter, which is limited, results in significant overestimation of total erythropoiesis from plasma iron turnover when turnover is normal or decreased but not when turnover is elevated.)

Effective erythropoiesis can be estimated from:

1. The reticulocyte index (see Chapter 2), which indicates the number of new RBCs entering the circulation.

2. The percent incorporation of radioactive iron into RBCs. Normally, about 85% of a tracer dose of ^{59}Fe will be incorporated into young circulating cells within 2 weeks. In disorders with impaired effective erythropoiesis, this value is markedly reduced.

Ineffective erythropoiesis represents the difference between total and effective erythropoiesis and normally comprises about 15% of total erythropoiesis. Conditions with markedly increased ineffective erythropoiesis are usually recognized clinically by a pattern of:

1. Marked erythroid hyperplasia in the bone marrow.
2. A disproportionately low reticulocyte index for the degree of erythroid hyperplasia found in the bone marrow.

When defective RBCs are formed, the most abnormal cells may be destroyed in the marrow or immediately on entering the circulation, whereas the remainder of the RBCs may circulate for an interval before they are destroyed. Thus, some anemias are characterized by evidence of both increased ineffective erythropoiesis and hemolysis. Such disorders include

1. Megaloblastic anemias.
2. Thalassemia syndromes.
3. Myelodysplastic syndromes with refractory anemia (see Chapter 11).

CLASSIFICATION OF HEMOLYTIC DISORDERS

Hemolytic states may be divided into two groups:

1. *Intrinsic hemolytic anemias,* in which hemolysis stems from a defect of the patient's RBCs. Therefore, normal RBCs are not destroyed rapidly when transfused into such a patient (Fig. 6-1). Most intrinsic hemolytic anemias are hereditary. Causes include:
   a. *Abnormal hemoglobins,* such as Hgb S, Hgb H, unstable hemoglobins, which result in hemolysis because the abnormal hemoglobin forms aggregates within the RBC, causing the cells to become rigid and lose the deformability necessary for survival in the microcirculation.
   b. *Enzyme abnormalities,* which may be divided into:
      (1) Deficiencies in enzymes in the main glycolytic pathway (Embden-Meyerhof pathway). *Pyruvate kinase deficiency* is the most common of this group of hemolytic anemias.

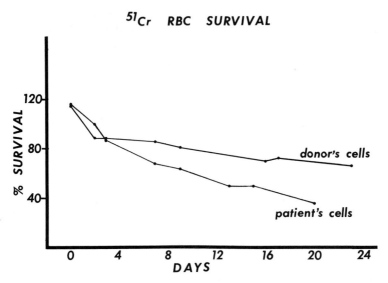

Fig. 6-1. Difference in survival between the patient's own cells labeled with ⁵¹Cr and normal donor cells labeled with ⁵¹Cr in a patient with an intrinsic hemolytic anemia (hereditary spherocytosis). Despite negative family studies, the diagnosis was established by osmotic fragility studies, the above RBC survival curves, and cessation of hemolysis following splenectomy.

(2) Deficiencies in enzymes of the hexose monophosphate shunt (or in other enzymes required for the synthesis or function of reduced glutathione). *Glucose-6-phosphate dehydrogenase (G6PD) deficiency* is the most common cause for this type of hemolytic anemia.

(3) Abnormalities of enzymes involved in nucleotide metabolism:

    (a) Pyrimidine-5′-nucleotidase deficiency, which results in the persistence of unwanted pyrimidine nucleotides in the RBC that compete metabolically with the adenine nucleotides.

    (b) *Increased activity* of adenosine deaminase, which results in the increased breakdown of adenosine to inosine rather than its salvage by conversion to adenosine monophosphate.

c. *Membrane abnormalities:*

(1) *Hereditary spherocytosis,* in which abnormalities of the cytoskeletal protein, spectrin, result in the formation of microspherocytes and hemolysis.

(2) *Hereditary elliptocytosis*, in which other abnormalities of spectrin and another membrane skeletal protein, called band 4.1, result in the formation of elliptical and other abnormally shaped RBCs and hemolysis of variable degree.

(3) *Paroxysmal nocturnal hemoglobinuria*, an acquired disorder in which an RBC membrane protein necessary for the normal decay of the activated complement component, C3b, is missing from the membrane, with resultant accumulation of C3b and increased sensitivity of the RBC to lysis by complement.

2. *Extrinsic hemolytic anemias*, in which the patient's RBCs are normal but become damaged by an external factor. In these disorders, transfused normal cells will be damaged as readily as the patient's own cells. Extrinsic hemolytic anemias are acquired and often secondary to identifiable underlying disease. Causes include:

a. *Damage by antibodies*. These may be:

(1) *Alloantibodies*, as can occur in transfusion of incompatible blood or in hemolytic disease of the newborn.

(2) *Autoantibodies*, which may develop either without other evidence of immunologic disease or as a complication of disease known to disturb immunologic mechanisms—systemic lupus erythematosus, lymphoma, chronic lymphocytic leukemia.

(3) *Drug-related antibodies*, which may cause hemolysis as a result of:

(a) A drug coming down on the RBC membrane where it then reacts with an antibody to the drug (penicillin type).

(b) A drug stimulating formation of antibody to an antigenic determinant on the RBC membrane formed as a result of binding of the drug to a membrane binding site (quinine type ?).

(c) A drug stimulating formation of autoantibodies (alpha-methyldopa type).

b. *Mechanical damage*, which produces a characteristic RBC morphology (see Fig. 2-12) and may result from:

(1) Trauma to RBCs as blood flows through small vessels containing deposits of fibrin, as in thrombotic thrombocytopenic purpura and hemolytic-uremia syndromes.

(2) Trauma to RBCs by a prosthetic heart valve or occasionally by other abnormalities in the heart or great vessels.

c. *Alterations in plasma lipids* leading to alterations in the lipid of the RBC membrane. This usually occurs as a complication of liver disease (Zieve's syndrome, spur cell anemia).
d. *Severe hypophosphatemia*, which impairs generation of RBC adenosine triphosphate (ATP).
e. *Infectious agents and toxins*:
   (1) Massive malarial infection.
   (2) Circulating clostridial exotoxin, as occasionally occurs after septic abortion.
   (3) Poisonous snake venoms.

SITES OF HEMOLYSIS

Damaged RBCs may breakdown within the circulation (*intravascular hemolysis*) or may be phagocytosed by macrophages in the spleen, liver, and bone marrow (*extravascular hemolysis*). The terms intravascular and extravascular hemolysis, which refer to where damaged RBCs are broken down, should not be confused with the terms intrinsic and extrinsic hemolytic anemia, which refer to how RBCs become damaged. The different pigment changes resulting from intravascular and extravascular hemolysis have been discussed in Chapter 2.

RBCs must be severely damaged to undergo intravascular hemolysis. Causes include:

1. Membrane lysis by *complement* (for example, ABO blood group transfusion reaction, paroxysmal nocturnal hemoglobinuria).
2. *Mechanical damage* (prosthetic heart valve, hemolytic-uremia syndrome, thrombotic thrombocytopenic purpura).
3. Damage by certain *infectious agents or toxins*, such as clostridial exotoxin, snake venoms.

The degree of cell damage also determines the primary site of extravascular hemolysis. All three organs—liver, spleen, and bone marrow—remove RBCs with extensive membrane damage or extensive membrane coating with antibody and complement. However, because liver blood flow exceeds blood flow through the other organs, the liver will remove most of the cells. RBCs with less extensive membrane changes may escape phagocytosis in the liver or bone marrow, but, because of the unique "percolation" of RBCs through the splenic pulp, the cells cannot escape entrapment and phagocytosis in the splenic cords. Thus, the spleen becomes the primary site of destruction of minimally altered RBCs.

SELECTED READING

1. Weiss, L and Tavassoli, M: Anatomical hazards to the passage of erythrocytes through the spleen. Semin Hematol 7:372, 1970.

7

RBC Metabolism: Relations to RBC Function and Hemolytic Anemias

RBC ENERGY METABOLISM

The mature RBC is the simplest cell in the human body, possessing neither a nucleus nor organelles nor mitochondria. It consists, essentially, of a cell membrane and underlying membrane skeleton (see Chapter 8) that encloses a cytosol containing a 33% solution of hemoglobin and a low concentration of the enzymes and other components of a limited number of metabolic reactions. These reactions generate four substances important for the cell's function:

1. Adenosine triphosphate (ATP), which provides the energy necessary for cation pumps to maintain normal intracellular cation concentrations and for other reactions that are poorly understood but allow the membrane to preserve its shape and deformability.
2. Reduced nicotinamide adenine dinucleotide (NADH), which is required to reduce methemoglobin (see Chapter 10).
3. Reduced glutathione (GSH), which serves as a reservoir of reducing power to protect hemoglobin from oxidative damage by hydrogen peroxide and other peroxides.
4. 2,3-Diphosphoglycerate (2,3-DPG), which facilitates the release of oxygen from hemoglobin at tissue oxygen tensions and which may also be involved in reactions with membrane skeleton proteins necessary for normal RBC membrane deformability.

The Embden-Meyerhof Pathway

Since the mature RBC does not contain mitochondria, it must depend solely on glycolysis for energy. The main glycolytic pathway (shown in incomplete form in Fig. 7-1) consists of a series of anaerobic reactions (the Embden-Meyerhof pathway) by which one molecule of glucose is converted into two molecules of pyruvate with the net formation of two molecules of ATP.

NADH is also generated. Pyruvate may either diffuse out of the cell or be converted into lactate. If the latter occurs, NADH is reoxidized to NAD.

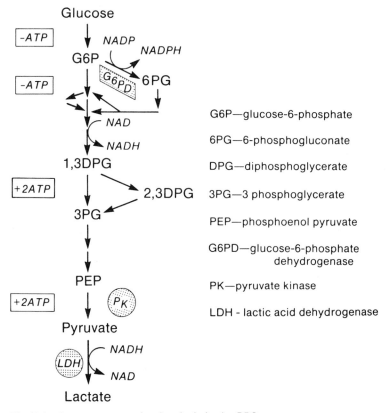

Fig. 7-1. Important steps in glycolysis in the RBC.

Hexose Monophosphate Shunt

An aerobic shunt (the hexose monophosphate or pentose phosphate shunt) bypasses early steps of the Embden-Meyerhof pathway (see Fig. 7-1). This shunt is important because glycolysis via this route generates reduced nicotinamide adenine dinucleotide phosphate (NADPH), which is required in the RBC to reduce glutathione (Fig. 7-2). The hexose monophosphate shunt is normally responsible for about 10% of glycolysis; however, when the level of GSH in the RBC falls, for example, after exposure to oxidant drugs, activity of the hexose monophosphate shunt increases markedly.

Impaired generation of GSH due to a defect of the first enzyme of the hexose monophosphate shunt—glucose-6-phosphate dehydrogenase (G6PD)—is a relatively common cause in black males in the United States for episodes of hemolytic anemia provoked by oxidant drugs or by infection. Hemolytic disorders due to defects in other enzymes necessary for the formation or function of GSH (for examples, glutathione reductase, glutathione peroxidase) are extremely rare.

2,3-Diphosphoglycerate Shunt

A second shunt (the Rapoport-Luebering shunt) is present further down the Embden-Meyerhof pathway (see Fig. 7-1). At first glance, it would seem to serve no useful purpose since it bypasses a reaction,

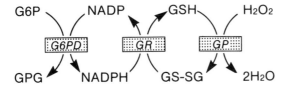

G6P-glucose-6-phosphate

GPG-6-phosphogluconate

G6PD-glucose-6-phosphate
dehydrogenase

GR-glutathione reductase

GP-glutathione peroxidase

Fig. 7-2.   Generation and function of GSH in the RBC.

the direct conversion of 1,3 diphosphoglycerate (1,3-DPG) to 3-phosphoglycerate (3-PG), that generates ATP. As a molecule of glucose is metabolized in the early steps of the Embden-Meyerhof cycle, two molecules of ATP are converted to ADP. If the two molecules of 1,3-DPG that are formed enter the 2,3-DPG shunt, they do not generate two molecules of ATP on conversion to 3-PG (see Fig. 7-1). The later generation of two molecules of ATP at the step of conversion of two molecules of phosphoenol pyruvate (PEP) to pyruvate then only replaces the two molecules of ATP initially lost. Glycolysis generates NADH but yields no net gain of ATP.

However, organic polyphosphates combine with hemoglobin to alter its oxygen affinity. Since 2,3-DPG accounts for over half of the phosphorus in the erythrocyte, its generation via the shunt plays an important regulatory role in tissue oxygen delivery. Each molecule of hemoglobin carries four molecules of oxygen. The globin chains of Hgb A are arranged in such a way that the β chains move apart slightly as the molecule begins to give up oxygen. This widens a central gap in the molecule and allows 2,3-DPG to enter and to bind to the β chain. The reaction between hemoglobin and 2,3-DPG may be thought of as follows:

$$HgbO_2 + 2,3\text{-}DPG \longleftrightarrow HgbDPG + O_2$$

Thus, an increase in the 2,3-DPG level of the RBC increases the amount of oxygen released from hemoglobin at a given partial pressure of oxygen, that is, 2,3-DPG shifts the oxygen dissociation curve to the right (Fig. 7-3).

When arterial blood supplies insufficient oxygen to the tissues, the body attempts to compensate by extracting more oxygen from each unit of blood. It must accomplish this with as little further fall in partial pressure of oxygen as possible in order to preserve the driving pressure that moves oxygen into the cells. Red cell levels of 2,3-DPG increase in patients with anemia, cardiac disease impairing tissue perfusion, or pulmonary disease interfering with oxygenation in the lungs—which permits such patients to release more oxygen from hemoglobin at a given tissue partial pressure of oxygen. The stimulus for increased production of 2,3-DPG in these circumstances may stem from an increased binding of 2,3-DPG to deoxyhemoglobin, which apparently diverts 1,3-DPG into the shunt pathway.

Hemoglobin F, which contains γ chains instead of β chains, binds 2,3-DPG less well than does hemoglobin A. This is an advantage for fetal RBCs, which must oxygenate hemoglobin, not at the high partial pressure of oxygen in the lungs, but at the lower partial pressure of oxygen in maternal blood flowing through the placenta.

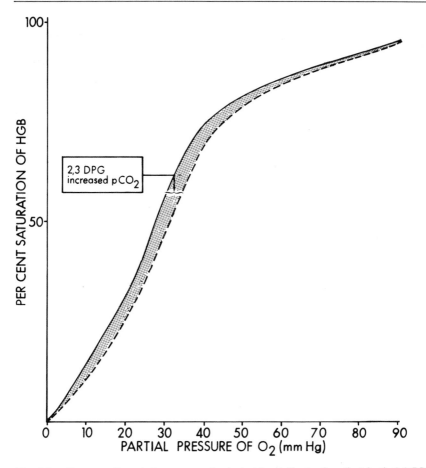

Fig. 7-3. Oxygen dissociation curve of whole blood illustrating that both 2,3-DPG and an increase in the partial pressure of CO_2 (Bohr effect) shift the curve to the right. This increases significantly the release of oxygen from hemoglobin at the partial pressure of oxygen normally present in the capillary bed.

2,3-DPG possibly serves another important function in the RBC in that it binds to spectrin and actin in the membrane skeleton (see Chapter 8). This weakens spectrin-actin crosslinks and so increases the lateral mobility of integral proteins of the membrane bilayer. Such lateral movement of integral proteins is required for the deformability that permits a RBC to squeeze through a capillary one half the diameter of the cell.

HEMOLYTIC ANEMIAS ASSOCIATED WITH IMPAIRED FORMATION OR FUNCTION OF ATP

Pyruvate Kinase Deficiency

Hereditary hemolytic anemias have been described in association with defects in each of the enzymes of the Embden-Meyerhof pathway. Except for pyruvate kinase deficiency, these disorders are very rare. Although uncommon, pyruvate kinase deficiency ranks behind G6PD deficiency as the second most frequent hereditary anemia due to an RBC enzymatic abnormality.

The individual with pyruvate kinase deficiency inherits a defective gene for pyruvate kinase from each parent. Many mutant forms of pyruvate kinase have now been described, and the affected person is usually a *double heterozygote* who has acquired a different mutant gene from each parent. Hemolysis may be mild or severe, depending upon the properties of the mutant enzymes.

Severely affected homozygotes are anemic and jaundiced at birth and may require repeated transfusions during infancy. Less severely affected patients may or may not require intermittent transfusions throughout life. Anemia often worsens at times of infection or other stress. Splenomegaly is present. The indirect bilirubin level may be mildly elevated. As in all lifelong hemolytic disorders, patients may develop pigment gallstones at an early age.

Typical spherocytes are not present on the blood smear, and osmotic fragility studies (see Chapter 8) are negative. However, a minor population of small, dense RBCs with spicules may be noted on the peripheral blood smear. Reticulocyte counts are elevated, and unusually high reticulocyte counts may be found after splenectomy. Splenectomy, which decreases but does not abolish hemolysis, is usually recommended for patients with severe anemia.

The differential diagnosis of a hereditary hemolytic anemia without distinctive RBC morphologic clues to the diagnosis (for example, spherocytes, elliptocytes, sickled cells) includes three disorders:

1. Pyruvate kinase deficiency.
2. A severe variant of G6PD deficiency with resultant continuous hemolysis (see below).
3. An unstable hemoglobin (see Chapter 5).

Screening tests help to differentiate between these possible diagnoses: simple spot tests based upon the fluoresence of NADPH for the detection of pyruvate kinase deficiency and G6PD deficiency and an isopropanol stability test for the detection of an unstable hemoglobin.

Acquired Hypophosphatemia

Profound hypophosphatemia may cause RBC phosphate concentration to fall to levels that substantially impair red cell glycolysis. If, as a consequence, red cell ATP levels fall to about 15% of normal, the red cells become rigid spherocytes and a patient may develop acute hemolytic anemia. Since diminished red cell glycolysis also causes 2,3-DPG levels to fall, decreased tissue release of oxygen from hemoglobin compounds the resultant hypoxia. Correcting the hypophosphatemia rapidly corrects both the hemolysis and the impaired tissue oxygenation due to lowered 2,3-DP levels.

Hemolytic Anemia with Increased Red Cell Adenosine Deaminase Activity

The adenine nucleotides—ATP, ADP, and AMP (adenosine monophosphate)—contain the purine base adenine, a ribose sugar, and one or more phosphate groups. In human red cells, some AMP is irreversibly deaminated to inosine monophosphate with resultant decrease in the adenine nucleotide pool. The mature red cell cannot replenish the pool by new synthesis from small precursor molecules and must rely, instead, upon salvage pathways. One pathway involves the taking up from plasma of adenosine (adenine plus ribose but without attached phosphate) formed in the liver and other tissues. Adenosine entering the RBC may either be phosphorylated to AMP, and so enter the adenine phosphate pool, or may be deaminated to inosine with resultant loss to the pool. The former reaction is catalyzed by the enzyme adenosine kinase; the latter reaction is catalyzed by the enzyme adenosine deaminase.

A large kindred has been described in which a hereditary hemolytic anemia, transmitted as an autosomal dominant disorder, is associated with a manyfold increase in red cell adenosine deaminase activity and reduced red cell ATP levels. Presumably, the low ATP levels reflect inadequate salvage of adenine nucleotides due to preferential deamination of adenosine to inosine. The disorder is noteworthy, not only because it results from *increased* rather than decreased activity of a red cell enzyme, but also because it provides evidence for the importance of the adenosine salvage pathway for normal RBC survival.

Pyrimidine-5'-Nucleotidase Deficiency

As the reticulocyte is converted into a mature RBC, its RNA is degraded into purine (adenine, guanine) and pyrimidine (cytosine, uracil) nucleotides. The pyrimidine nucleotides must be disposed of to prevent their competing with ATP and ADP in metabolic reactions. An enzyme, pyrimidine-5'-nucleotidase splits off phosphate from pyrimidine nucleotides and the resulting pyrimidine nucleosides can then diffuse out of the RBC.

A number of families have now been recognized in which an autosomal recessive hemolytic anemia stems from hereditary pyrimidine-5'-nucleotidase deficiency. Finding many RBC on the blood smear with coarse basophilic stippling provides a clue to the diagnosis. Such basophilic stippling reflects impaired ribosomal RNA degradation resulting from the accumulation of pyrimidine nucleotides within the RBC. Presumably, the hemolysis reflects successful competition of pyrimidine nucleotides with adenine nucleotides in important steps of the Embden-Meyerhof pathway.

Finding stippled RBC on a blood smear should also alert one to the possibility of lead poisoning (see Fig. 2-8). The basophilic stippling of lead poisoning results from inhibition by lead of pyrimidine-5'-nucleotidase activity.

GLUCOSE-6-PHOSPHATE DEHYDROGENASE DEFICIENCY

In the 1950s, an unstable variant of glucose-6-phosphate dehydrogenase (G6PD) was found to be the cause of hemolytic anemia in black males sensitive to the antimalarial drug primaquine. Since then, more than 150 variants of G6PD have been identified by such properties as electrophoretic mobility, heat stability, and activity against substrates under various experimental conditions. These variants result from mutations affecting the gene coding for the amino acid sequence of G6PD. In some variants, enzymatic activity is severely deficient. In others, enzymatic activity is only moderately impaired; for example, the A⁻ variant (see below) has normal initial enzymatic activity that decreases as the RBC ages. In a few variants, discovered because of altered physical properties, enzymatic activity is normal.

The vast majority of G6PD variants are rare. The common variants associated with an increased risk of hemolysis are found in persons from tropical or subtropical countries. The high gene frequency in such populations represents another example of *balanced polymor-phism* in which the disadvantage conferred by the G6PD variant is offset by a selective advantage, possibly protection against falciparum malaria.

Clinical manifestations depend upon the degree of G6PD deficiency that a variant produces:

1. In the A^- (African) variant, an individual is asymptomatic until he is exposed to oxidant drugs or develops a serious infection. The African variant may also be associated with an increased incidence of neonatal jaundice in premature infants.
2. In Mediterranean variants, a group of variants found in Sardinians, Sicilians, Greeks, Sephardic and Oriental Jews, and Arabs, G6PD deficiency is more severe than in the African variant. Nevertheless, an affected person is usually asymptomatic until a drug or infection precipitates acute hemolysis. Some individuals also develop a fulminant hemolytic anemia after exposure to the fava bean (*favism*).
3. In variants producing the most profound G6PD deficiency, a mild continuous hemolysis is present. Infection or exposure to oxidant drugs triggers an acute, severe exacerbation. These rare variants are usually encountered in persons of northern European extraction.

Electrophoretic Mobility

G6PD from Caucasians migrates a certain distance on starch gel electrophoresis. G6PD with this electrophoretic mobility is called Type B. About 70% of blacks in the United States also have Type B G6PD. The remaining 30% have a G6PD with a more rapid electrophoretic mobility that is called Type A. In about two thirds of individuals with Type A G6PD, the G6PD has normal enzyme activity and is therefore called Type A^+. In the remaining one third, the Type A G6PD is unstable and deteriorates as the RBC ages. This variant, called Type A^- or the African variant, is responsible for hemolytic anemia in blacks due to G6PD deficiency.

Genetics of G6PD

The structural gene for G6PD is located on the X chromosome. Since a man is a hemizygote with only one X chromosome, he can have only one type of G6PD. A woman may be either a homozygote or a heterozygote with a different G6PD gene on each of her X chromosomes. If she is a heterozygote, her blood and other tissues will contain two types of G6PD.

Although a woman has two X chromosomes, she does not make twice as much G6PD as a man. In each cell of her body, only one X chromosome is active. Inactivation of one X chromosome occurs randomly in early embryonic life when each organ and tissue is represented by only a small number of precursor cells. Each organ and tissue of the female is thus a mosaic—a mixture of cells containing an active X chromosome from one parent and cells containing an active X chromosome from the other parent. Thus, whereas electrophoresis of a lysate of blood from a black woman who is a heterozygote for Type A and Type B G6PD will yield a band with Type A mobility and a band with Type B mobility, each individual RBC in the blood sample contains either Type A G6PD or Type B G6PD but not both.

It is important to emphasize that genetic mosaicism occurs only for traits on the X chromosome. For example, the structural gene for the β chain of hemoglobin is located on an autosomal chromosome. In a person who has one gene for hemoglobin A and one gene for hemoglobin S (sickle cell trait), each mature RBC arises from an erythroid precursor in which both autosomal chromosomes are active, and therefore each RBC must contain both Hgb A and Hgb S.

G6PD as a Cell Marker

Because single cells from a female heterozygous for Type A and B G6PD will contain only Type A or Type B G6PD, the characterization of G6PD in tumor tissue from such a heterozygote provides evidence for the monoclonal or polyclonal origin of the tumor. If the tumor tissue contains only one type of G6PD, then it is of monoclonal origin. If the tumor tissue contains both Type A and Type B G6PD, then it is of polyclonal origin. Such G6PD marker studies played a major role in establishing that, with rare exceptions (for example, early stages of fatal lymphoproliferative disorders related to Epstein-Barr viral infection, see Chapter 21), hematologic malignancies are monoclonal proliferative processes. G6PD marker studies have also helped to identify the cell of origin of a hematologic malignancy. For example, in heterozygotes for G6PD with chronic myelogenous leukemia, not only granulocytic cell lines, but also erythroid precursors, megakaryocytes, and B-lymphocytes were found to contain only a single type of G6PD. This provided important evidence that chronic myelogenous leukemia results from malignant transformation of a multipotent hematopoietic stem cell.

Clinical Manifestations of the A⁻ Variant

Hemolysis in black patients with the A⁻ variant is the only common manifestation of G6PD deficiency seen in the United States. Because the locus for G6PD is on the X chromosome, the patient is usually a male. However, hemolysis can also occur in females in two circumstances:

1. With an 11% gene frequency in the black population, occasional females will be homozygous for the A⁻ variant.
2. Since a female heterozygous for the A⁻ variant is a genetic mosaic, she will have a population of RBCs just as deficient in G6PD as the G6PD-deficient cells of a male. What part of her whole RBC population these deficient cells make up depends upon the chance inactivation of X chromosomes in the embryonic cells that become the hematopoietic stem cells. In some heterozygous women, the proportion of deficient cells is high enough to give rise to clinically significant hemolysis.

An affected individual may notice weakness, dark urine, and scleral icterus within several days of the onset of an infection or of starting to take an oxidant drug (for example, nitrofurantoin, certain sulfa drugs). Physical examination may reveal only mucosal pallor and scleral icterus. Splenomegaly is unusual.

Laboratory examination discloses:

1. *Evidence of hemolysis*
   a. A peripheral blood smear with numerous polychromatophilic macrocytes. If the RBC injury is severe enough to produce intravascular hemolysis, ghost cells may occasionally be noted on the smear. Spherocytosis is usually not prominent.
   b. A falling hematocrit despite an elevated reticulocyte count.
   c. Pigment changes
      (1) Increased bilirubin in the serum and urobilinogen in the urine.
      (2) Hemoglobinemia, methemalbuminemia, and hemoglobinuria if intravascular hemolysis occurs.
2. *Heinz bodies* (see Fig. 2-15), which are clumps of denatured hemoglobin that become attached to the RBC membrane, will usually, but not invariably, be found in the RBCs during the he-

molytic reaction. They are often first noticed when the reticulo-cytes are being counted because the dyes used to precipitate RNA as a reticulin network also stain Heinz bodies. The discovery of Heinz bodies may be the first clue to the diagnosis. (Heinz bodies may also be found in patients with hemolysis caused by an unstable hemoglobin.)

3. *An abnormal screening test for G6PD activity.* A commonly used spot test measures the fluorescence of NADPH generated in a reaction mixture in which the patient's lysed RBCs provides the G6PD needed for the reaction.

Hemolysis results from the impaired ability of the G6PD deficient RBC to provide the GSH needed to detoxify hydrogen peroxides and other peroxides formed within or entering the RBC (see Fig. 7-2). Consequently, these materials cause oxidative damage to hemoglobin that leads to its precipitation and crosslinking to the RBC membrane as Heinz bodies. Cells containing such precipitates are usually phagocytosed by mononuclear phagocytes but can become so rigid that they are also destroyed intravascularly.

Hemolysis ceases when use of an offending drug is stopped. In some patients, hemolysis slows down even though the drug is continued because the older, G6PD-deficient RBCs are replaced by young RBCs having more adequate levels of G6PD activity.

SELECTED READING

1. Beutler, E.: Glucose-6-phosphate dehydrogenase deficiency. In Stanbury JB, Wyngaarden JB, Fredrickson DS, Goldstein JL, and Brown MS (eds): The Metabolic Basis of Inherited Disease, 5th ed. New York, McGraw-Hill, 1983.
2. Jacob HS, and Amsden T: Acute hemolytic anemia with rigid red cells in hypophosphatemia. N Engl J Med 285:1446, 1971.
3. Valentine WN: The Stratton lecture. Hemolytic anemia and inborn errors of metabolism. Blood 54:549, 1979.

8

Hemolytic Anemias Caused by RBC Membrane Abnormalities

STRUCTURE OF THE RBC MEMBRANE

Red blood cell membranes are obtained by lysing RBCs in hypotonic saline and separating by centrifugation the heavier membranes from the released cytosolic proteins. Membranes are composed of *lipids*, which are arranged in a bilayer, and *proteins*, some of which are embedded within or traverse the lipid bilayer and others which adhere to its cytoplasmic surface. Several of the proteins at the cytoplasmic surface persist as a proteinaceous reticulum after RBC membranes are treated with a nonionic detergent (Triton). This proteinaceous network is called the *membrane skeleton*. The membrane may be considered to consist of two interacting parts:

1. An outer membrane bilayer of lipids and embedded proteins.
2. The underlying membrane skeleton.

The lipids of the bilayer consist of almost equal quantities of phospholipid and cholesterol plus a small amount of a glycolipid (a lipid containing a carbohydrate side chain) called ceramide. The choline-containing phospholipids (lecithin and sphingomyelin) are located in the outer layer of the bilayer with their hydrophilic heads oriented toward the exterior surface of the membrane; the amino-containing phospholipids (phosphatidyl ethanolamine and phospha-

130

tidyl serine) are located in the inner layer with their hydrophilic heads oriented toward the cytoplasmic surface of the membrane. The hydrophobic tails of both layers are oriented toward the interior of the membrane. Membrane cholesterol is in the free, non-esterified form and exchanges readily with plasma cholesterol. It is inserted between the inner and outer bilayer leaflets and is oriented perpendicular to the bilayer plane. An increase in the ratio of cholesterol to phospholipid decreases the fluidity of the membrane.

Techniques have been developed to extract the proteins from the membrane and to separate them on gel electrophoresis according to their size. The protein bands so obtained were initially identified numerically, beginning at the top of the gel—band 1, band 2, and so on. Today, many have more definitive names, that is, bands 1 and 2 are the two chains of spectrin and band 5 is erythrocyte actin, but some, such as band 3, retain their original numerical name.

Two of the proteins embedded within the bilayer traverse the bilayer, with their NH_2-terminal extending beyond the external surface and their carboxy-terminal extending beyond the cytoplasmic surface. One protein, glycophorin, is rich in carbohydrate; its functions are not yet known. The second protein, band 3, forms an anion channel in the membrane, through which chloride ions enter and leave the RBC as intracellular bicarbonate ion concentration varies with the carbon dioxide content of the blood. The carboxy-segment of band 3 is a key site of attachment to the membrane of hemoglobin, of certain enzymes, and of the membrane skeleton.

The major proteins of the membrane skeleton are spectrin, actin, band 4.1, and band 4.9. A fifth protein, ankyrin, although not strictly a component of the membrane skeleton since it may not persist after treatment of membranes with Triton, binds the membrane skeleton to the membrane bilayer. Spectrin is composed of two polypeptide chains (an α chain and a β chain) that intertwine to form a heterodimer. In the intact red cell, spectrin dimers associate head to head to give rise to tetramers or possibly higher oligomers (Fig. 8-1). At their tail ends, spectrin dimers are attached to the protein band 4.1 and to short filaments of actin, with resultant formation of a cross-linked, two-dimensional network of spectrin just beneath the lipid bilayer. Band 4.9 (not shown in Fig. 8-1) is also located in the membrane skeleton in association with actin; it may function to stabilize short actin oligomers. Ankryin binds to the β chain of spectrin heterodimers near the NH_2-terminal, or head end, and also to the carboxy-terminal of the integral membrane protein, band 3. This links the membrane skeleton to the membrane bilayer.

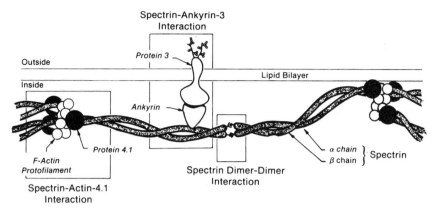

Fig. 8-1. A schematic model of the RBC membrane skeleton. A key integral membrane protein traversing the lipid bilayer, band 3, to which spectrin is bound at its head end through ankyrin, is shown. Another group of integral proteins traversing the bilayer, the glycophorins, to one of which spectrin may be attached at its tail end, are not shown in this figure. (Wolfe LC, John KM, Falcone JC, Byrne AM, Lux SE: A genetic defect in the binding of protein 4.1 to spectrin in a kindred with hereditary spherocytosis. N Engl J Med 307:1367, 1982, reproduced by permisson of the New England Journal of Medicine.)

Thus, as shown schematically in Figure 8-1, three interactions have been identified to date as required for the normal structure and function of the RBC membrane skeleton. They are:

1. The head-to-head interaction of spectrin dimers to form spectrin tetramers.
2. The binding of spectrin tails to actin through protein 4.1.
3. The binding of spectrin through ankryin to band 3 of the membrane bilayer.

Through as yet poorly understood interactions with the membrane bilayer, the membrane skeleton maintains the normal RBC membrane plasticity that allows RBCs to squeeze through the capillaries without loss of membrane or fragmentation and to return to their normal biconcave shape in the larger vessels. As described below, molecular alterations in the membrane skeleton can cause hereditary hemolytic anemias in which the RBC have abnormal shapes and unstable membranes.

HEMOLYTIC ANEMIAS DUE TO HEREDITARY MEMBRANE ABNORMALITIES

Hereditary Spherocytosis

Hereditary spherocytosis encompasses a group of hereditary hemolytic disorders of varying severity characterized by the following:

1. Autosomal dominant genetic transmission. (A very rare recessive form with life-threatening hemolysis has also been described.)
2. Spherocytes on the peripheral blood smear.
3. Correction of the anemia by splenectomy.

PATHOGENESIS

All patients with hereditary spherocytosis apparently have some degree of reduced spectrin content of the membrane skeleton; in the rare, recessive form of the disease this may amount to 50%. Since the molecular basis for the disorder remains undefined in most patients, we do not know whether only a few or many different spectrin defects will eventually be found to produce the syndrome of hereditary spherocytosis. In a minority of kindreds, a defect in spectrin that impairs its binding to protein 4.1 has been demonstrated.

Whatever its molecular bases, an abnormality of the membrane skeleton in hereditary spherocytosis causes the RBCs to lose membrane and so change from biconcave discs to spheres (spherocytes). This decreases their deformability. As a result, the spherocytes are delayed within the red pulp of the spleen as they work their way through the fenestrations of the splenic cords to enter the splenic sinusoids. In this metabolically deprived environment with its low glucose concentration, the RBCs are particularly susceptible to further membrane loss. After an unknown number of passages through the spleen, the RBCs become so damaged that they are phagocytosed selectively by mononuclear phagocytes of the red pulp. Therefore, splenectomy, although not affecting the underlying abnormality in the RBC membrane skeleton, corrects the anemia of hereditary spherocytosis.

CLINICAL MANIFESTATIONS

In some families, hereditary spherocytosis causes marked anemia that requires splenectomy in early childhood. In other families, episodes of anemia and jaundice are so mild that they may escape detection until late in life. Frequently, the patient is a young adult who seeks medical attention because of unexplained slight jaundice that may or may not be associated with weakness. Because patients with hereditary spherocytosis have an increased excretion of bilirubin, they have a high incidence of pigment gallstones. Gallstones or biliary colic in a youngster alerts one to the possibility of underlying hereditary spherocytosis that would require splenectomy at the time of cholecystectomy.

Because it is an autosomal dominant disorder, the work up of a patient with suspected hereditary spherocytosis should include study of both parents and of all siblings and children of the patient.

Physical examination usually reveals slight scleral icterus. A palpable spleen is found consistently.

Laboratory findings include:

1. The presence of spherocytes on the peripheral blood smear.
2. An elevated reticulocyte count.
3. A mildly elevated indirect reacting serum bilirubin level.
4. Increased osmotic fragility of the RBC. Sometimes the osmotic fragility of unincubated RBCs is nearly normal, with only a small tail of abnormally fragile cells; however, the osmotic fragility of RBCs that have been incubated for 24 hours at 37°C is markedly increased (Fig. 8-2).
5. A negative antiglobulin (Coombs') test result.

CRISES

Many patients with hereditary spherocytosis can maintain a normal hemoglobin level because increased red cell production keeps up with increased red cell destruction (compensated hemolytic anemia). However, crises of anemia may interrupt this state of compensation at unpredictable intervals. The patient in crisis may present:

1. With increased reticulocytosis, bilirubinemia, and splenomegaly. Presumably, infection or other stress has stimulated splenic mononuclear phagocytic activity with resultant increased hemolysis as the cause for the falling RBC count (hemolytic crisis).
2. With a markedly depressed reticulocyte count, diminished or absent erythroid precursors in the bone marrow, and no increase in bilirubinemia or splenomegaly. Something, such as a parvovirus infection, has temporarily curtailed RBC production and produced an aplastic crisis. During recovery from such a

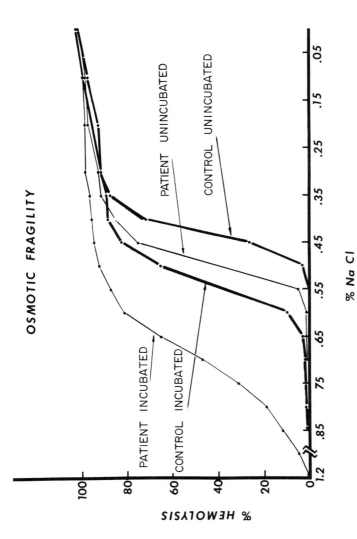

Fig. 8-2. Osmotic fragility of unincubated and incubated RBCs from a normal individual and from a patient with hereditary spherocytosis. The striking increase in fragility produced by incubation of hereditary spherocytosis RBCs is obvious.

135

crisis, marked erythroid hyperplasia and a high reticulocyte count are found. If the patient is first seen at this stage, it may be impossible to distinguish between increased hemolysis and earlier aplasia as the cause for the anemic crisis.

THERAPY

Since splenectomy abolishes clinically significant hemolysis, splenectomy is usually recommended once the diagonsis is established. Exceptions are:

1. An infant or young child. Splenectomy increases the risk of serious pneumococcal septicemia, particularly during the early years of life. Therefore, unless anemia is very severe, one delays splenectomy until a child is older.
2. An older patient with a mild form of the disease in whom the morbidity and risk of the procedure may outweigh its benefit, which, in such a patient, consists primarily of the prevention of pigment gallstones.

If significiant hemolysis persists after splenectomy, the diagnosis of hereditary spherocytosis should be abandoned and another cause for the hemolysis should be sought.

Hereditary Elliptocytosis

Hereditary elliptocytosis consists of a heterogenous group of disorders in which large numbers of ellipitcal RBCs are found on the peripheral blood smear. The elliptical shape reflects failure of RBCs deformed by shear stress in the microcirculation to return to a normal biconcave shape in the larger vessels.

Several forms of hereditary elliptocytosis have been described and undoubtedly more will be found. Most appear to result from defects in spectrin that impair its self-association to form tetramers. Types of hereditary elliptocytosis include:

1. An asymptomatic form, which is essentially an autosomal dominant "cosmetic" disorder. Many elliptocytes are found on the blood smear, yet hemolysis is absent or very mild. The affected individual is a heterozygote. This is the common form of hereditary elliptocytosis seen in the United States.
2. A hybrid disorder combining features of mild hereditary elliptocytosis and mild hereditary spherocytosis. Both elliptocytes and spherocytes are seen on the blood smear and the RBCs, particularly after incubation, have increased RBC fragility. Most pa-

tients have evidence of compensated, mild hemolysis. This disorder is also relatively common in the United States.

3. Rare forms with moderately severe hemolytic anemia and a peripheral blood smear on which one finds elliptical RBCs, spherocytes, and RBC fragments (Fig. 8-3). Some of these patients are homozygote members of kindreds in which heteroygotes have the asymptomatic "cosmetic" disorder; however, in some families, the disorder appears to stem, not from a defect in spectrin, but from a defect in the binding of ankyrin to band 3 or from an absence of protein 4.1.

Hereditary Pyropoikilocytosis

Hereditary pyropoikilocytosis is a moderate to severe hemolytic disorder which resembles severe forms of hereditary elliptocytosis in

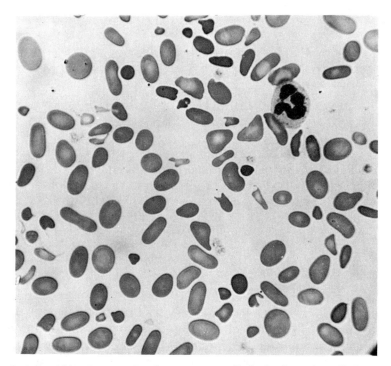

Fig. 8-3. Peripheral blood smear showing numerous elliptical cells and small pieces of fragmented RBCs. This patient, who was seen many years ago, was then thought to have an unusual form of hereditary elliptocytosis. The correct diagnosis is probably hereditary pyropoikilocytosis but would require a heat precipitation test for confirmation.

that elliptocytes, spherocytes, and RBC fragments are seen on the peripheral smear. It differs from the latter in that:

1. The large numbers of microspherocytes and other small RBC fragments that are formed as a consequence of shear stress in the microcirculation give rise to a striking microcytosis (MCV 55–75 fL).
2. The RBCs exhibit abnormal sensitivity to heat. Whereas normal RBCs fragment at temperatures exceeding 49°C, the RBCs in hereditary pyropoikilocytosis fragment at 45 to 46°C.

The dimer-dimer association of spectrin in the RBCs of patients with hereditary pyropoikilocytosis is defective. The molecular basis for the abnormality has yet to be delineated.

The patient is a presumed double heterozygote. In at least one parent, mild elliptocytosis will be found. The other parent may have no identifiable morphologic or biochemical RBC abnormality but special tests of red cell deformability will demonstrate a defect.

HEMOLYTIC ANEMIAS DUE TO ACQUIRED MEMBRANE DEFECTS

Paroxysmal Nocturnal Hemoglobinuria

PATHOGENESIS

Paroxysmal nocturnal hemoglobinuria (PNH) is characterized by an acquired intrinsic abnormality of RBC membranes that increases their sensitivity to lysis by complement. The disorder arises as a somatic mutation in a pluripotent hematopoietic stem cell that differentiates to form not only RBCs but granulocytes and platelets, which are also abnormal in this disorder. Occasionally, PNH develops after an obvious earlier marrow-damaging event, for example, idiopathic or drug-induced marrow aplasia (see Chapter 11).

Mechanism of the Membrane Abnormality. The underlying cause for the blood cell membrane defects of PNH is unknown but related to one way in which cell membrane proteins are affixed to the membrane. Certain proteins, located primarily on the outer surface of the lipid bilayer, are attached to the membrane by a glycolipid tail. This glycolipid tail begins at the COOH-terminal of the protein and ends linked to inositol on phosphatidyl inositol, a phospholipid found in the outer layer of the lipid bilayer. Treating membranes with phospholipase C, an enzyme that cleaves inositol from phosphatidyl inositol, releases these proteins from membranes. Two RBC membrane proteins whose activity in PNH is markedly decreased are attached to the membrane through such a glycolipid linkage to phosphatidyl inositol. One of these proteins is the enzyme, acetylcholinesterase; the second is a protein called decay-accelerating factor (DAF).

Although deficiency of RBC acetylcholinesterase in PNH may be an epiphenomenon, diminished DAF activity appears at least partly responsible for the increased sensitivity to complement that causes hemolysis in PNH. DAF functions like factor H, a known regulator of complement activation in soluble systems, to facilitate proteolytic inactivation of the key intermediate of complement activation, C3b, by an inhibitor called factor I. The RBCs in PNH accumulate C3b on their surface as a result of the normally slow, spontaneous activation of C3 by the alternative pathway of complement plus the impaired inactivation of C3b in the absence of DAF. This allows the complement activation sequence to proceed to completion on the membrane, with resultant formation of the terminal C5b,6,7,8,9 complex, the so-called membrane attack complex.

However, impaired ability to prevent formation of the membrane attack complex does not fully explain the increased sensitivity of the membrane of the PNH red cell to complement. Exposing PNH red cells to formed membrane attack complex damages the red cells more extensively than does exposing normal RBC to formed membrane attack complex. The possibility exists that an as yet unrecognized protein that dampens the ability of the membrane attack complex to open holes in the RBC membrane may also be missing from the RBC membrane in PNH.

Disturbed Hematopoiesis in Paroxysmal Nocturnal Hemoglobinuria. When RBCs from a patient with PNH are exposed to increasing amounts of activated complement, one finds a population of RBCs very sensitive to lysis by complement, sometimes a second, smaller population of RBCs with moderately increased sensitivity to lysis by complement, and a third population of cells that require as much complement for lysis as do normal cells. Studies of a patient with PNH who was also a heterozygote for G6PD revealed that the cells with increased sensitivity to complement contained only a single G6PD isoenzyme, and therefore were of monoclonal origin. In contrast, the cells with normal responsiveness to complement contained both isoenzymes, and therefore represented the polyclonal progency of residual normal stem cells. Apparently, the mutation of PNH confers an advantage that allows the descendents of the mutated stem cell to "take over" hematopoiesis to a large extent but not completely.

Indeed, as distinct from a somatic hematopoietic stem cell mutation that leads to uncontrolled overproliferation and, therefore, a hematologic malignancy (see Chapter 15), the mutation of PNH is frequently associated with a variable degree of marrow *hypoproliferation*. Thus, reactive erythroid hyperplasia in response to increased erythropoietin production may not be as prominent in PNH as in patients with the same degree of anemia due to other causes for hemolysis. Hypoproliferation is not confined to patients in whom PNH arises after known marrow aplasia and presumably reflects aberrant growth properties of the PNH clone.

Leukopenia is common in PNH. It is not known whether it results from impaired granulocyte production, from an effect of increased sensitivity of granulocyte membranes to damage by complement, or from both. As in patients with other syndromes in which somatic mutations result in aberrant hematopoiesis and abnormal differentiated cells (myelodysplastic syndromes, Chapter 11), in a small number of patients with PNH, the disease, at some point in its course, transforms into an acute myeloblastic leukemia.

Thrombocytopenia sometimes occurs in PNH. The platelets, which also lack DAF on their surface, are unusually susceptible to damage by platelet antibodies in in vitro test systems. Whether this mechanism or hypoproliferation is primarily responsible for the thrombocytopenia is not known.

CLINICAL MANIFESTATIONS

PNH usually begins insidiously in a previously healthy person. Occasionally, as already mentioned, it develops in a patient with idiopathic or drug-induced marrow aplasia. The patient is frequently aware of increased fatigue due to anemia. Hemolysis is often increased at night because carbon dioxide retention during sleep leads to a slight fall in plasma pH that facilitates activation of complement. Nocturnal hemoglobinuria may result and cause the patient's urine to be very dark in color (hence the disease's name, paroxysmal nocturnal hemoglobinuria). However, some patients may have been unaware of dark morning urine.

Abnormal physical findings may be limited to pallor, slight jaundice, or both. Splenomegaly is not prominent and is often absent.

Laboratory findings include:

1. Anemia with reticulocytosis and occasional nucleated RBCs on the blood smear but *without spherocytosis* or other distinctive alterations in RBC morphology.

2. Moderate leukopenia and variable thrombocytopenia.
3. Plasma and urine pigment abnormalities that reflect the severity of the intravascular hemolysis:
   a. When intravascular hemolysis is severe, the plasma will contain hemoglobin, methemalbumin, and an elevated indirect-reacting bilirubin level. When intravascular hemolysis is low grade, plasma abnormalities may be limited to a low haptoglobin level and an elevated indirect-reacting bilirubin level.
   b. When intravascular hemolysis is severe, the urine will be "coffee colored" because it contains hemoglobin. When hemoglobinuria is absent, the urine still contains evidence of chronic intravascular hemolysis in the form of hemosiderin granules in the sediment.
4. Evidence of increased susceptibility of the RBC to hemolysis by complement in the form of a positive acid hemolysis test (Ham test) or a positive sucrose hemolysis test. The latter is a simple test in which 9 mL of a 10% sucrose solution is added to 1 mL of the patient's blood taken in citrate or oxalate anticoagulant (but not EDTA, which will block complement activation). This creates an isotonic environment with low ionic strength in which RBCs become coated with complement. After 30 minutes, the sensitive population of cells in PNH will have lysed (giving the sucrose solution a red color), whereas other RBCs remain intact.

SCREENING TESTS

Because its clinical manifestations need not be distinctive, PNH must be ruled out in any patient with an unexplained chronic hemolytic anemia. Two simple screening tests are used:

1. Staining of the urine sediment for hemosiderin to look for evidence of chronic intravascular hemolysis.
2. The sucrose hemolysis test to look for evidence of increased sensitivity of RBC to lysis by complement.

If these simple tests are negative, the diagnosis of PNH is excluded.

COURSE, COMPLICATIONS, AND THERAPY

PNH is a disorder in which a chronic anemia, with intermittent exacerbations of acute hemolysis, persists until the patient's death. Infection, by increasing activation of C3, may trigger a hemolytic episode. Complications of PNH include:

1. *Thrombosis*, which is a major cause of death. The patient with PNH is peculiarly susceptible to venous thrombosis at unusual sites, including the hepatic veins with resultant development of the Budd-Chiari syndrome. The cause for the thrombotic tendency is unknown.
2. *Iron deficiency.* The chronic intravascular hemolysis of PNH may result in sufficient iron loss in the urine to deplete iron stores and produce a complicating iron deficiency anemia.
3. *Development of acute leukemia.*

No definitive treatment is available for PNH except possibly the high-risk procedure of bone marrow transplantation in a young patient with an HLA-compatible sibling. If transfusions are needed during an exacerbation of hemolysis, leukocyte and platelet poor, washed RBCs should be used to avoid reactions to antigens on WBCs or platelets that may activate complement. Oral iron will correct secondary iron deficiency anemia but may provoke increased hemolysis. Presumably, this results from an increased output of new complement-sensitive RBCs in response to the iron therapy. Androgens have been used to stimulate erythropoiesis in patients with marrow hypoplasia but may also provoke increased hemolysis for the same reason. Adrenal glucocorticoids have been reported to benefit some patients. Their mechanism of action is not clear, and their possible benefits must be balanced against the deleterious effects of the long-term use of glucocorticoids. Patients who have experienced one thrombotic episode probably deserve a trial of long-term therapy with an oral anticoagulant.

Spur Cell Anemia

An anemia with striking acanthocytosis, called spur cell anemia, may develop in patients with advanced chronic liver disease. An increase in the ratio of cholesterol to phospholipid in the RBC membrane plays an important role in the pathogenesis of this anemia, which is discussed further in Chapter 12.

SELECTED READING

1. Goodman SR, and Shiffer K: The spectrin membrane skeleton of normal and abnormal human erythrocytes: a review. Am J Physiol 244:C121. 1983.
2. Palek J, and Lux SE: Red cell membrane skeletal defects in hereditary and acquired hemolytic anemias. Semin Hematol 20:189, 1983.

3. Pangburn MK, Schreiber RD, and Muller-Eberhard HJ: Deficiency of an erythrocyte membrane protein with complement regulatory activity in paroxysmal nocturnal hemoglobinuria. Proc Natl Acad Sci USA 80:5430, 1983.

4. Rosse WF: Paroxysmal nocturnal hemoglobinuria—present status and future prospects: Tenth Annual Paul M. Aggeler Memorial Lecture, Medical Staff Conference, University of California, San Francisco. West J Med 132:219, 1980.

9

Hemolytic Anemias Caused by Antibodies

An understanding of hemolytic anemias caused by antibodies requires a review of RBC antigens and of the properties of IgM and IgG RBC antibodies.

RBC ANTIGENS

About 400 RBC antigens have been identified by serologic means. Their immunologic specificity is derived from structural differences in the carbohydrates, lipids, and proteins of the RBC membrane. These may be minor differences. For example, blood group A antigen differs from blood group B antigen only in that the carbohydrate chain of group A antigen ends in N-acetyl-galactosamine, whereas the carboydrate chain of group B antigen ends in galactose.

RBC antigens that are peptides are under direct genetic control, that is, the gene products are polypeptide chains whose amino acid sequences determine their antigenic specificity. RBC antigens that are carbohydrates are under indirect genetic control. The gene products are enzymes called *transferases* that catalyze attachment to carbohydrate chains of the monosaccharides responsible for antigenic specificity.

Those antigens controlled by genes at the same locus (alleles) or closely linked loci are classified together as a blood group system, for example, the ABO system or the Rh system. Some of the more important of the 21 established blood group systems are discussed briefly below.

144

ABO System

The ABO system, discovered in 1900, remains the most important of the blood group systems. For simplification, an individual's ABO phenotype may be thought of as being determined by three allelic genes (Table 9-1). However, additional alleles at the ABO locus are known to exist because two subgroups of A (A_1 and A_2) that differ in some serologic properties have been identified.

The ABO antigens are not confined to RBCs but are found on most, if not all, cells. Moreover, about 80% of individuals have glycoproteins with ABO antigenic specificities in secretions (saliva, gastric juice). These individuals, who are referred to as secretors, have a gene designated as Se and may be of genotype Se/Se or Se/se. Nonsecretors have the genotype se/se.

Certain cattle serum samples were found to contain antibodies that react preferentially with group O RBCs. Group O individuals who are secretors were found to have a substance in their secretions that neutralizes these antibodies. Individuals of blood groups A, B, or AB who are secretors also have this substance in their secretions in lesser amounts. Since an individual of blood type AB cannot possess an O gene (see Table 9-1), this neutralizing substance cannot require the product of the O gene for its formation. Therefore, it was not called O substance but was given the name *H substance.*

It is now known that:

1. *Production* of H substance requires a gene called the H gene (the inactive allele is the h gene).
2. *Secretion* of H substance into body fluids requires the Se gene (the inactive allele is the se gene).
3. *Conversion of H substance into A or B antigens* requires the presence of an A or B gene (the inactive allele is the O gene).

Table 9-1. The Relation between ABO Phenotypes and Genotypes

PHENOTYPE	GENOTYPE	AGGLUTINATION OF RBCS	
		By Anti-A Serum	By Anti-B Serum
A	A/A	+	−
A	A/O	+	−
B	B/B	−	+
B	B/O	−	+
AB	A/B	+	+
O	O/O	−	−

Steps in the formation of the A and B antigens on the RBC membrane are summarized in Figure 9-1.

H antigen is found, not only on group O RBCs, but in lesser amounts (since not all H substance is converted into A or B substance) on the RBCs of the other ABO blood groups. Very rare individuals, homozygous for the inactive h allele, have no H antigen on their RBCs and, since H is the precursor, no A or B antigen either. Individuals with this rare genotype, called the Bombay genotype, develop naturally occurring antibodies to the A and B antigens and to the H antigen. Therefore, they cannot be transfused except with Bombay genotype blood.

Lewis System

The Lewis antigens differ from all other RBC antigens in that they are not synthesized within the RBC but are absorbed onto the RBC. The allelic genes of the Lewis system are Le and le. An individual who is le/le does not make a Lewis antigen. An individual who has an Le gene (Le/Le or Le/le) makes an antigen called Le^a which differs from H substance only in the position of its fucose group. Le^a is either absorbed onto the RBC membrane or modified, by addition of a second fucose group, to form Le^b before absorption. Conversion of Le^a to Le^b requires the presence of an Se gene. Thus, an individual's Lewis phenotype results from an interaction of Le and Se genes in one of the following possible combinations:

LE GENE	SE GENE	PHENOTYPE
+	+	Le^{a-b+}
+	−	Le^{a+b-}
−	+ or −	Le^{a-b-}

Ii System

The name anti-I was given to an IgM antibody from the serum of a patient with cold agglutinin disease (see below). This antibody reacted with the RBCs of many thousands of individuals who were therefore said to have the I antigen. It failed to react with blood from rare adults who, therefore, lacked the I antigen and had, instead, an i antigen.

The Ii antigens are carbohydrate antigens related to the ABO blood group antigens, and, like the ABO antigens, are present on many cells other than RBCs. Adult RBCs, with rare exception, have many I antigen sites and few i antigen sites. In contrast, cord blood has primarily i antigen sites. The conversion to the adult pattern is

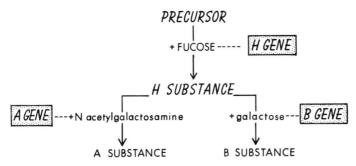

Fig. 9-1. Steps in the synthesis of A and B antigen on the RBC membrane.

completed by age 2 or 3 years. In hereditary disorders with abnormal erythropoiesis (for example, thalassemia) and in some acquired conditions with abnormal erythropoiesis (for example, aplastic anemia), adult patients may make RBCs that retain features of fetal erythropoiesis, including increased amounts of i antigen. The Ii system is of clinical interest because the antibodies responsible for most instances of IgM cold agglutinin disease have anti-I specificity.

Rh System

When RBCs from Rhesus monkeys are injected into rabbits, an antiserum is produced that reacts with RBCs from most humans. Reactive individuals are Rh (Rhesus) positive. Unreactive individuals (15% of Caucasians, 5% of blacks, 1% of Asians) are Rh negative. Rh positive RBCs have an antigen that is called Rh_o in one nomenclature and D in another. An Rh-positive person is of either homozygous (D/D) or heterozygous (D/d) genotype. An Rh-negative person must be of d/d genotype.

The Rh system contains antigens besides D and d and, for simplicity, may be thought of as consisting of three pairs of allelic genes, C/c, D/d, and E/e, located so close together on the chromosome that they are inherited from each parent as a unit. Certain resultant patterns of antigens are more common than others. For example, with few exceptions, the Rh-negative individual is not only d/d but cde/cde.

The D antigen is highly immunogenic and D incompatibility is a major cause of hemolytic disease of the newborn. Approximately 80% of Rh-negative individuals given Rh-positive blood will develop anti-D antibodies. The other Rh antigens are much less immunogenic; they produce antibodies after transfusion in only a few individuals.

Other Blood Group Systems

Several other blood group systems (Kidd, Duffy, Kell, MNSs) are clinically important because the antigens possess sufficient immunogenicity to sensitize occasional patients after transfusion, with the resultant risk of hemolysis after a later transfusion.

The *Kidd system* has two allelic antigens, Jk^a and Jk^b, and three major phenotypes: Jk(a + b −), Jk(a − b −), and Jk(a + b +). Antibodies to Jk^a may cause a severe transfusion reaction and yet be difficult to demonstrate in vitro. If good typing serum were readily available, typing for the Jk^a antigen to prevent sensitization would probably be added to the routine typing procedure for blood transfusion (see Chapter 30).

The *Duffy system* has two major antigens, Fy^a and Fy^b. Three phenotypes are found in whites: Fy(a + b −), Fy(a − b +), and Fy(a + b +). A fourth phenotype, Fy(a − b −) represents homozygosity for an allele producing no Fy antigen and is common in blacks. Fy(a − b −) RBCs resist invasion by the malarial parasite *Plasmodium vivax*, which suggests that the Fy antigen is part of an RBC surface receptor for the parasite. The selective advantage of protection against vivax malaria may explain the increased prevalence of the Fy(a − b −) phenotype in blacks.

The *Kell system,* like the Rh system, has several sets of antigens of which one allelic pair, the K and k antigens, possess the most immunogenicity. A rare variant phenotype, named *McLeod* after the first patient, has been described in which the RBCs lack a precursor material for the Kell antigens, called K$_x$. Persons with the McLeod phenotype have a compensated hemolytic anemia and a blood smear showing RBC with numerous irregular or blunt surface projections (acanthocytes, see Fig. 12-1). This suggests that the Kell system antigens are present on structural components of the RBC membrane whose deletion impairs membrane stability. Of further interest, but unclear meaning, is the discovery that males with X-linked chronic granulomatous disease (see Chapter 14) lack K$_x$ on their granulocytes and may also have a decreased expression of Kell antigens on their RBCs.

RBC ANTIBODIES

RBC antibodies are of two classes: IgM antibodies and IgG antibodies. (The structure of the various classes of antibodies is discusssed in Chapter 20.)

IgM Antibodies

When RBCs are suspended in saline, the repulsion of their like negative charges keeps individual red cells many Ångstrom units apart. Because IgM antibodies are large molecules (molecular weight, 900,000 daltons) with ten antigen combining sites per molecule, IgM antibodies can span the space between individual RBCs and bind to antigen sites on more than one RBC. Therefore, IgM antibodies can agglutinate RBCs suspended in saline. Cooling enhances the interaction of IgM antibodies with RBC membrane antigens; thus, IgM antibodies bind more readily to RBCs at temperatures below body temperature.

IgM antibodies activate complement on the RBC membrane. Complement activation by the classic pathway requires binding of a complement component called Clq to a site that becomes available on the carboxy-terminal portion (Fc fragment, see Chapter 20) of an antibody molecule after its antigen binding site reacts with antigen. A Clq molecule must bind to not just one but two Fc fragment binding sites spaced just the right distance apart (a doublet) for the activation of Clq. Because IgM antibodies usually have specificity for antigens with many RBC membrane sites and because each antibody molecule has ten antigen combining sites and five Clq binding sites, the reaction between a single IgM molecule and RBC membrane antigen sites can activate a Clq molecule on the RBC membrane.

Clinically important IgM antibodies include:

1. The naturally occurring ABO alloagglutinins.
2. The cold agglutinins that may develop after infection or as a manifestation of an immunologic disorder.

IgG Antibodies

IgG antibodies are much smaller molecules (molecular weight, 160,000 daltons) than IgM antibodies. Although each antibody molecule has two antigen combining sites, a single molecule usually cannot react with two RBCs suspended in saline; therefore, with rare exceptions, IgG antibodies coat but do not agglutinate RBCs in saline.

IgG antibodies may or may not bind complement to the RBC membrane. This depends upon the number and IgG subclass (see Chapter 20) of antibody molecules that attach to the RBC membrane. Unlike IgM antibody, many molecules of IgG antibody must attach to the membrane to favor the probability of forming a doublet and, therefore, of activating Clq.

Clinically important IgG antibodies include:

1. The alloantibodies responsible for hemolytic disease of the newborn.
2. The antibodies responsible for the warm type of autoimmune hemolytic anemia.

The Antiglobulin Test

Special techniques are necessary to demonstrate IgG antibody on RBCs. The test usually used is the antiglobulin test (Coombs' test), which uses rabbit anti-human globulin antiserum (Coombs' serum). There are two kinds of antiglobulin tests:

1. *The direct antiglobulin (direct Coombs') test,* which tests for IgG antibody coating circulating RBCs. A drop of antiglobulin serum is added to a saline suspension of the patient's washed RBCs. If the RBCs are coated with IgG, it reacts with the anti-human globulin antiserum and the red cells agglutinate.
2. *The indirect antiglobulin (indirect Coombs') test,* which tests for IgG *antibody in the patient's serum* capable of binding to RBC antigens. The patient's serum is incubated with a mixture of group O test RBCs that contain most of the known RBC antigens. Then, the RBCs are washed, suspended in saline, and reacted with the anti-human globulin antiserum. If the patient's serum contains free antibody that comes down onto the test RBCs during the preliminary incubation, then the RBCs will agglutinate on the addition of the antiglobulin antiserum.

The above interpretations of positive tests are true when the antiglobulin antiserum reacts only with IgG. Because the antiglobulin test is mainly used for cross matching for blood transfusion, most laboratories use a broad-spectrum antiglobulin serum, which reacts both with IgG and with complement components. Therefore, when a patient is discovered to have a positive direct antiglobulin test, further tests are required with IgG-specific antiglobulin serum and with complement-specific antiglobulin serum to characterize the protein coating the RBCs.

HEMOLYSIS CAUSED BY ALLOANTIBODIES

An RBC alloantibody is an antibody that will react with RBCs from the same species but not with RBCs from the individual producing the antibody. Hemolysis due to alloantibodies is seen in two clinical circumstances: in hemolytic blood transfusion reactions and in hemolytic disease of the newborn.

Hemolytic Transfusion Reactions

ABO REACTIONS

Antibodies to the A and B antigens develop naturally in early infancy. All individuals of blood type A possess anti-B antibodies; all individuals of blood type B possess anti-A antibodies; and all individuals of blood type O possess both anti-A and anti-B antibodies. Therefore, a patient may have a severe hemolytic reaction the first time he or she is given blood of the wrong ABO blood group. The plasma will contain agglutinins that destroy the transfused RBCs, that is, he or she will have a *major side* transfusion reaction.

Theoretically, group O donor blood should be safe for any recipient, because group O cells possess neither the A nor the B antigen and, therefore, will not be destroyed by either anti-A or anti-B antibodies in a recipient's plasma. However, group O donor blood may contain a high titer of anti-A and anti-B antibodies in its plasma. When such group O blood is given as a whole blood transfusion, the antibodies in the transfused plasma may hemolyze the recipient's RBCs. This is called a *minor side* hemolytic transfusion reaction. Consequently, except for ABO hemolytic disease of the newborn (in which a group A infant acquires maternal anti-A antibodies transplacentally and will, therefore, hemolyze group A blood), it is safest to transfuse only with ABO group-specific blood.

Rh REACTIONS

Because of the powerful immunogenicity of the D antigen, hemolysis due to Rh incompatability occurs primarily in the Rh-negative (no D antigen) patient who is mistakenly given Rh-positive blood. However, since anti-D antibodies do not develop naturally, the patient must first have been sensitized by an earlier exposure to RBCs containing the D antigen. In a man, this can happen only from the prior administration of Rh-positive blood or blood components (for example, platelet concentrates) contaminated with RBCs. In a woman, this can also result from sensitization by fetal Rh-positive RBCs that gain access to the maternal circulation at delivery or at the time of an abortion.

Despite the large number of RBC antigens, the recipient of a blood transfusion is usually typed only for the ABO blood group and the presence or absence of the D antigen (Rh type). One relies upon screening for antibodies in both the recipient's plasma and the donor's plasma to prevent hemolysis by alloantibodies to other RBC antigens (see Chapter 30). However, this practice does not prevent occasional patients from developing an alloantibody after exposure to foreign RBC antigens in transfused blood. When this happens, it may be hard to find compatible blood for further transfusions if:

1. The antibody develops to an antigen present in the vast majority of donors.
2. Alloantibodies develop to several RBC antigens.

MANIFESTATIONS AND TREATMENT OF
HEMOLYTIC TRANSFUSION REACTIONS

The findings and management of hemolytic transfusion reactions are discussed in Chapter 30.

Hemolytic Disease of the Newborn

Rh HEMOLYTIC DISEASE

Pathogenesis. Hemolytic disease of the newborn due to Rh incompatibility usually results from the following events:

1. The fetus receives from the father the D antigen, which the mother does not possess.
2. The mother has been sensitized to the D antigen from a previous pregnancy or exposure to blood products. Therefore, she makes an IgG type of anti-D antibody in response to booster antigenic stimuli from tiny amounts of fetal RBCs that leak across the placenta during the pregnancy.
3. Since the mother's RBCs do not possess the D antigen, they do not react with the antibody. However, the IgG antibody crosses the placenta and reacts with fetal RBCs with resultant hemolysis.

Manifestations and Treatment. If intrauterine RBC production lags too far behind intrauterine RBC destruction, the fetus becomes severely anemic and may die of heart failure with massive edema (hydrops fetalis). When severe Rh incompatibility has occurred with an earlier pregnancy or if the mother has a rising titer of anti-D antibody, amniocentesis is performed to measure amniotic fluid bilirubin concentration, which reflects the severity of intrauterine hemolysis. This is used to decide whether to recommend transuterine transfusion of RBCs into the peritoneal cavity of the fetus. Labor is induced after the 34th week if the analysis of the ratio of lecithin to sphingomyelin in the amniotic fluid indicates sufficient maturity of the fetal lung to lessen the risk of the respiratory distress syndrome associated with prematurity.

If intrauterine RBC production can match RBC destruction, the infant will be born alive and without significant anemia. The main clinical problem is prevention of cerebral damage due to a rising level of bilirubin (kernicterus) in the first days of life. The findings at birth are:

1. *Physical examination.* The infant is not jaundiced at birth, but jaundice may become apparent within hours. Hepatosplenomegaly is found.
2. *Laboratory examination.*
    a. Peripheral blood count.
       (1) The hemoglobin level is lower than the expected normal of 16 to 19 g per dL at birth but need not be markedly depressed. A relatively high cord blood hemoglobin level, for example, 15 g per dL, provides no assurance that the infant will not develop marked hyperbilirubinemia.
       (2) Polychromatophilic macrocytes and nucleated RBC are found in large numbers on the blood smear and the reticulocyte count is markedly elevated.
       (3) Spherocytes are not present or not prominent on the blood smear (which reflects phagocytosis of entire RBCs rather than of pieces of RBC membrane).
       (4) The WBC count is high.
       (5) Thrombocytopenia, with a platelet count below 50,000 per µL, sometimes occurs.
    b. Serologic studies.
       (1) *The infant's cord blood cells have a positive direct antiglobulin test.* This finding alone permits a presumptive diagnosis of Rh hemolytic disease.
       (2) *The mother's RBCs have a negative direct antiglobulin test,* but the mother's serum contains anti-D as demonstrated by a *positive indirect antiglobulin test.*

(3) The mother will be Rh negative and the infants cord blood cells will be Rh positive. (Rh typing of the infant's cells may be difficult if the Rh antigen sites are heavily coated with anti-D from the mother.)

c. Bilirubin. Levels may be only slightly higher than the upper limit of normal (3 mg per dL) at birth because the excess bilirubin load is disposed of by way of the placenta during intrauterine life. Bilirubinemia increases rapidly within hours after birth because hemolysis continues and the liver cells of the newborn cannot bind and conjugate bilirubin efficiently.

Hemolysis persists with decreasing intensity for a number of days until all maternal antibody has been consumed. The goal of treatment is to prevent non-conjugated bilirubin, which is lipid soluble, from rising to a level (about 20 mg per dL) that can damage the lipid-rich tissue of the central nervous system. If the serum level is above 7 mg per dL at birth, one begins treatment with an exchange transfusion without delay. If the bilirubin is in the 4 to 5 mg per dL range and rising slowly, one often begins treatment with phototherapy (exposure to ultraviolet light), which converts bilirubin into water-soluble products excreted in the urine and bile.

Prevention. Sensitization of an Rh-negative woman as a result of a first pregnancy can now be prevented. Studies utilizing a stain for Hgb F that permits recognition of fetal cells on the mother's blood smear revealed that the sensitizing exposure during a first pregnancy occurs at the time of delivery (or abortion), when 1 to 10 mL of fetal RBCs may enter the maternal circulation. The fetal RBCs must circulate in the mother to act as an antigenic stimulus. The injection of anti-D antibody will destroy the fetal RBCs before they can stimulate maternal antibody production. Therefore, an Rh-negative mother, unless she is already sensitized, should be given an intramuscular injection of high titer anti-D gamma globulin (RhoGam) within 72 hours of delivery, abortion, or genetic amniocentesis. This practice has markedly reduced the incidence of Rh hemolytic disease of the newborn.

ABO HEMOLYTIC DISEASE

ABO hemolytic disease is less common than would be expected from the high incidence of ABO incompatibility between mother and infant. It usually occurs in a group A infant whose mother is group O. Every group O mother will have anti-A and anti-B in her serum, but these natural agglutinins are IgM antibodies that cannot cross the placenta. However, an occasional group O mother also makes anti-A of the IgG type, which can cross the placenta and react with the group A cells of the fetus.

Severe anemia is rare. Unlike Rh-hemolytic disease, spherocytes are prominent on the infant's blood smear, and the direct antiglobulin test is often only weakly positive. Jaundice developing during the first day usually provides the earliest clue to the diagnosis. The major risk is failure to recognize and correct hyperbilirubinemia before the central nervous system is damaged. If exchange transfusion is used, group O blood is given to prevent hemolysis of transfused RBCs by anti-A in the infant's plasma.

HEMOLYSIS CAUSED BY AUTOANTIBODIES

An RBC autoantibody is an antibody that reacts with an antigen on the RBCs of the individual making the antibody. It violates the immunologic rule that one does not make antibodies that react with one's own antigens. Autoantibodies that associate best with antigens at body temperature (warm type) produce different clinical syndromes from autoantibodies that associate best with RBC antigens at 4°C (cold type).

Hemolytic Disease Due to Warm-Reactive Autoantibodies

Autoimmune hemolytic disease of the warm type is caused by IgG autoantibodies in about 90% of patients. The disorder may be:

1. *Idiopathic,* in which an individual, usually over the age of 40 years, develops persistent hemolysis without evidence of underlying disease.
2. *Secondary.*
   a. As a frequent complication of certain diseases associated with altered immunologic reactivity: systemic lupus erythematosus, malignant lymphomas, chronic lymphocytic leukemia.
   b. As an infrequent complication of other diseases in which immunologic reactivity may be disturbed: multiple myeloma, a variety of malignant neoplasms, ulcerative colitis, demyelinating disease of the central nervous system.
   c. After use of drugs (for example, alpha methyldopa) that can stimulate RBC autoantibody formation (Chapter 22).

Warm-reactive autoantibodies usually behave like panagglutinins, that is, they react with RBCs of all blood commonly available for testing. Nevertheless, many idiopathic autoantibodies and all autoantibodies arising in patients taking alpha methyldopa have an Rh-related antigenic specificity; they fail to react when tested against RBCs of the rare Rh_{null} type (which possess no Rh antigens). How a drug like alpha methyldopa causes a patient to make an antibody to one of his or her own RBC antigens is unknown but obviously important to an understanding of the pathogenesis of all acquired autoimmune hemolytic anemia.

MECHANISM OF HEMOLYSIS

Incubating warm IgG autoantibodies with RBCs in vitro does not appear to damage the cells. However, if the RBCs, which become coated with IgG, are transfused into an experimental subject, they are rapidly cleared from the circulation. The RBCs adhere to macrophages in the spleen, liver, and bone marrow which have membrane receptors for the Fc fragment of IgG. The macrophages may then engulf the whole RBC or phagocytose pieces of the RBC membrane. The latter causes formation of spherocytes, which are less flexible cells that are more readily engulfed on subsequent contact with macrophages, particularly in the slowed circulation of the red pulp of the spleen.

If enough antibody can attach to antigen sites to form doublets, warm type IgG autoantibodies may also fix complement on the RBC membrane. Warm IgG autoantibodies rarely activate the entire complement sequence, with resultant intravascular hemolysis, but may cause binding of C3b to the RBC membrane. RBCs coated with both IgG and C3b adhere to both Fc and C3b receptors on macrophages and so are phagocytosed more efficiently than are RBCs coated only with IgG.

RBCs coated lightly with IgG are usually removed by macrophages in the spleen because its circulation favors intimate contact of macrophages with RBCs as they filter through the red pulp. RBCs coated heavily with IgG or with both IgG and C3b are removed preferentially by the Kupffer cells lining the sinusoids of the liver because liver blood flow far exceeds splenic blood flow.

The functional status of the mononuclear phagocytic system influences the severity of the hemolysis. A process activating macrophages, such as infection, usually intensifies hemolysis. Moreover, as increasing numbers of RBCs are destroyed in the spleen, the spleen enlarges and movement of RBCs through the red pulp is further slowed, with consequent increased trapping of RBCs and phagocytosis by the macrophages of the red pulp.

CLINICAL MANIFESTATIONS

The patient frequently seeks medical attention because of sudden weakness and malaise. He or she may have fever, tachycardia, and slight jaundice. The spleen is usually palpable. Patients with secondary autoimmune acquired hemolytic anemia may have additional physical findings due to the underlying disorder.

Laboratory examination discloses:

1. Peripheral blood count.
   a. Anemia, which is often severe and usually characterized by *spherocytes* on the blood smear.
   b. Evidence of increased RBC production: polychromatophilic macrocytes and, usually, nucleated RBCs on the blood smear (Fig. 9-2) and a markedly elevated reticulocyte count. (In a rare patient, RBC production is not enhanced and the reticulocyte count is low. Such a patient is desperately ill because the hemoglobin level falls rapidly to extremely low values.)
   c. WBC count that is usually elevated but is occasionally normal or reduced.
   d. Normal or elevated platelet count. (Infrequently, a patient may present with the combination of an idiopathic autoimmune hemolytic anemia and idiopathic thrombocytopenic purpura, a combination referred to as Evans' syndrome.)
2. The direct antiglobulin test is positive with broad-spectrum antiglobulin serum. Further testing with specific sera may reveal different patterns:
   a. Only IgG on the RBCs in many patients with idiopathic disease and in all patients with alpha methyldopa-related disease.
   b. Both IgG and C3b on the RBCs in some patients, particularly patients with systemic lupus erythematosus.
   c. Only C3b on the RBCs in unusual patients who have amounts of IgG on the RBCs below the threshold of sensitivity of the antiglobulin test.
   The indirect antiglobulin test may or may not be positive, depending upon whether antibody in excess of that coating the cells is circulating free in the plasma.
3. The serum bilirubin is elevated, usually in the 2 to 4 mg per dL range, because of an increase in indirect-reacting bilirubin.

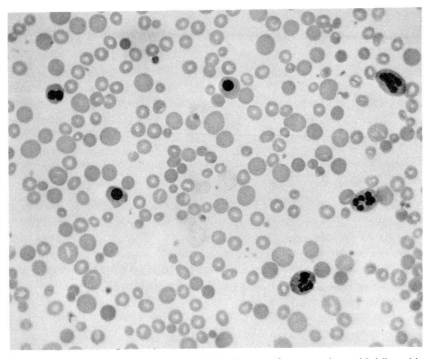

Fig. 9-2. Low-power view of peripheral blood smear from a patient with idiopathic autoimmune hemolytic anemia. Note spherocytes, polychromatophilic macrocytes, and nucleated RBCs.

TREATMENT

Autoimmune hemolytic anemia is frequently an *emergency.* If the *indirect* antiglobulin test is positive, it is usually impossible to find compatible blood for transfusion because the panagglutinin in the patient's serum coats the RBCs of all available donor bloods. If the patient is critically ill, one must occasionally transfuse with incompatible packed RBCs. The color of the patient's plasma must be checked after 50 mL of packed cells are given, and again later during the transfusion, to look for free hemoglobin indicative of rapid intravascular hemolysis.

Large doses of an adrenal glucocorticosteroid (for example, 50 mg of prednisone twice daily) are given without delay. Glucocorticosteroids have two therapeutic actions:

1. An immediate therapeutic effect due to suppression of macrophage function and resultant decreased phagocytosis of IgG-coated RBCs.

2. A delayed therapeutic effect due to suppression of autoantibody synthesis and a fall in levels of circulating antibody.

Most patients respond to adrenal steroid therapy with a progressive rise in the hematocrit that begins within several days. Over days to weeks, the reticulocyte count falls; the indirect antiglobulin test becomes negative, amd finally, in some patients, the direct antiglobulin test also becomes negative.

As the patient responds, one begins to reduce the dose of adrenal steroid. However, many patients with idiopathic disease will require chronic steroid therapy. If the dosage needed to control hemolysis exceeds 15 mg per day, other measures must be considered. These include:

1. Splenectomy, which may particularly help the patient whose RBCs are being preferentially removed by splenic macrophages. Splenectomy also has a potential adverse effect; the splenectomized patient has an increased risk of severe infection with encapsulated microorganisms, for example, pneumococcal septicemia.
2. A trial of an immumosuppressive agent such as azothioprine (Immuran^R).

Hemolysis Caused by IgM Cold-Reactive Autoantibodies

Most people have low titers of IgM cold agglutinins. These antibodies do not cause hemolysis because they do not bind to RBC membrane antigens at the temperature to which blood falls in exposed body areas. Cold agglutinin titers may rise in certain infections, particularly infection with *Mycoplasma pneumoniae*, in which a high titer is often used as a presumptive diagnostic test. Why infection should stimulate production of antibodies that can react with antigens (usually of the Ii system) on the RBC membrane is unknown. With few exceptions, the thermal amplitude of the agglutinin remains low, and, therefore, despite their high titer, the antibodies do not react with RBCs in vivo.

If, however, an individual makes IgM cold agglutinins that do react with RBCs at temperatures reached in the capillaries of the skin and subcutaneous tissues, then hemolysis may occur. This is seen in two very different clinical situations, both uncommon:

1. As an acute hemolytic episode complicating infection, usually mycoplasmal infection but occasionally infectious mononucleosis or cytomegalovirus infection. The cold agglutinins are heter-

ogenous, containing both kappa and lambda light chains on immunoelectrophoresis (see Chapter 20), and reflect polyclonal production of IgM antibodies in response to infection. The antibodies disappear as the patient recovers.

2. In *cold agglutinin disease*, a disorder of older patients characterized by chronic hemolysis and, usually, a high titer of cold agglutinins. The patient continues to make the cold agglutinin for years and probably never ceases to form it. The cold agglutinin is homogenous on immunoelectrophoresis, containing either kappa or lambda light chains but not both. Thus, the cold agglutinin is produced by a single clone of cells, that is, the antibody is *monoclonal* in origin. In many patients, further investigation uncovers evidence of an underlying lymphocytic lymphoma and, indeed, every patient with idiopathic cold agglutinin disease should be evaluated periodically for this possibility. Occasional patients have later developed findings of a particular lymphoma in which large amounts of monoclonal IgM antibody are made, macroglobulinemia of Waldenström (see Chapter 20).

MECHANISM OF HEMOLYSIS

Cold-reactive IgM antibodies cause hemolysis through the following sequence of events:

1. As blood flows through cooler body areas, IgM antibody binds to RBC membrane antigens and brings Clq down onto the membrane with it.
2. As the RBCs return to warmer body regions, the IgM antibody comes off the RBC membrane, but activation of complement on the RBC membrane progresses.
3. If large amounts of Clq have come down onto the RBCs, as may occur when a patient becomes chilled, then complement activation may progress to formation of the membrane-attack complex (C5b,6,7,8,9), with resultant intravascular hemolysis.
4. If, as is usual, lesser amounts of Clq have come down onto the RBCs, then activation of complement stops with the binding of C3b to the RBC membrane.
5. Two things may happen to RBCs coated with C3b:
   a. They may undergo hemolysis because of adherence to C3b receptors on macrophages and subsequent phagocytosis. Because of the high rate of liver blood flow, this occurs primarily in the Kupffer cells of the liver sinusoids.

b. The C3b on the RBC surface may be cleaved by factor I of the complement sequence to form C3d. Although C3d remains attached to the RBC membrane, macrophages have no receptor for C3d and the RBC escapes hemolysis. This probably explains why only a mild hemolytic anemia is found in many patients with chronic cold agglutinin disease.

MANIFESTATIONS AND TREATMENT

Acute Postinfectious Cold Agglutinin-Induced Hemolysis. As mentioned, hemolysis is transient but may be severe. On examination of the blood smear, clumps of agglutinated RBCs may be noted along with variable numbers of polychromatophilic macrocytes and spherocytes. A cold agglutinin test will be positive in high titer, and the agglutinin will react with RBCs in the cold and at room temperature or above. The antiglobulin test with broad-spectrum antiglobulin serum will be positive due to binding of C3b and C3d to the RBCs. Occasionally, blood transfusion may be required; typing and crossmatching is usually difficult because of interference by the cold agglutinin. An "in-line warmer" should be used to warm the blood as it is being administered.

Chronic Cold Agglutinin Disease. Patients frequently complain of mottling and numbness of the skin of the fingers, toes, and face in colder weather. Chilling may induce an episode of hemoglobinuria. Symptoms due to anemia may or may not be present. In the idiopathic disorder, the physical examination may be entirely normal. The spleen is usually not enlarged. Finding lymphadenopathy or splenomegaly suggests the presence of an underlying lymphoma. Anemia is usually mild to moderate, with a modest increase in the reticulocyte count. As described above for acute cold agglutinin-induced hemolysis, clumps of agglutinated RBCs may be noted on the blood smear, the cold agglutinin test will be positive in high titer, and the antiglobulin test will usually be positive with broad-spectrum antiglobulin serum.

The patient should be protected against exposure to cold. If the patient has a lymphoma, an alkylating agent, such as chlorambucil or cyclophosphamide, is usually given, and this may improve the anemia by suppressing production of the cold agglutinin. Adrenal glucocorticosteroids have rarely proved of benefit. Splenectomy is valueless, since the RBCs are removed primarily in the liver.

Paroxysmal Cold Hemoglobinuria

Very rarely, usually as a complication of a viral infection, a patient may develop profound intravascular hemolysis after exposure to cold due to an IgG antibody that preferentially reacts in the cold. Unlike postinfectious IgM cold agglutinins, which have specificity for the Ii antigen system, the IgG cold antibody has specificity for the P antigen system of the red cell membrane. The antibody activates complement so effectively that when blood is chilled in vitro, RBC aggregates are formed that do not return to normal appearance on warming the blood (as in the usual test for a cold agglutinin). Instead, the aggregates undergo hemolysis. This forms the basis for a test called the Donath-Landsteiner test, which is diagnostic of paroxsymal cold hemoglobinuria.

SELECTED READING

1. Frank MM, Schreiber AD, Atkinson JP, and Jaffe CJ: NIH conference. Pathophysiology of immune hemolytic anemia. Ann Intern Med 87:210, 1977.
2. Petz LD, and Garratty G: Acquired Immune Hemolytic Anemias. New York, Churchill Livingstone, 1980.
3. Polesky HF: Diagnosis, prevention and therapy in hemolytic disease of the newborn. Clin Lab Med 2:107, 1982.

10

Methemoglobinemia

Methemoglobin is hemoglobin whose ferrous iron has been oxidized to ferric iron. Small amounts of methemoglobin form continuously in normal RBCs from the interaction of hemoglobin with traces of superoxide ion. However, the methemoglobin level of normal RBCs does not exceed 1% of total hemoglobin because the methemoglobin is rapidly reduced back to hemoglobin, primarily by a reducing system catalyzed by the enzyme NADH dehydrogenase (also called NADH cytochrome b_5 reductase). Ascorbic acid and glutathione may also directly reduce minor amounts of methemoglobin in the RBC. An additional potential reducing mechanism involving the enzyme NADPH dehydrogenase is present in the RBC but cannot function in the absence of an added, exogenous electron carrier.

The enzymatic mechanisms for reducing methemoglobin in the RBC are illustrated in Figure 10-1 and may be summarized as follows:

1. *The mechanism utilizing NADH dehydrogenase.* NADH is formed in the RBC during anaerobic glycolysis (see Chapter 7). The hydride ion (H^-) of NADH provides an electron that is transferred to cytochrome b_5 in an enzymatic reaction catalyzed by NADH dehydrogenase. (This is why NADH dehydrogenase is now often called *NADH cytochrome b_5 reductase*). Reduced cytochrome b_5, in a nonenzymatic reaction, then transfers the electron to methemoglobin, with consequent reduction of the ferric iron of methemoglobin to the ferrous iron of hemoglobin.
2. *The potential mechanism utilizing NADPH dehydrogenase.* NADPH is formed during aerobic glycolysis via the pentose

163

NADH Dehydrogenase Catalyzed, Naturally Active System

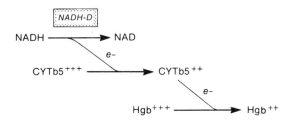

NADPH Dehydrogenase Catalyzed System, Requires Exogenous Electron Carrier

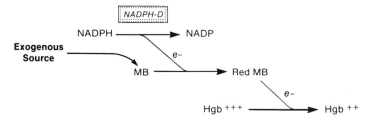

Fig. 10-1. Schematic representation of NADH dehydrogenase-linked and NADPH dehydrogenase-linked methemoglobin reduction. Note that the latter cannot function without an exogenously added electron carrier such as methylene blue. Abbreviations: CYT b_5, cytochrome b_5; e, electron; HGB, hemoglobin; and Red MB, reduced methylene blue.

phosphate shunt (see Chapter 7). Although the RBC contains a second dehydrogenase, NADPH dehydrogenase, that can catalyze reduction of NADPH, it normally does not function because an acceptor for the electron is not present in the RBC. A gap exists in the chain for transferring the electron to methemoglobin. However, if an exogenous electron carrier is provided, for example, by methylene blue, then the NADH-linked methemoglobin-reducing mechanism functions very effectively. This is why methylene blue is given clinically to treat methemoglobinemia.

Methemoglobin cannot carry oxygen, therefore, the patient with methemoglobinemia is *cyanotic*. The life span of the RBC is normal and anemia does not develop. Indeed, in some patients with hereditary methemoglobinemia, slight polycythemia may be found as the result of chronic mild anoxia.

Clinical states associated with methemoglobinemia are:

1. *Acquired.* Acquired methemoglobinemia may develop in three circumstances:

    a. In a normal adult after accidental ingestion of a large amount of an oxidant material capable of forming methemoglobin, for example, the ingestion of an antifreeze compound during a drinking bout. The markedly enhanced formation of methemoglobin overwhelms the normal NADH-linked methemoglobin-reducing system, which is limited by the concentration of cytochrome b_5 in the RBC.

    b. In infants under the age of 3 months, in whom the red cell's methemoglobin-reducing capacity is not yet fully developed. Nitrates in well water used to prepare infant formula (which are reduced by intestinal flora to nitrites) and oxidant material in disinfectants used to wash diapers or in dyes used to mark diapers have been implicated in acquired methemoglobinemia in the newborn.

    c. In heterozygotes for hereditary NADH dehydrogenase deficiency (see below). Heterozygotes do not ordinarily develop methemoglobinemia but may do so after taking oxidant drugs, for example, the malarial chemoprophylactic agents primaquine and chloroquine, that would not induce significant methemoglobinemia in normal individuals.

    Concentrations of 20% to 30% methemoglobin cause cyanosis but require no treatment. However, higher concentrations may lead to stupor and even death from anoxia. The intravenous injection of 1 to 2 mg of methylene blue per kg of body weight activates the NADPH dehydrogenase-linked reducing system and will rapidly correct the methemoglobinemia. Repeated doses may be needed until the offending agent has been cleared from the body.

2. *Hereditary.* The hereditary methemoglobinemias may result from:

    a. Homozygosity for an abnormal gene for NADH dehydrogenase. This enzyme is found in many tissues, including brain, embedded by a hydrophobic tail in endoplasmic reticulum. However, in the mature RBC, it is found in the soluble fraction of cytoplasm, its hydrophobic tail having been cleaved off during maturation of the RBC. Different abnormal allelic genes cause NADH dehydrogenase deficiency. Usually, the abnormal allele causes decreased activity of only the soluble enzyme in the RBC. The homozygote has persisting methemoglobinemia in the 20% to 45% range, with a peculiar slate-gray cyanosis but no other evidence of disease. Treatment (oral methylene blue, ascorbic acid) is given only for cosmetic effect. However, a minority of patients with homozygous NADH dehydrogenase deficiency develop severe neurologic dysfunction in infancy. In these patients, the abnormal allele affects not only the soluble enzyme in the RBC but also the insoluble enzyme in other tissues, including the central nervous system, where NADH dehydrogenase participates in essential reactions of lipid metabolism.

b. Hemoglobins M. In this group of abnormal hemoglobins, an amino acid substitution in either the α or β chain in the region of the heme pocket causes the formation of an abnormally stable methemoglobin. M hemoglobins may be identified by their abnormal absorption spectrum. Homozygosity for Hgb M is lethal. Heterozygotes have about 20 to 30% methemoglobin and are asymptomatic except for cyanosis.

SELECTED READING

1. Schwartz JM, Reiss AL, and Jaffe ER: Hereditary methemoglobin with deficiency of NADH cytocyome b₅ reductase. In Stanbury JB, Wyngaarden JB, Fredrickson DS, Goldstein JL, and Brown MS (eds): The Metabolic Basis of Inherited Disease, 5th ed. New York, McGraw-Hill, 1983.

11

Anemias Due to Failure of Erythropoiesis

This chapter is concerned with five partially overlapping marrow disorders or groups of disorders in which anemia results from a serious failure of RBC production: aplastic anemia (marrow aplasia), pure red cell aplasia, myelodysplastic syndromes, sideroblastic anemias, and congenital dyserythropoietic anemias. Other anemias caused by impaired erythropoiesis are discussed in earlier chapters: anemias due to impaired hemoglobin synthesis are discussed in Chapters 3 and 5 and anemias due to impaired DNA synthesis are discussed in Chapter 4. Anemias that occur secondary to nonhematologic disorders causing a diminished marrow response are discussed in Chapter 12. Failure of erythropoiesis also causes anemia in the hematologic malignancies, which are discussed in later chapters.

APLASTIC ANEMIA

The patient with aplastic anemia (marrow aplasia) has pancytopenia (reduced numbers of circulating RBCs, granulocytes, and platelets) and a hypocellular bone marrow. The marrow hypocellularity can result from two pathogenetic mechanisms:

1. Depletion of hematopoietic stem cells by an agent or event that kills stem cells.
2. Suppression of proliferation and maturation of stem cells by an immunologic (lymphocyte-mediated) mechanism.

Conceivably, both mechanisms could operate in a given patient. A cytotoxic event could initiate hypocellularity by destroying the majority of the stem cells; then, T-lymphocytes, in an autoimmune response to antigens liberated from damaged stem cells or simply as an expression of their normal regulatory function, could perpetuate hypocellularity by preventing the remaining stem cells from repopulating the marrow.

In most patients, a preceding event initiating the aplastic anemia cannot be identified, and the aplastic anemia is called idiopathic. In some patients a cause can be found:

1. *Genetic or congenital abnormalities.* These are a cause for marrow aplasia in infants or small children, usually in association with other constitutional defects—stunted growth, limb deformities, skin pigmentation, microphthalmia (Fanconi's anemia).
2. *Toxins or ionizing radiation.* The most important toxins are benzene and related cyclic hydrocarbons (found in solvents prepared from petroleum distillates, rubber cement, airplane glues, certain insecticides, and so on).
3. *Drugs.* These fall into two categories:
   a. Drugs that can cause aplasia in any patient if given in excess:
      (1) Alkylating agents, busulfan, and nitrosourea compounds. These drugs, which damage resting stem cells as well as cells in cycle, may cause prolonged and even irreversible aplasia.
      (2) Other cancer chemotherapeutic agents that affect only cells in cycle (for example, methotrexate). Although aplasia may be profound, it is usually reversible within days.
   b. Drugs that cause aplasia in a rare, sensitive patient. Aplasia need not be related to the amount of drug given. The most important drug in this group is chloramphenicol (Chloromycetin). Others include the anti-inflammatory agents, phenylbutazone (Butazolidin) and sulindac (Clinoril); gold compounds used to treat rheumatoid arthritis; the sulfa drugs; tolbutamide; and the antiepileptic drugs phenytoin (Dilantin), methylphenylethylhydantoin (Mesantoin), trimethadione (Tridione), and carbamazepine (Tegretol).
4. *Infection.* Aplastic anemia following non-A, non-B viral hepatitis is well documented. Instances of aplastic anemia after infectious mononucleosis have also been reported. Whether human parvovirus infection, a principal cause for acute red cell aplasia (see below), can also cause chronic marrow aplasia is presently unknown. Many patients with aplastic anemia give a history of a

poorly characterized, presumably viral illness preceding the discovery of the aplasia.
5. *Pregnancy.* Aplastic anemia occasionally develops during or shortly after a pregnancy. The reason for the association is unknown.

A few patients may present initially with findings of aplastic anemia—pancytopenia and a hypoplastic marrow—and then develop clear-cut evidence of *acute leukemia* within days or months. Such patients probably have acute leukemia from the onset. A rare patient develops acute leukemia after many years of known marrow aplasia. As discussed in Chapter 8, a rare patient with aplastic anemia may later develop *paroxysmal nocturnal hemoglobinuria* and, conversely, a patient with paroxysmal nocturnal hemoglobinuria may develop increasing evidence of marrow hypoplasia.

Clinical Findings

The typical clinical findings of aplastic anemia are:

1. Symptoms attributable to bone marrow failure: weakness and cardiovascular and cerebral symptoms secondary to severe anemia; susceptibility to infection secondary to granulocytopenia; and abnormal bleeding secondary to thrombocytopenia.
2. A physical examination with negative findings except for pallor and, frequently, scattered petechiae or ecchymoses. The patient has no fever unless infection is present. The liver, spleen, and lymph nodes are not enlarged since the death or suppression of stem cells prevents compensatory extramedullary hematopoiesis in these organs.
3. A pancytopenia with:
   a. Severe normochromic to macrocytic anemia and reticulocytopenia.
   b. Leukopenia with severe granulocytopenia and without immature granulocytes in the peripheral blood.
   c. Marked thrombocytopenia.
4. A hypocellular bone marrow. In many patients, a histologic section of a bone marrow particle (Fig. 11-1) or a bone marrow biopsy shows almost total replacement of cells by fat. The few remaining cells are histiocytes, plasma cells, lymphocytes, and tissue mast cells. In some patients, residual islands of cellularity, containing erythroid and myeloid elements, may be found.

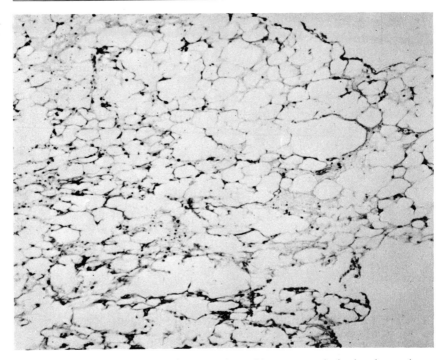

Fig. 11-1. Bone marrow particle from a patient with marrow aplasia showing replacement of hematopoietic cells by fat.

Course and Management

Aplastic anemia is a very serious diease. In previous years up to 50% of patients with "severe" aplastic anemia at the time of diagnosis—a granulocyte count of less than 500 per μL, a platelet count of less than 20,000 per μL, and a reticulocyte count of less than 10,000 per μL—died of infection or hemorrhage within 3 months. Moreover, patients initially presenting with less severe pancytopenia often worsen over weeks to several months; their prognosis then becomes equally grim.

Possible approaches to therapy include the following:

1. Bone marrow transplantation.
2. Immunosuppression with antilymphocyte globulin.
3. Administration of androgens.

Since no method yet exists to distinguish aplastic anemia due to stem cell death from aplastic anemia due to immunosuppression of stem cells, one must recommend treatment without knowing the mechanism of a patient's aplasia. Currently, if the patient is under 30 years of age and has a willing, HLA-identical sibling donor, he or she is usually referred to a center for bone marrow transplantation. Therefore, in a young patient newly discovered to have aplastic anemia, it is important:

1. To obtain HLA typing of the patient and all siblings quickly to identify a potential histocompatible donor. Since an individual's HLA antigens are transmitted as a haplotype (linked group of allelic antigens) from each parent, the patient has a 25% chance of being HLA-identical with each sibling.
2. To withhold blood transfusions if at all possible, since random blood transfusions may sensitize the patient to minor histocompatibility antigens of the potential donor and so increase the risk of graft rejection. When blood products must be given, for example, platelet concentrates to control life-threatening hemorrhage, the transfusion of blood from a family member who may serve as a potential marrow donor should be avoided.

BONE MARROW TRANSPLANTATION

Although the rationale for bone marrow transplanation is to supply donor stem cells to replace the patient's destroyed stem cells, the immunosuppression given to prepare the patient for transplantation (very large doses of cyclophosphamide sometimes supplemented by total body irradiation or cyclosporine) may also play a key role in restoring hematopoiesis. In some instances in which an *identical twin* has served as the donor, transplantation without initial immunosuppression (which in identical twins is unnecessary to prevent rejection of foreign tissue) has failed to restore hemopoietic function, whereas a second transplantation preceded by immunosuppressive measures has restored hemopoietic function.

For a bone marrow transplant to be successful;

1. Donor stem cells must reconstitute the recipient's bone marrow, that is, the transplant must not be rejected.
2. Stem cells and other lymphocytic elements from the donor marrow must reconstitute the recipient's immune system, which, depending upon the immunosuppressive measures used, has been partially to totally wiped out.

The two major hazards to survival after bone marrow transplant are:

1. *Graft-versus-host disease*, which is the name for the syndromes that develop when immunocompetent lymphocytes of donor origin attack the tissues of the recipient. Graft-versus-host disease occurs in some 35% to 60% of recipients and is seen in two forms:

   a. Acute graft-versus-host disease, which develops within 30 to 100 days of transplantation and is manifested by skin rash, diarrhea, liver abnormalities, and increased susceptibility to infection due to profoundly depressed immunologic function. It is frequently fatal.

   b. Chronic graft-versus-host disease, a debilitating disorder of long-term survivors with features of both immunodeficiency and autoimmunity. Patients develop scleroderma-like skin involvement and have frequent infections due to impaired immunity.

2. *Infection*, which represents a serious risk not only while the patient is severely granulocytopenic immediately after the transplant but during the weeks to months needed for donor stem cells and other lymphocytic elements to restore immune function. Viral interstitial pneumonias, probably related to impaired T-cell function in the recipient, are particularly feared and may have a 50% rate of mortality.

The incidence of both infection and chronic graft-versus-host disease increases with the age of the recipient. Therefore, patients over the age of 40 years are not candidates for bone marrow transplantation, and in some institutions anti-lymphocyte globulin is tried first in the patient between 30 and 40 years of age. However, for patients under 30 years of age who have not received blood transfusions prior to transplantation, a survival rate after transplantation has been reported of over 70%.

IMMUNOSUPPRESSION WITH ANTI-LYMPHOCYTE GLOBULIN

Anti-lymphocyte globulin is antiserum made in an animal (usually a horse) to human lymphocytes. Such antiserum is as yet poorly characterized, and different batches may differ in the properties of their anti-lymphocyte antibodies and, therefore, in their therapeutic effectiveness. Anti-lymphocyte globulin is given to patients with aplastic anemia in the hope of eliminating T-cells or other lymphocytes that may be suppressing the proliferation and differentiation of stem cells.

Although still considered experimental therapy, administration of anti-lymphocyte globulin has improved survival in several published series of patients. The antiserum is given intravenously, over several hours each day, for 4 to 10 days. Occasional patients may develop severe anaphylactic reactions; all patients develop serum sickness, for which most require treatment with adrenal glucocorticoids. Already thrombocytopenic, most patients become more severely thrombocytopenic after receiving the antiserum and require transfusion of platelet concentrates to protect against hemorrhage.

No method currently exists to predict who will respond to therapy. A rise in reticulocyte count or in the number of circulating neutrophilic granulocytes is the first evidence of response. It is first noted some 4 to 12 weeks after completion of therapy. Responses are often incomplete but of sufficient magnitude to raise the platelet and granulocyte counts to levels compatible with survival and to diminish or abolish the need for RBC transfusions. Many patients are also given androgen therapy in an attempt to supplement the effect of the anti-lymphocyte globulin. Occasional patients have responded, only to relapse several months later.

At this writing, the Aplastic Anemia Study Group in the United States believes that controlled comparisons would show anti-lymphocyte globulin therapy and histocompatible bone marrow transplantation to be equivalent with respect to survival of patients with aplastic anemia. Anti-lymphocyte globulin is clearly the preferred treatment for the older patient and may also be superior for younger patients who have received multiple transfusions and, therefore, have a high risk of graft rejection.

ANDROGEN THERAPY

A small but not negligible number of patients with aplastic anemia have responded to large daily doses of an oral androgen (for example, oxymetholone, 2–3 mg per kg). Again, no method of identifying the patient who will respond exists. Several months may elapse before the first evidence of a response is noted. In the responding patient, androgens should be continued in full doses for about 2 years and then gradually discontinued. If the blood count then begins to fall, androgens should be given again in the minimum dose required to maintain the blood count at a safe level.

Up to one third of patients taking oral androgens develop hepatic toxicity, which necessitates substitution of an intramuscularly injected preparation (with some risk of hematoma in thrombocytopenic patients) for the oral agent. An occasional patient receiving long-term oral therapy may develop hepatic peliosis (vascular lacunae in the liver that may rupture and bleed), hepatic adenoma, or hepatocellular carcinoma.

GENERAL MEASURES

Patients with aplastic anemia should not be exposed to solvents, sprays, paints, insecticides, and other potential bone marrow toxins. Only drugs that are essential should be given. Aspirin-containing drugs should not be used because aspirin interferes with platelet function and so increases the risk of thrombocytopenic bleeding. Infection should be treated promptly with antibiotics after smears and cultures are taken for bacteriologic diagnosis. Transfusions of packed RBCs are usually limited to the amounts necessary to correct distressing manifestations of anemia. Platelet concentrates are rarely given prophylactically but are reserved for use at the first sign of acute, life-threatening bleeding.

PURE RED CELL APLASIA

Pure red cell aplasia differs from aplastic anemia in that granulocytopoiesis and thrombocytopoiesis are normal. Therefore, pure red cell aplasia is not a disorder of stem cells, but a disorder in which a process or processes specifically suppresses differentiation of erythroid progenitors without impairing differentiation of progenitors of the other blood cell lines.

Acute Pure Red Cell Aplasia

Acute pure red cell aplasia usually goes unrecognized because a brief period of suppressed erythropoiesis has little effect upon the RBC count when the RBC life span is normal. If a patient has a hemolytic anemia, for example, sickle cell anemia or hereditary spherocytosis, then a temporary cessation of erythropoiesis can cause a substantial fall in the RBC count and an *aplastic crisis*. An aplastic crisis has often followed acute viral illness, and it is now thought that a particular virus, the human parvovirus, is responsible for the majority of such occurrences. The virus is cytotoxic for erythroid progenitor cells and can be demonstrated by electron microscopy within the nucleus of the infected cell. Acute red cell aplasia may also develop as a reaction to drugs (chloramphenicol, phenytoin).

Prolonged or Chronic Forms of Pure Red Cell Aplasia

INFANTS AND CHILDREN

Two forms of chronic pure red cell aplasia have been described in infants and children. In both, the patient has a severe anemia and reticulocytopenia but normal WBC and platelet counts. Overall bone marrow cellularity appears normal because of normal myeloid elements and megakaryocytes, but erythroid precursors are virtually absent. In some patients, very young pronormoblasts may be present in the marrow without more differentiated erythroid forms. The two disorders are:

1. *Transient erythroblastopenia of childhood,* a disorder usually of older infants and small children that spontaneously remits within a few months. At the time of diagnosis, the RBC are of normal size and the fetal hemoglobin and i-antigen content of the RBCs are not elevated. Washed bone marrow mononuclear cells from such patients will form erythroid colonies on in vitro culture in the presence of normal serum from another individual but not in the presence of the patient's own serum. An immunoglobin (IgG) in the patient's serum is thought to be responsible for suppressing erythropoiesis.

2. *Congenital hypoplastic anemia* (Diamond-Blackfan anemia), a disorder usually recognized within the first year of life. In this condition, the RBCs are usually macrocytic and contain elevated levels of fetal hemoglobin and increased amounts of i-antigen. Minor congenital abnormalities are often also present (thumb deformities, strabismus) but major defects, such as those seen in Fanconi's syndrome, are not found. It is suggested but not yet proved that the disorder is transmitted as an autosomal recessive defect. In vitro studies reveal no evidence of an inhibitor of erythropoiesis but, rather, diminished numbers and diminished sensitivity to erythropoietin of both early and late erythroid progenitor cells in the patient's marrow (BFU-E and CFU-E, see Chapter 1). Remissions of varying extent and duration follow administration of adrenal glucocorticoids. The prognosis is much more serious than for transient erythroblastopenia of childhood since some patients respond inadequately to adrenal steroids and require lifelong support with transfusions.

Moreover, children with this disorder appear to have an increased risk for acute leukemia.

ADULTS

Primary Red Cell Aplasia. Primary chronic pure red cell aplasia in adults is a rare disorder that usually presents with symptoms referable only to anemia and negative findings on physical examination except for pallor. A peripheral blood count shows a severe, normocytic anemia with a reticulocytopenia but a normal WBC and platelet count. Erythroid precursors in the bone marrow are markedly diminished to absent, whereas myeloid elements and megakaryocytes are normal. Serologic evidence suggestive of abnormal immune function—hypogammaglobulinemia or a positive test for antinuclear antibody—is sometimes found.

In a small proportion of patients, primary red cell aplasia will be associated with a *thymoma*, and every patient with primary red cell aplasia should have radiologic studies of the chest to search for a thymoma. If found, it should be removed, both because of the possibility of its malignant degeneration and because aplasia sometimes remits following the surgery. However, the thymoma does not cause the aplasia, since late relapses after thymectomy may occur and, indeed, patients have been described in whom a thymoma was removed years before the development of aplasia. Thymectomy is without effect upon red cell aplasia in the patient without a thymoma.

A cytotoxic immunoglobulin (IgG) that impairs differentiation or maturation of erythroid precursors in culture has been demonstrated in the serum of about one half of patients with primary red cell aplasia who have been tested. Therefore, immunosuppression of erythropoiesis is thought to represent a major mechanism for primary pure red cell aplasia. In such patients, large numbers of erythroid colonies are formed when the patient's marrow, washed free of autologous plasma, is cultured in vitro.

If thymectomy fails to induce remission and in the patient without a thymoma, immunosuppressive therapy is given, beginning with large doses of adrenal corticosteroids. If a remission is induced, small doses of adrenal corticosteroids are often required indefinitely to maintain the remission. If steroids fail to induce or maintain a remission, cytotoxic drugs are added, usually azothioprine or cyclophosphamide, with variable success. A small number of patients may develop a spontaneous remission. Whatever the mechanism of remission, recurrences are frequent. They may or may not respond to the same regimen that induced the initial remission.

Secondary Red Cell Aplasia. Secondary red cell aplasia may develop —with a frequency that has probably been underestimated—in patients with chronic lymphocytic leukemia or lymphocytic lymphoma. In chronic lymphocytic leukemia, T-lymphocytes in the marrow of a particular subset bearing Fc receptors on their membrane for IgG (so-called Tγ cells) have been implicated in the suppression of erythropoiesis.

Pure red cell aplasia has also been described as a complication of long-standing rheumatoid arthritis and of systemic lupus erythematosus. An IgG serum inhibitor of erythropoiesis has been demonstrated in some patients with pure red cell aplasia secondary to these disorders and an expanded Tγ cell clone in other patients.

MYELODYSPLASTIC SYNDROMES

Manifestations and Classification

Refractory myelodysplastic anemia is a prominent manifestation of a group of disorders of hematopoietic stem cells referred to as the myelodysplastic syndromes. These disorders have two features in common:

1. Cytopenias of one or more cell lines in the peripheral blood.
2. Increased but abnormal-appearing (dysplastic) hematopoiesis in the bone marrow.

Thus, whereas anemia in aplastic anemia and pure red cell aplasia results from absent marrow erythroid activity, anemia in the myelodysplastic syndromes usually results from ineffective erythropoiesis.

In some patients with a myelodysplastic syndrome, erythroid abnormalities predominate, whereas in other patients, granulocytic abnormalities predominate. The latter are sometimes referred to as having "preleukemia."

MYELODYSPLASIA WITH PREDOMINANT ERYTHROID ABNORMALITIES

The patient, usually over 50 years of age and most often a man, has a chronic anemia of insidious onset and gradually increasing severity. Physical examination is often negative, but infrequently, the liver, spleen, or both may be palpable.

Laboratory examination reveals:

1. *In the peripheral blood*—an anemia with a normocytic to macrocytic MCV and a low reticulocyte count, a low-normal to slightly below normal WBC count, and a platelet count that is normal or slightly reduced. Even when mean RBC size is normal, frequent macrocytes, often round rather than teardrop shaped and occasionally of very large size, are seen on the blood smear. Polychromatophilia and RBCs with coarse basophilic stippling may also be seen. In a subgroup of patients, two distinct populations of RBC are found, one normochromic and the other hypochromic (dimorphic RBC morphology).

2. *In the marrow*—erythroid hyperplasia and evidence of dyserythropoiesis with asynchrony of nuclear and cytoplasmic maturation leading to "megaloblastoid" changes, nuclear fragmentation, normoblasts with lobulated nuclei (so-called popcorn cells), and occasional binucleated late normoblasts. If patients have hypochromic cells in the peripheral blood, a significant population of ring sideroblasts (Fig. 11-2) will also be noted as morphologic evidence that some subclones of erythroid precursors cannot synthesize hemoglobin normally despite plentiful amounts of intracellular iron.

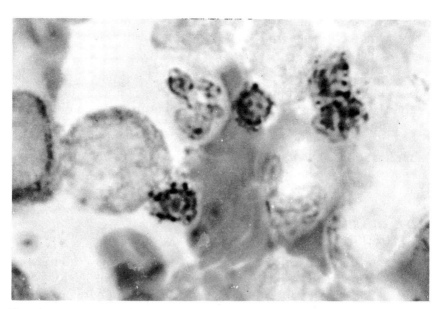

Fig. 11-2. Iron stain of a bone marrow smear showing ring sideroblasts with coarse granules of iron in mitochondria encircling the nuclei of normoblasts.

MYELODYSPLASIA WITH PREDOMINANT GRANULOCYTIC ABNORMALITIES

In these patients, dysplastic maturation of granulocytes, often accompanied by abnormalities of megakaryocytic maturation, overshadows the erythroid abnormalities. Leukopenia is characteristic. Most patients will also have an anemia and a moderate to severe reticulocytopenia. Hypogranular granulocytes, segmented neutrophilic granulocytes with only two lobes (the acquired Pelger-Huët anomaly), small numbers of circulating myelocytes and promyelocytes, and even occasional myeloblasts may be seen on the blood smear. A few patients will have increased absolute numbers of circulating monocytes. Most patients will also have a moderate thrombocytopenia.

Dysplastic myeloid hyperplasia, with increased numbers of myeloblasts and of promyelocytes with prominent nucleoli and coarse azurophilic granules, is the most impressive bone marrow abnormality. Erythropoiesis is also dsyplastic and occasionally is strikingly diminished. (This pattern should not be confused with primary red cell aplasia where granulocytic precursors and megakaryocytes are normal.) Dysplastic megakaryocyte maturation, micromegakaryocytes with a single nucleus and megakaryocytes with multiple, small separated nuclei, is frequently prominent.

CLASSIFICATION OF MYELODYSPLASTIC SYNDROMES INTO MULTIPLE SUBGROUPS

In place of the two broad categories described above, a French-American-British cooperative group has recently proposed criteria for classifying the myelodysplastic syndromes into five subgroups as follows:

1. *Refractory anemia.* Anemia, erythroid hyperplasia, and dyserythropoiesis are present without or with only minimal abnormalities of granulocytes or platelets and of their precursors in the bone marrow. Blast cells in the marrow are less than 5%.
2. *Refractory anemia with ring sideroblasts.* Findings are similar to the above but, in addition, a population of hypochromic RBCs are present in the peripheral blood and ring sideroblasts make up more than 15% of all nucleated cells in the bone marrow.
3. *Refractory anemia with excess of blasts (RAEB).* Abnormalities of the WBC and platelets accompany the anemia and up to 5% of circulating WBCs may be blasts. In addition to dyserythro-

poiesis, dysgranulopoiesis and abnormalities of megakaryocyte maturation are present in the bone marrow. Blast cells make up 5% to 20% of nucleated marrow cells. Ring sideroblasts may or may not be seen.

4. *RAEB in transformation.* The findings are similar to RAEB but, in addition, one or more of the following is noted: more than 5% circulating blasts in the peripheral blood; between 20% and 40% blasts in the bone marrow; Auer rods (see Chapter 15) in granulocyte precursors.

5. *Chronic myelomonocytic leukemia.* This represents a group of disorders whose defining feature is an absolute peripheral blood monocytosis (>1000 per μL). Other features resemble RAEB except that in some but not all patients a significant increase of monocyte precursors (promonocytes) is also found in the bone marrow.

Not all hematologists have accepted this classification. For example, the author believes that classifying patients with RAEB with associated monocytosis as chronic myelomonocytic leukemia blurs the meaning of that diagnosis, which seems better reserved for a myeloproliferative disorder in which the leukocyte count is high due to a substantial monocytosis, the spleen is enlarged, and the urinary lysosome level is markedly increased. Opinion also differs as to how many blasts must be found in the bone marrow to conclude that RAEB has become acute leukemia.

Regardless of how one choses to classify the myelodysplastic syndromes, observers generally agree upon the following:

1. A small but not insignificant fraction of patients whose abnormalities appear initially confined to the erythroid series develop increasing evidence with time of abnormalities of myeloid and megakaryocytic cell lines.

2. When myeloid findings predominate, the patient has a substantially increased risk of developing acute leukemia.

Course and Management

The myelodysplastic syndromes are ultimately fatal disorders. The patients are usually elderly (the exception being patients who develop a myelodysplastic syndrome following cytotoxic therapy for malignant disease). Other underlying disease is often present, for example, heart disease or diabetes, which magnifies the tissue hypoxia of an increasingly severe anemia or the susceptibility to infection of an increasingly severe leukopenia. Death usually results from debility, infection, or bleeding—either as a complication of myelo-dysplasia or of its leukemic transformation.

Folate, vitamin B_{12}, and androgens have no effect upon the anemia. For reasons discussed in the next section, patients with hypochromic RBCs and ring sideroblasts are often given pharmacologic doses of pyridoxine. Although anemia has improved with pyridoxine therapy in some patients, in the majority it has not. At some point, most patients become dependent upon repeated transfusions for survival.

Median survival times have been reported of 4 years for patients presenting with a refractory anemia without evidence of dysmyelopoiesis and of 1 year in patients presenting with both dyserythropoiesis and dysmyelopoiesis. This partially reflects a differing risk for leukemic transformation, which is about 10% for patients with predominantly erythroid findings, about 30% for patients with evidence of dysmyelopoiesis as well, and essentially 100% for patients in whom a myelodysplastic syndrome develops after cytotoxic therapy for a malignant disorder (for example, after therapy with an alkylating agent in multiple myeloma).

Leukemia arising in the setting of myelodysplasia has usually proved resistant to aggressive chemotherapy, which most often only hastens the patient's death. Therefore, most physicians have not begun chemotherapy in patients whose disease appears to be transforming into leukemia, and many physicians delay chemotherapy even after findings of acute leukemia are unequivocable. However, improved tolerance to chemotherapy and a small number of complete remissions have recently been described with prolonged administration of low doses of chemotherapeutic agents. It is too early to know whether a wider experience will substantiate these early reports.

SIDEROBLASTIC ANEMIAS

Possibly because ring sideroblasts are so striking a morphologic finding (see Fig. 11-2), anemias in which hypochromic RBCs are noted in the peripheral blood and large numbers of ring sideroblasts are present in the bone marrow have been grouped together in the past as the sideroblastic anemias. These anemias, which are of diverse pathogenesis and prognosis, have one common feature—defective heme synthesis in RBCs containing plentiful amounts of iron. The result is accumulation of coarse granules of ferritin in the mitochondria that encircle the nucleus, that is, the formation of ring sidero-blasts. The defect in heme synthesis may be the principal abnormality (as in hereditary sideroblastic anemias) or may be only one of multiple abnormalities responsible for impaired erythropoiesis.

The sideroblastic anemias include the following disorders:

1. *Hereditary sideroblastic anemia.* With few exceptions, patients with this rare disorder (or disorders) are males, and the disease seen in most kindreds is clearly transmitted by a defective gene on the X chromosome. Hemoglobin synthesis is markedly impaired and the MCV and MCHC are both decreased. Occasional siderocytes are found on the blood smear. The reticulocyte count is low but erythroid hyperplasia is present in the marrow (ineffective erythropoiesis). The serum iron is high, the marrow is loaded with iron (reflecting the increased iron absorption associated with chronic ineffective erythropoiesis, see Chapter 3), and ring sideroblasts are found in large numbers. In about one half of kindreds patients have responded at least partially to the administration of pharmacologic doses of pyridoxine. Its use is based upon a premise that the disease results from a defect in δ-amino-levulinic acid synthetase, the enzyme catalyzing the first and rate-limiting step in protoporphyrin synthesis (see Fig. 1-2)—and that flooding the body with pyridoxine, the precursor of the coenzyme for the reaction (pyridoxal phosphate), may partially overcome the defect.

2. *Acquired sideroblastic anemias,* which may be divided into
   a. Primary or idiopathic sideroblastic anemia. This is the same disease as refractory anemia with ring sideroblasts, which has been discussed in the preceding section. As mentioned, a small number of these patients have also responded to administration of pyridoxine but the majority have not.
   b. Secondary sideroblastic anemias. These usually result from exposure to drugs or toxins but may also occur for unknown reasons in uncommon patients with a variety of chronic neo-plastic and inflammatory disorders. The drugs and toxins include:
      (1) Alcohol. A bone marrow examination performed on admission of a patient with severe alcoholism frequently shows megaloblasts, vacuolated normoblasts, and ring sidero-blasts. The ring sideroblasts disappear within a few days of withdrawal of alcohol.
      (2) Antituberculous drugs—particularly isoniazid, but also possibly cycloserine and pyrazinamide. Isoniazid inhibits

pyridoxine metabolism, and this inhibition is undoubtedly important for the development of the anemia. The use of isoniazid is common but its association with sideroblastic anemia is uncommon, and so a second factor predisposing to anemia in certain patients is probably also involved. The anemia may respond to administration of pyridoxine even though the use of isoniazid is continued.

(3) Chloramphenicol, which may induce multiple abnormalities in hematopoiesis, including ring sideroblasts.
(4) Lead, which can impair heme synthesis at several steps, including the incorporation of iron into protoporphyrin, and so can result in the formation of ring sideroblasts.

CONGENITAL DYSERYTHROPOIETIC ANEMIAS

The congenital dyserythropoietic anemias are a group of rare hereditary disorders in which one finds the combination of:

1. A refractory normochromic anemia, often with impressive anisocytosis and poikilocytosis. Basophilic stippling may be noted. The reticulocyte count is normal or only minimally elevated.
2. Ineffective erythropoiesis with marked erythroid hyperplasia in the bone marrow characterized by the presence of many *multinucleated erythroid precursors*.

The most common form of congenital dyserythropoietic anemia is called Type II and is also often referred to by the acronym HEMPAS (Hereditary Erythroblastic Multinuclearity with a Positive Acidified-Serum lysis test). The anemia is of variable severity. Hepatosplenomegaly and some degree of jaundice is usually present. (The latter reflects an increased bilirubin load for excretion secondary to the ineffective erythropoiesis and resultant intramedullary hemolysis.) Numerous binucleated late polychromatophilic normoblasts are typically noted on a stained smear of a bone marrow aspirate.

The RBCs in HEMPAS have abnormalities in the types of carbohydrate molecules attached to the erythrocyte membrane proteins. The RBCs also have a surface antigen not found on normal cells that reacts with an IgM antibody absent from the patient's own serum but present in ABO group-compatible sera from some other individuals. At an acid pH, this antigen-antibody reaction activates complement by the classic pathway with consequent lysis of the patient's RBCs. This helps to confirm the diagnosis. In contrast to the RBCs of paroxysmal nocturnal hemoglobinuria, which also have a positive acidified-serum lysis test, the RBCs in HEMPAS have a negative sucrose hemolysis test. (The latter results from activation of complement not by the classic pathway but by the alternate pathway.)

Because of a chronically increased excretion of bilirubin, the patient with HEMPAS has an increased risk of forming bilirubin gallstones. Moreover, as in other patients with anemias associated with lifelong ineffective erythropoiesis, the patient with HEMPAS persistently absorbs increased amounts of dietary iron and may develop secondary hemochromatosis after many years.

SELECTED READING

1. Bennett JM, Catovsky D, Daniel MT, Flandrin G, Galton DAG, Gralnick HR, and Sultan C: The French-American-British (FAB) Cooperative Group: Proposals for the classification of the myelodysplastic syndromes. Br J Haematol 51:189, 1982.
2. Bottomley SS: Sideroblastic anemia. Clin Haematol 11:389, 1982.
3. Camitta B, O'Reilly RJ, Sensenbrenner L, Rappeport J, Champlin R, Doney K, August C, Hoffmann RG, Kirkpatrick D, Stuart R, Santos G, Parkman R, Gale RP, Storb R, and Nathan D: Antithoracic duct lymphocyte globulin therapy of severe aplastic anemia. Blood 62:883, 1983.
4. Camitta BM, Storb R, and Thomas ED: Aplastic anemia. Pathogenesis, diagnosis, treatment, and prognosis. N Engl J Med 306:645 and 712, 1982.
5. Champlin RE, Feig SA, Sparkes RS, and Gale RP: Bone marrow transplantation from identical twins in the treatment of aplastic anemia: implication for the pathogenesis of the disease. Br J Haematol 56:455, 1984.
6. Clark CA, Dessypris EN, and Krantz SB: Studies on pure red cell aplasia. XI. Results of immunosuppressive treatment of 37 patients. Blood 63:277, 1984.
7. Koeffler HP: Myelodysplastic syndromes (preleukemia). Semin Haematol 23:284, 1986.
8. Najaen Y for Joint Group for the Study of Aplastic and Refractory Anemias: Long-term follow-up in patients with aplastic anemia. A study of 137 androgen-treated patients surviving more than two years. Am J Med 71:543, 1981.

12

Secondary Anemias in Nonhematologic Disorders

ANEMIA OF CHRONIC DISEASE

Pathogenesis

A patient with a chronic infection, a chronic inflammatory condition, or a malignancy will develop a moderate (for example, Hgb 10 g per dL) but persistent anemia which does not respond to hematinics and improves only when the underlying disorder improves. The anemia stems from the combination of:

1. Moderately increased RBC destruction secondary to an unknown extrinsic factor—possibly stimulation by disease of macrophage phagocytic activity.
2. A failure to increase RBC production to compensate for the increased RBC destruction. RBCs continue to be made at a normal rate, which is abnormal, since production should increase to correct the anemia.

One reason erythropoiesis fails to increase is that iron release from mononuclear phagocytes, which is the primary source of iron for making new RBCs, does not increase. Thus, restricted iron availability limits erythropoiesis despite a normal total iron body content. Body responses to infection or tissue injury that could impede rapid mobilization of iron from macrophages include:

1. Release from activated macrophages of *interleukin 1*, the soluble factor (monokine) now known to mediate the metabolic

185

changes referred to as the acute phase response. Interleukin 1 causes a rapid fall in plasma iron level when injected experimentally into an animal.

2. Release of *lactoferrin* from the specific granules of neutrophilic granulocytes during chemotaxis and phagocytosis. Lactoferrin binds iron tightly and, at the acid pH of inflammatory sites, can remove iron from transferrin. Iron bound to lactoferrin is phagocytosed by macrophages. Thus, release of lactoferrin could shunt plasma iron away from its delivery by transferrin to the normoblasts and back to the macrophages.

3. Increased apoferritin synthesis by tissue cells. An increase in macrophage apoferritin could facilitate retention as ferritin of iron liberated from the phagocytosis of senescent RBCs.

It is not clear whether mechanisms in addition to limited iron availability impede erythropoiesis significantly in the anemia of chronic disease. Some evidence exists that:

1. Synthesis of erythropoietin is inadequate for the degree of anemia in some but not all patients.

2. Activated bone marrow monocytes/macrophages from patients with disseminated fungal infection (and so, presumably, from other chronic systemic infections) liberate materials that impede proliferation and differentiation of erythroid progenitor cells in in vitro cultures.

Manifestations

The anemia of chronic disease has the following characteristics:

1. The RBCs are normocytic to moderately microcytic with a normal or moderately reduced MCV (75 to 90 fL range). RBC morphology is otherwise normal.

2. The reticulocyte count is not elevated.

3. The free erythrocyte protoporphyrin level (FEP) is increased (reflecting the restricted iron availability for erythropoiesis, see Chapter 3).

4. The serum ferritin level is increased (reflecting both increased primary apoferritin synthesis by tissue cells and increased accumulation of iron in ferritin in macrophages).

5. Both the serum iron and the total iron binding capacity (TIBC) are reduced.

6. Bone marrow macrophages contain increased amounts of iron on Prussian blue stains of a bone marrow preparation (see Fig.

3-2). (The bone marrow is examined for iron stores less frequently now that serum ferritin assays are generally available.)

ALCOHOLISM

Moderate macrocytosis (MCV, 100–110 fL) may be a clue to unsuspected alcoholism in a patient who drinks heavily but eats well and appears healthy. On reviewing the blood smear, one sees only uniform-appearing, round macrocytes; the oval macrocytes, anisocytosis, and hypersegmented neutrophils that characterize the blood smear of a megaloblastic anemia are not seen. The patient is not anemic, the serum folate level is normal, and no evidence of decompensated liver disease is found. The macrocytosis, which apparently reflects a direct effect of alcohol upon erythropoiesis, disappears within 2 to 4 months if the patient stops drinking.

Patients hospitalized for the consequences of acute and chronic alcoholism are frequently anemic and may exhibit evidence of impaired erythropoiesis and sometimes of hemolysis. If performed early, a bone marrow examination may reveal erythroid precursors containing cytoplasmic vacuoles and also ring sideroblasts. These findings disappear within 3 to 4 days after alcohol withdrawal. If the patient has been eating poorly and drinking heavily for several weeks to months, megaloblastic changes are usually also found. These stem not just from diminished folate stores caused by a poor diet but from a block in folate metabolism induced by alcohol. Megaloblasts also begin to disappear from the marrow after hospitalization because alcohol intake is stopped and the patient receives folate in the hospital diet.

Alcoholic patients may also develop a brisk hemolytic anemia as a complication of worsening liver disease (see discussions of Zieve's syndrome and spur cell anemia, below).

LIVER DISEASE

Cirrhosis

USUAL CAUSES OF ANEMIA

A moderate macrocytic anemia, with a hematocrit in the 30% range, is commonly found in the patient with cirrhosis, portal hypertension, and congestive splenomegaly. Three factors contribute to the low hematocrit:

1. Increased plasma volume.
2. Mild to moderate hemolysis as evidenced by a shortened RBC life span; an accumulation of excessive radioactivity from labeled RBCs over the spleen in some but not all patients; and increased fecal excretion of urobilinogen.
3. Impaired RBC production, causing an inability to compensate for the hemolysis.

The relative importance of each factor varies from patient to patient. The anemia does not respond to treatment with liver extract, folic acid, or vitamin B_{12} and improves only as the patient's general condition improves.

A more severe anemia may be found in some patients as the result of one or more of the following complications:

1. Acute gastrointestinal bleeding from esophageal varices or a peptic ulcer.
2. Iron deficiency secondary to chronic gastrointestinal bleeding. Such a patient may have an MCV that is normocytic rather than macrocytic, hypochromic cells on the blood smear, a low saturation of transferrin, and no iron stores in the bone marrow.
3. Folic acid deficiency caused by a poor diet and alcoholism. This complication is suspected when hypersegmented neutrophils and oval macrocytes (instead of the usual round macrocytes of liver disease) are seen on the blood smear.

SPUR CELL ANEMIA

An occasional patient with far-advanced cirrhosis develops a severe hemolytic anemia with bizarre, spiculated red cells present on the peripheral blood smear (Fig. 12-1). RBCs with such thorny projections are called acanthocytes. When they arise in the setting of advanced cirrhosis, they are also called spur cells.

Spur cells form as a consequence of the following sequence of events:

1. Severe liver disease leads to impaired esterification of plasma cholesterol with a resultant rise in free plasma cholesterol. Since plasma free cholesterol can exchange with cholesterol in the red cell membrane, both the amount of cholesterol and the ratio of cholesterol to phospholipid in the membrane rises.
2. This causes the red cell to acquire excessive surface area and to lose membrane fluidity. The RBC then passes through an intermediate stage in which it flattens and acquires a scalloped con-

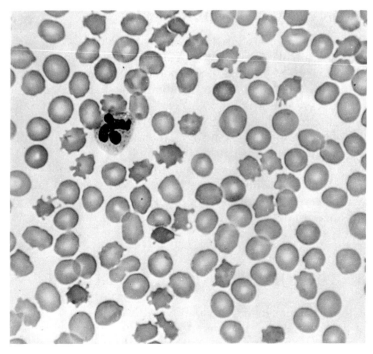

Fig. 12-1. Peripheral blood smear from a patient with far-advanced alcoholic cirrhosis and a severe hemolytic anemia associated with many spur cells.

tour. This intermediate stage is seen when normal RBCs are incubated in vitro with serum from a patient with spur cell anemia.

3. However, RBCs in the intermediate stage are not seen on the patient's blood smear either before or after transfusion of normal RBC. As blood flows through the enlarged, congested red pulp of the spleen, the rigid, cholesterol-laden RBC loses surface area and is transformed into a distorted, spiculated cell. On subsequent passage through the spleen, these distorted cells are trapped and phagocytosed by macrophages in the red pulp.

Studies of a patient with spur cell anemia who underwent splenectomy substantiate that this two-step process occurs in vivo. After splenectomy, the patient's spur cells disappeared and hemolysis subsided. Only RBCs with scalloped contours were seen on the blood smear. (Although splenectomy causes hemolysis to subside, it is generally not indicated because of advanced, life-limiting liver disease.)

Hemolytic Anemia with Lipemia

Occasional patients are seen after a heavy drinking spree with a combination of fever, hepatomegaly, jaundice, lipemia, and brisk hemolysis (Zieve's Syndrome). Splenomegaly is unusual. Spherocytes are found on the blood smear in about one half of the patients. The reticulocyte count is high and erythroid hyperplasia is found in the bone marrow. Plasma triglyceride levels are markedly elevated, and the plasma appears very turbid. However, no evidence exists that the hypertriglyceridemia causes the hemolysis.

Patients with this syndrome have acute alcoholic hepatitis but not advanced cirrhosis. Liver biopsy shows marked fatty infiltration without much fibrosis. As the patient's condition improves with abstinence from alcohol, a good diet, and bed rest, the hemolysis subsides.

ANEMIA OF CHRONIC RENAL FAILURE

Although acute hemolytic anemia with fragmented RBCs and acute, oliguric renal failure occur together in the hemolytic-uremic syndromes (see Chapter 25), patients with other causes of acute renal failure are generally not anemic. In contrast, patients with chronic uremic failure virtually always develop a severe anemia. The anemia is normocytic; the majority of the red cells look normal on the peripheral blood smear, but small numbers of RBCs with irregularities of contour (burr cells) are also seen. The reticulocyte count is not elevated and the marrow fails to show erythroid hyperplasia, despite a hematocrit that may fall to the 15% to 20% range.

Although the life span of normal RBC transfused into patients with chronic renal failure is usually somewhat shortened, the anemia stems primarily from depressed erythropoiesis. Hypoproliferation results from two abnormalities:

1. Inappropriately low production of erythropoietin because of damage or destruction of the cells in the kidney that make erythropoietin.
2. Retention in plasma of a material, possibly a polyamine called spermine, that inhibits erythropoiesis.

The contribution of each factor varies in different patients. For example, occasional patients, primarily patients with polycystic kidney disease, make enough erythropoietin so that their hematocrit will rise to normal after they are changed from hemodialysis to continuous ambulatory peritoneal dialysis (which more effectively removes the inhibitory material). Conversely, despite presumed continued retention of the inhibitory material, erythrocytosis replaced anemia in two patients being maintained on long-term dialysis for chronic glomerulonephritis who developed acquired cystic disease of end-stage kidneys and overproduction of erythropoietin by the cells lining the cysts.

Iron deficiency secondary to blood loss may also contribute to the anemia of patients undergoing chronic hemodialysis. Therefore, such patients are usually monitored with serum ferritin levels and given iron when the serum ferritin level falls below 35 μg per L. Patients are also routinely given folic acid to replace folate cleared from plasma during dialysis.

ENDOCRINE DEFICIENCY DISEASES

Patients with hypopituitarism or hypothyroidism are moderately anemic. The anemia is normochromic and normocytic without poikilocytosis or reticulocytosis. Tissue metabolism is reduced in these disorders, and the tissues need less oxygen than normal. Presumably, the output of erythropoietin falls as a reflection of the decreased need for oxygen-carrying capacity of the blood. This "physiologic anemia" is corrected as metabolism quickens under the influence of hormonal replacement therapy.

SELECTED READING

1. Cooper, RA: Hemolytic syndromes and red cell membrane abnormalities in liver disease. Semin Hematol 17:103, 1980.
2. Lee, GR: The anemia of chronic disease. Semin Hematol 20:61, 1983.
3. Radtke HW, Rege AB, LaMarche MB, Bartos D, Bartos F, Campbell RA, and Fisher JW: Identification of spermine as an inhibitor of erythropoiesis in patients with chronic renal failure. J Clin Invest 67:1623, 1981.
4. Shalhoub RJ, Rajan U, Kim VV, Goldwasser, E, Kark JA, and Antoniou, LD: Erythrocytosis in patients on long-term hemodialysis. Ann Intern Med 97:686, 1982.
5. Zappacosta AR, Caro J, and Erslev A: Normalization of hematocrit in patients with end-stage renal disease on continuous ambulatory peritoneal dialysis. The role of erythropoietin. Am J Med 72:53, 1982.

13

Polycythemias

The term polycythemia usually refers to an increase in RBC *concentration* in the blood. A patient deserves study for polycythemia when the following values are obtained consistently:

	MEN	WOMEN
Red blood cells ($\times$ 10^6 per μL)	>6.0	>5.7
Hemoglobin (g per dL)	>18	>17
Hematocrit (%)	>54	>51

When these measurements of RBC concentration are very high (hematocrit over 60%), one safely assumes that they reflect an increase in the total number of RBCs in the circulating blood, that is, an increased RBC mass. When these values are only moderately elevated (hematocrit less than 60%), it is possible that a contracted plasma volume has produced a relative polycythemia (Fig. 13-1), and RBC mass and plasma volume should be determined.

RBC MASS AND PLASMA VOLUME

RBCs labeled with ^{51}Cr are used to measure RBC mass. A known amount of radioactive cells is injected, and, after allowing time for mixing, the radioactivity of the RBCs in a sample of the patient's blood is determined. RBC mass will be directly proportional to the dilution of the label, that is, the fewer radioactive RBCs in the sample, the greater the total number of RBCs with which the labeled cells

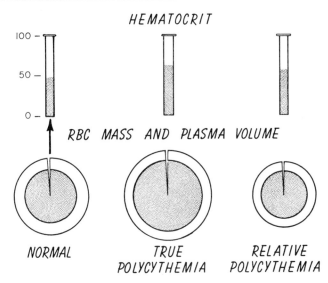

Fig. 13-1. Illustration of how an elevated hematocrit could result from either a true increase in RBC mass or a decrease in plasma volume with a normal RBC mass.

must have mixed. Albumin labeled with ^{125}I is used to measure plasma volume by the same principle.

Normal values for RBC mass are given as 26 to 32 mL per kg body weight for men and 23 to 29 mL per kg body weight for women. Normal values for plasma volume are 36 to 44 mL per kg body weight for both men and women. These normal values, obtained from studies of young adults, may be invalid for older, overweight patients because fatty tissue contains less blood than lean tissue. Thus, finding a high-normal value for RBC mass in mL per kg in an obese patient with an elevated hematocrit leaves one suspicious that the RBC mass may, in fact, be elevated in that patient.

TYPES OF POLYCYTHEMIA

The polycythemias may be divided into three groups:

1. Polycythemia vera or primary polycythemia: a hematologic stem cell disease of clonal origin characterized by increased production not only of RBCs but also of granulocytes and platelets.

2. Secondary polycythemia: a complication of a variety of disorders in which increased production of erythropoietin leads to an increased RBC mass.
3. Relative polycythemia (stress polycythemia, spurious polycythemia): a common syndrome of probably more than one pathogenesis in which a chronic, mild polycythemia may stem from a decreased or low-normal plasma volume and a normal or modestly increased RBC mass.

Polycythemia Vera

Polycythemia vera was established as a hematologic stem cell disorder of clonal origin from studies of women with the disease who are heterozygotes for Type A and Type B G6PD (see Chapter 7). Only one type of G6PD is found in the RBCs, granulocytes, and platelets of these women. Thus, their circulating blood cells cannot be of polyclonal origin—derived both from stem cells containing Type A G6PD and stem cells containing Type B G6PD—but are derived instead from a single clone of stem cells.

The abnormal clone apparently requires only minimal amounts of erythropoietin for erythroid differentiation. Plasma erythropoietin levels are low in polycythemia vera and do not rise after the RBC mass is reduced by venisections. Moreover, unlike normal stem cells, the stem cells of a patient with polycythemia vera will differentiate into erythroid colonies on culture in vitro without added erythropoietin.

When marrow from a G6PD heterozygote with polycythemia vera is cultured in vitro without added erythropoietin, the erythroid colonies formed contain only a single type of G6PD. If erythropoietin is added to the culture, then a mixture of Type A erythroid colonies and Type B erythroid colonies is found. This means that the marrow still contains normal stem cells. They are suppressed in vivo by whatever confers a proliferative advantage to the abnormal clone. As the disease progresses, the number of normal stem cells in the marrow demonstrable in vitro diminishes.

The mean age of onset of polycythemia vera is 60 years. Only 5% of patients are under 40 years of age at the time of diagnosis.

HISTORY AND PHYSICAL FINDINGS

The patient frequently complains of symptoms referable to an *increased blood volume*: dizziness, fullness in the head, headache, dyspnea, lethargy, and weakness. *Epigastric distress* is a common complaint that may result from engorgement of the gastric mucosa and possibly also from increased gastric secretion due to an elevated blood histamine level. *Itching of the skin, paticularly after bathing, may be severe.* This is not due to engorgement of the skin alone since it is not a prominent complaint in other polycythemias. Symptoms related to *peripheral vascular insufficiency,* for example, numbness or burning of the toes may be present.

The patient is often thin, a reflection of the hypermetabolic state associated with chronically increased hematopoiesis. The following abnormalities are frequently found on physical examination:

1. Plethora and suffusion of mucous membranes.
2. Distention of veins on funduscopic examination and, rarely, papilledema.
3. An enlarged spleen in about 75% of patients. Early in the disease, only the tip may be palpated; late in the disease, an occasional patient develops marked splenomegaly.
4. An enlarged liver in about 50% of patients.
5. Nondescript eruptions and excoriations of the skin.

Important negative findings include the absence of pulmonary abnormalities, of cyanosis, and of clubbing of the fingers.

LABORATORY FINDINGS

1. *Peripheral blood count.*
   a. The RBC count, hemoglobin level, and hematocrit will be elevated. A hemoglobin level above 20 g per dL is not infrequent in an untreated patient. RBC morphology on the peripheral blood smear is not distinctive although the RBCs are often slightly microcytic.
   b. A moderate leukocytosis (11,000–20,000 per μL) will be found in about two thirds of patients. Increased numbers of band forms and a slight absolute basophilia are frequently noted.
   c. The platelet count will be moderately elevated (450,000–800,000 per μL) in about two thirds of patients. An occasional patient may have a platelet count of over 1,000,000 per μL.
2. *RBC mass.* Values are definitely elevated (greater than 36 mL per kg body weight in men and greater than 32 mL per kg body weight in women).
3. *Bone marrow.* Whereas smears of aspirated marrow may provide little useful information, histologic sections of marrow particles from an aspirate or of marrow obtained by needle biopsy will demonstrate:

    a. Hypercellularity with a moderate to marked increase in the ratio of cells to fat (Fig. 13-2).

    b. Increased numbers and clusters of megakaryocytes, a finding often helpful in differentiating polycythemia vera from other polycythemias (Fig. 13-3).

    c. Absence of stainable iron, which reflects use of storage iron for increased hemoglobin synthesis.

4. *Other tests.*

    a. Leukocyte alkaline phosphatase, which is estimated from the intensity of staining for alkaline phosphatase of granulocytes on a blood smear, is usually high.

    b. The serum vitamin B_{12} level is elevated (greater than 900 pg per mL) in about 25% of patients, and the capacity of the serum to bind added vitamin B_{12} is increased (greater than 2,200 pg per mL) in about 75% of patients. This reflects increased production of the vitamin B_{12} binding protein transcobalamin I by granulocytes participating in the proliferative process.

    c. The serum uric acid level is high in about one third of patients.

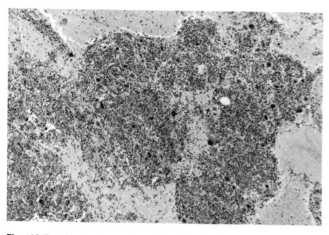

Fig. 13-2. Low-power view of a histologic section of two marrow particles held together by fibrin clot (light gray material surrounding the particles). Note intense hypercellularity of particles in this patient with polycythemia vera. The single, small white area represents the only remaining fat in either particle. Numerous megakaryocytes stand out because of their large, dark nuclei.

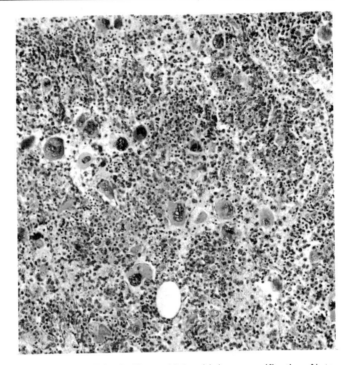

Fig. 13-3. Portion of one of the particles in Figure 13-2 at higher magnification. Note striking megakaryocytic hyperplasia.

COMPLICATIONS

Paradoxically, the patient has an increased risk of both *thrombosis* and *abnormal bleeding*. Presumably, the tendency for thrombosis results from:

1. Altered flow patterns of the viscous, thick blood.
2. The marked thrombocytosis found in some patients.

The causes for the bleeding tendency are not understood well. Possibly, the increased ratio of RBCs to fibrin in the whole blood clot affects its stability. Marked engorgement of capillaries and venules secondary to a greatly expanded blood volume could also contribute to excessive bleeding. Moreover, in some patients, the platelets behave abnormally in platelet function tests, which suggests an impaired ability of the platelets to form hemostatic plugs.

Because of the risks of thrombosis and hemorrhage, *elective surgery must not be performed* until the RBC mass has been reduced to normal and, if thrombocytosis is marked, until the platelet count has been lowered.

Five percent to 10% of patients with polycythemia vera develop gout because of the overproduction of uric acid resulting from increased cellular proliferation. Peptic ulcer occurs in an estimated 10% of patients. This, plus the abnormal bleeding tendency, results in a substantial incidence of serious *gastrointestinal bleeding.*

EVOLUTION

As the disease progresses, about 15% of patients with polycythemia vera drift into a syndrome referred to as "spent polycythemia vera," which is characterized by the following:

1. Anemia due to an increasing failure of erythropoiesis. Teardrop-shaped RBCs and occasional nucleated RBCs will be seen on the peripheral blood smear. (Treatable iron deficiency secondary to phlebotomies must be ruled out as a contributing cause for the anemia.)
2. A rising WBC count with increased numbers of immature granulocytes on the blood smear. Rarely, the WBC count may exceed 50,000 per μL and resemble the WBC count of chronic myelogenous leukemia (from which it is readily distinguished by the high alkaline phosphatase content of the granulocytes).
3. Increasing splenomegaly, which may produce severe discomfort due to symptoms of pressure.
4. Increased amounts of reticulin and fibrous tissue in a bone marrow biopsy section.

If a patient is first seen in the "spent" phase, the findings may be difficult to distinguish from those of myelofibrosis with extramedullary myeloid metaplasia (see Chapter 16).

A patient with polycythemia vera may also suddenly develop *acute non-lymphocytic leukemia.* In a cooperative study of treatment carried out by a polycythemia vera study group, acute leukemia developed in 1.5% of patients treated by phlebotomy alone. Leukemia developed in over 10% of patients treated by irradiation with ^{32}P or with the oral alkylating agent, chlorambucil. The interval until onset of acute leukemia was less than 5 years for most patients developing acute leukemia after chlorambucil and 6 to 10 years for most patients developing acute leukemia after [32]P.

TREATMENT

Failure to treat patients with polycythemia vera results in a median survival of less than 2 years, primarily because of fatal thrombosis or hemorrhage. In the study cited above, cumulative survival (close to 60% at 10 years) did not differ significantly for patients treated only with repeated phlebotomy and patients treated with ^{32}P. Excessive early deaths due to thrombosis in the phlebotomy group balanced later deaths due to acute leukemia in the ^{32}P group.

Therefore, whether to manage a patient with phlebotomy alone or phlebotomy followed by a myelosuppressive agent depends on assessment of a patient's risk for an early thrombotic event. One approach to treatment may be summarized as follows:

1. Initial phlebotomies at 2- to 3-day intervals to reduce RBC mass.
2. Management by continued phlebotomy alone in the patient under the age of 50 years unless findings arousing concern of incipient thrombosis are present—platelet count over 700,000 per μL plus a history of an earlier thrombotic event, angina, or neurologic symptoms suggestive of transient episodes of cerebral ischemia. If myelosuppression is needed, hydroxyurea, which is an antimetabolite and therefore may have less risk for inducing secondary leukemia than an alkylating agent or ^{32}P, may be the best agent to use. (Insufficient data are as yet available to be sure.)
3. Myelosuppressive therapy with hydroxyurea or with ^{32}P (whose long-term effects are known and which is easier to use than daily oral hydroxyurea in that a single intravenous injection may control the disease for months) in the patient between the ages of 50 and 70 years if one believes that the likelihood of a thrombotic episode within the ensuing 5 years is substantial. (Uncontrollable itching may be another indication for myelosuppressive therapy.)
4. Administration of ^{32}P after initial phlebotomies to most patients over age 70, because of the known increased risk for arterial thrombotic disease in the elderly.

Secondary Polycythemia

Secondary polycythemia results from increased erythropoiesis due to increased production of erythopoietin. Proliferation of granulocytes and platelets is not increased. Augmented production of erythropoietin may be:

   a. Physiologically appropriate, that is, a response to tissue hypoxia. This is the usual cause for secondary polycythemia.

   b. Physiologically inappropriate, that is, secondary to:

     (1) Secretion by a neoplasm (hypernephroma or hepatoma).

     (2) Other poorly understood effects of a cerebellar hemangioblastoma or a pheochromocytoma.

     (3) Secretion by the cells lining the cysts in polycystic kidney disease.

The *clinical manifestations* of secondary polycythemia may be summarized as follows:

1. In most patients, evidence is readily found of an underlying disease accounting for enhanced synthesis of erythropoietin (pulmonary disease, right-to-left cardiac shunt, tumor). Chronic anoxia can often be documented easily by demonstrating that the arterial oxygen saturation is below 90%.
2. The spleen is not enlarged.
3. The RBC count, hemoglobin level, and hematocrit are elevated due to an increased RBC mass (which should be measured if the hematocrit is below 60%).
4. The WBC and platelet counts are normal (unless some other cause for leukocytosis exists).

If a measurement of arterial oxygen saturation is normal, one considers the following possible reasons for secondary polycythemia:

1. Recurring *intermittent* arterial oxygen desaturation, for example, sleep apnea, a disorder in which arterial oxygen saturation falls only during sleep.
2. An impaired ability of hemoglobin to release oxygen to the tissues. One screens for this by measuring the p50—the partial pressure of oxygen at which the hemoglobin in a blood sample releases 50% of its oxygen. Finding a p50 below normal (27 mmHg) represents evidence that the oxygen dissociation curve of hemoglobin (see Fig. 7-3) is shifted to the left. With a left-shifted dissociation curve, hemoglobin may take up oxygen normally at the high partial pressure of oxygen found in the lungs, yet fail to release oxygen normally at the lower partial pressure of oxygen present in peripheral capillary beds (about 40 mmHg). Accumulation of carboxyhemoglobin in blood from smoking (see below) is a common cause for a reduced p50. An hereditary hemoglobinopathy that increases oxygen affinity is a rare cause but should be considered when polycythemia is discovered in a child or in several members of a family.

3. Increased erythropoietin synthesis secondary to a renal lesion (hypernephroma, renal cysts, hydronephrosis).

Relative Polycythemia

Relative polycythemia, stress polycythemia, spurious polycythemia, and Gaisböck's syndrome are names that have been used for the same syndrome. It is seen primarily in middle-aged males. The patient usually has a history of tension or anxiety, fatigue, headache, and smoking. He is frequently overweight. Slight plethora and, often, mild to moderate hypertension are noted on physical examination. The spleen is not palpable. The RBC count, hemoglobin level, and hematocrit are slightly to moderately elevated (hematocrit range, 54% to 60%) and the values do not increase over time. The WBC and platelet counts are normal as is arterial oxygen saturation.

Measurements of *RBC mass* and *plasma volume* do not reveal a consistent pattern. RBC mass is above the upper limit of normal (32 mL per kg) in some patients and within the normal range in other patients. (However, as mentioned, a high-normal value may be an elevated value in an overweight patient.) Plasma volume is *below normal* in many but not all patients. The terms "relative polycythemia" and "spurious polycythemia" stem from the patient in whom an elevated peripheral blood hematocrit results from a "normal" RBC mass and a reduced plasma volume (see Fig. 13-1).

Smoking has recently been recognized as a major cause for this syndrome. Inhaled carbon monoxide in cigarette or cigar smoke binds tightly to hemoglobin, yielding carboxyhemoglobin, whose intravascular half-life is 3 to 5 hours. In a heavy smoker, carboxyhemoglobin accumulates in the blood to levels of 4% to 20% as the day progresses. Carboxyhemoglobin compromises tissue oxygen delivery in two ways:

1. Binding of carbon monoxide to the iron of heme prevents that heme molecule from carrying oxygen until the carbon monoxide is released.
2. Binding of carbon monoxide to one or more of the four heme molecules contained within each hemoglobin molecule interferes with the normal movement of the polypeptide chains of the molecule that facilitates oxygen unloading from the other heme molecules, and so shifts the oxygen dissociation curve to the left.

Moreover, for unknown reasons, the experimental inhalation of a low concentration of carbon monoxide is associated with an acute reduction in plasma volume. Thus, smoking could also account for the contracted plasma volume found in many patients with relative polycythemia. In heavy smokers with relative polycythemia, the polycythemia disappears after the patient stops smoking.

DIAGNOSTIC APPROACH

The evaluation of a patient with an elevated hematocrit may be simplified by focusing initial attention on two questions:

1. Is a cause for chronic hypoxia obvious, for example, chronic obstructive pulmonary disease? If so, further hematologic study is rarely indicated.
2. Is there evidence suggestive of proliferation of other cell lines besides the RBCs, for example,
   a. An enlarged spleen on physical examination.
   b. A high WBC and platelet count.

If so, the patient probably has polycythemia vera and further work up is directed toward confirming that diagnosis.

If both of these questions are answered negatively, the hematocrit is between 54% and 60%, and the patient smokes, one should convince the patient to stop smoking and observe the hematocrit over the next several weeks. If the value falls to normal, the diagnosis of polycythemia secondary to smoking is established. If an elevated hematocrit persists, RBC mass and plasma volume should be measured. Arterial oxygen saturation should also be measured.

If the RBC mass is elevated and arterial oxygen saturation is reduced, one's attention turns to tracking a not initially obvious cause for arterial anoxemia. If RBC mass is elevated but arterial oxygen saturation is not reduced, then, as mentioned earlier, one needs to:

1. Rule out a cause for intermittent arterial anoxemia (for example, sleep apnea).
2. Measure p50 to screen for impaired oxygen release from hemoglobin.
3. Perform an ultrasound examination of the kidneys to look for evidence of an erythropoietin-producing renal lesion (for example, a renal tumor or renal cysts).
4. Consider the possibility of an unusual presentation of polycythemia vera without evidence in the peripheral blood of increased proliferation of granulocytic or megakaryocytic cell lines. Measuring plasma erythropoietin by radioimmunoassay will distin-

guish a patient in whom the level is not elevated from a patient with secondary polycythemia in whom the level is elevated. Unfortunately, this assay is still not generally available, and one is usually limited to looking further for evidence of granulocytic and megakaryocytic hyperplasia by:

a. Examining a histologic section of the bone marrow for evidence of increased myeloid activity and megakaryocytic hyperplasia (Fig. 13-2 and Fig. 13-3).
b. Measuring serum vitamin B_{12} and unsaturated B_{12} binding capacity.

SELECTED READING

1. Berk PD, Goldberg JD, Donovan PB, Fruchtman SM, Berlin NI, and Wasserman LR: Therapeutic recommendations in polycythemia vera based on Polycythemia Vera Study Group protocols. Semin Hematol 23: 132, 1986.
2. Berlin NI: Diagnosis and classification of the polycythemias. Semin Hematol 12:339, 1975.
3. Golde DW, Hocking WG, Koeffler HP, and Adamson JW: Polycythemia: mechanisms and management. Ann Intern Med 95:71, 1981.
4. Pearson TC, and Wetherley-Mein G: Vascular occlusive episodes and venous haematocrit in primary proliferative polycythaemia. Lancet 2: 1219, 1978.
5. Smith JR, and Landaw SA: Smokers' polycythemia. N Engl J Med 298:6, 1978.

14

Leukocytes: Properties, Production, and Functions

The leukocytes of blood (white blood cells, WBCs) normally consist of granulocytes, lymphocytes, and monocytes. They are recognized on a Wright's stained peripheral blood smear by the following morphologic features:

1. Granulocytes have a segmented nucleus with dense, clumped chromatin. The cytoplasm contains granules, which are fine and yellow-pink in the neutrophilic granulocyte (neutrophil), large and bright orange in the eosinophilic granulocyte (eosinophil), and large and purplish-black in the basophilic granulocyte (basophil). (Because most granulocytes are neutrophilic granulocytes, one often uses the term "granulocyte" as synonymous for neutrophilic granulocytes and the terms "eosinophil" and "basophil" for the other granulocytes.)

2. Most of the lymphocytes are small, quiescent cells with a round nucleus containing partially condensed, "smudgy-appearing" chromatin and limited amounts of light blue-staining cytoplasm. An occasional larger lymphocyte has an irregularly shaped or indented nucleus and increased amounts of cytoplasm containing areas of more deeply blue-staining cytoplasm. These are circulating stimulated lymphocytes, usually activated T-lymphocytes. An infrequent large lymphocyte may be seen with light blue cytoplasm and prominent azurophilic granules (large granular lymphocyte). This is a natural killer cell (discussed later).

3. Monocytes are large cells with an oval, indented, or "folded"

nucleus possessing lacy to strand-like chromatin and with plentiful, gray-blue cytoplasm containing fine azurophilic granules.

In the normal adult, 50% to 75% of the circulating WBC are neutrophilic granulocytes, 20% to 45% are lymphocytes, and the remaining 5% to 10% are monocytes and eosinophils. Basophils are uncommon.

The granulocytes and monocytes flow in one direction only. New cells are produced in the bone marrow, are released from the marrow into the circulating blood, and, after a brief stay in the blood, pass into the tissues. Once in the tissues, they do not return to the blood. In contrast, lymphocytes, particularly T-lymphocytes, constantly move back and forth between the circulating blood and the peripheral lymphoid tissues (described later).

Granulocytes are required for the phagocytic killing of many types of microorganisms and for the accompanying tissue inflammatory response. Lymphocytes are required for the body's cellular and humoral immune responses to antigens, that is, materials not recognized as self. Monocytes participate both in the phagocytic killing of certain types of microorganisms and in immune responses.

NEUTROPHILIC GRANULOCYTES

Granulocyte Maturation

Neutrophilic granulocytes and monocytes have a common progenitor cell that can give rise, depending upon in vitro culture conditions, to colonies containing mainly neutrophilic granulocytes or to colonies containing mainly macrophages. This progenitor cell does not have characteristic morphologic features permitting its recognition on a bone marrow smear stained with Wright's stain.

During maturation, the granulocyte acquires the biochemical reaction systems, the locomotor apparatus, and the surface membrane properties it needs to function as a phagocyte, that is, to ingest and kill bacteria. The morphologically recognizable stages of granulocyte maturation on a stained marrow smear have been defined as follows:

1. *Myeloblast.* This is the earliest morphologically identifiable member of the granulocytic series. It has a large round nucleus containing fine, stippled chromatin and one or more nucleoli. Its cytoplasm is blue and lacks granules.
2. *Promyelocyte.* The nuclear chromatin is beginning to condense,

but nucleoli are still visible. The cytoplasm is still blue; however, primary granules, which stain as azurophilic granules, are now present.

3. *Myelocyte.* The nucleus is still round, but nucleoli are no longer visible, and the chromatin is further condensed. The blue color of the cytoplasm of the immature cell is giving way to the yellow-pink color of the mature cell. Azurophilic granules may still be visible but are less prominent. Secondary granules, that is, fine neutrophilic granules, are also present.

4. *Metamyelocyte.* The nucleus has become indented and its chromatin is heavily condensed. The cytoplasm is uniformly yellow-pink and filled with secondary granules. Although still present, the primary granules are now no longer visible.

5. *Band.* The nucleus has become so indented that it has assumed a crescent shape. With further maturation, constrictions appear in the nucleus.

6. *Segmented granulocyte.* This is the mature granulocyte. The constrictions of the band's nucleus have narrowed to fine filaments of chromatin that separate the nucleus into two to four lobes.

The granules of the neutrophilic granulocyte serve different functions. The *primary granule* is a lysosomal granule, a package of powerful lytic enzymes (elastase, nonspecific collagenase, glycosidases) that break down proteins, nucleic acids, and carbohydrates. Primary granules also contain the enzyme *myeloperoxidase*, which catalyzes oxidation by H_2O_2 of halide ions with the resultant formation of microbicidal oxidized halides, for example, hypochlorite (OCl^-). These enzymes are released intracellularly after phagocytosis to breakdown bacteria or other ingested material. Primary granule enzymes also escape extracellularly during phagocytosis where they may dampen the inflammatory response by inactivating chemoattractants (see below) but where they may also attack and damage surrounding tissues.

The *secondary granules* function to translocate materials from the cytoplasm to the cell surface during granulocyte migration and activation. When present on the surface membrane, these materials can then participate in the reactions responsible for granulocyte adherence, chemotaxis, and the initiation of the "respiratory burst" (described later), essential events for effective phagocytosis and bacterial killing. These materials include:

1. Lactoferrin, an iron-chelating protein thought to be involved in neutrophil adherence.

2. A receptor for an inactivated complement component fragment called C3bi. This receptor also appears to serve as an essential surface recognition site for normal granulocyte adherence and chemotaxis.
3. A receptor for N-formylated methionyl peptides (chemoattractants formed from the breakdown of bacterial proteins and of mitochondrial proteins from damaged tissue cells).
4. Cytochrome b, an electron acceptor that completes the electron transfer chain needed for superoxide anion production in the surface membrane during the respiratory burst induced by some stimuli.

In addition, the secondary granules contain a cobalamin binding protein, transcobalamin I, which is released into the extracellular fluid and whose function is unknown (see Chapter 4). An enzyme called lysozyme, a mucopeptidase that attacks certain bacteria, is present in both primary and secondary granules.

The mature neutrophilic granulocyte also contains the enzyme alkaline phosphatase. Although its physiologic function is unknown, staining for leukocyte alkaline phosphatase has proved clinically valuable in distinguishing chronic myelogenous leukemia, wherein the granulocytes are deficient in this enzyme (see Chapter 16) from leukocytoses of other causes.

Kinetics of Production and Distribution

PRODUCTION

The granulocytic elements of the bone marrow may be divided into:

1. A *mitotic pool* consisting of myeloblasts, promyelocytes, and myelocytes.
2. A *postmitotic or maturation pool* consisting of metamyelocytes, bands, and segmented cells.

The total maturation time—the time from the first appearance of the cell as a myeloblast to its entrance into the circulation as a segmented granulocyte—is 12 to 13 days. Approximately one half of this time is spent in the mitotic pool. For each myeloblast in a bone marrow preparation, there are about three promyelocytes and thirteen myelocytes. Granulocytic precursors are thought to undergo one division at the myeloblast stage, one or two divisions at the promyelocyte stage, and two divisions at the myelocyte stage.

The postmitotic pool contains about twice the number of cells as the mitotic pool and provides a reserve of granulocytes of increasing maturity available for rapid release. For example, the leukocytosis associated with bands on the peripheral blood smear, which one finds within hours of the onset of an acute inflammatory process (for example, acute appendicitis), results from an increased release of cells from the postmitotic pool.

A sustained demand for increased numbers of granulocytes alters the kinetics of granulopoiesis in at least two ways:

1. Myelocytes undergo an increased number of divisions.
2. The time cells spend in the postmitotic pool is reduced to about 2 days.

PERIPHERAL DISTRIBUTION AND LIFE SPAN

When a normal subject is infused with radiolabeled granulocytes, only about one half of the expected radioactivity is recovered in a blood sample drawn after equilibration. This is because intravascular granulocytes are about equally divided between freely circulating cells (the circulating pool) and cells adherent to and moving slowly along the endothelium of the microcirculation (the marginal pool). Individual granulocytes move back and forth freely between these two pools, which, therefore, behave kinetically as a single pool. Stimuli that alter blood flow through the microcirculation (for example, strenuous exercise) cause cells to shift from the marginal pool into the circulating pool, with a resultant transient leukocytosis.

Radiolabeled granulocytes disappear from the intravascular pool with a half-time of only 12 hours. From this number and values for an average normal granulocyte count and total blood volume, one can calculate that an enormous number of granulocytes, about 2.5 billion cells in a 70-kg man, enter and leave the blood each hour. The life span of granulocytes in the tissues is unknown but is thought to be short.

MARROW GRANULOCYTE RESERVE

A patient given a large dose of a chemotherapeutic agent, such as cyclophosphamide, that temporarily blocks proliferation of cells in the mitotic pool develops a temporary granulocytopenia. Its time course reflects the status of the marrow granulocyte reserve, since granulocytes will continue to enter the blood from the post mitotic pool until it is exhausted. Normally, the nadir of the granulocytopenia will be found about 10 days after the drug is given. If marrow disease or damage has markedly reduced the marrow reserve, severe granulocytopenia will develop within a day or two after the drug is given.

Regulation of Granulopoiesis

Little is yet known about the physiologic regulation of granulopoiesis. Progenitor cells will not form colonies in vitro unless the culture contains a growth factor called granulocyte, macrophage-colony stimulating factor (GM-CSF). GM-CSF is also required for granulopoiesis in vivo. Cells of the marrow microenvironment produce GM-CSF; one stimulus for this is a fall in the number of granulocytes in the bone marrow. A two-step mechanism modulating GM-CSF release has been identified in which the initial step is release of interleukin 1 (see later) from marrow monocytes and macrophages. The interleukin 1 then stimulates the release of GM-CSF from other cells in the marrow microenvironment—endothelial cells, fibroblasts, and possibly, T-lymphocytes.

Monocytes synthesize and release prostaglandins of the E series (PGE). PGE decreases the sensitivity of progenitor cells to GM-CSF in vitro. Acidic isoferritins, compounds which were first identified in leukemic bone marrow and later in small amounts in normal bone marrow, inhibit the in vitro growth of normal granulocytic precursors but not of leukemic cells. It is not yet known whether PGE, acidic isoferritins, or both function as physiologic modulators of granulopoiesis. Continued proliferation in the presence of acidic isoferritins could be one mechanism allowing leukemic cells to overgrow normal granulocytic precursors in the leukemias.

Function of Neutrophilic Granulocytes

Neutrophilic granulocytes have only one known function in health—to engulf and kill bacteria that have penetrated the skin or mucosal barriers of the body. When granulopoiesis is markedly impaired and the concentration of neutrophilic granulocytes in the blood falls below about 500 per µL, an individual is at high risk of serious infection by organisms that may be normally found in the colon, the mouth, or on the skin. In certain pathologic conditions, neutrophilic granulocytes also ingest immune complexes or precipitates of crystalline material (for example, urate crystals in gout).

For effective phagocytic function, granulocytes must adhere to and emigrate through the endothelium of postcapillary venules; accumulate and aggregate at a tissue site; generate mediators that both recruit new granulocytes to the site and participate in microbial killing; ingest microorganisms or other materials; and undergo degranulation. An inflammatory tissue response accompanies these events; the effectors of phagocytosis and microbial killing are also the effectors of inflammation. Although the inflammatory response helps to contain microbial infection, in some circumstances it may also result in serious tissue damage as toxic oxygen metabolites and powerful lysosomal enzymes, escaping from activated granulocytes, attack constituents of the surrounding tissues. An example is the acute vasculitis with hemorrhagic tissue necrosis that follows the accumulation and activation of granulocytes around and within blood vessel walls after either an antigen-antibody reaction or the precipitation of immune complexes within blood vessel walls.

CHEMOATTRACTANTS

Binding of ligands to receptors on the granulocyte surface initiates the phagocytic defense reactions. Ligands that stimulate granulocytes to migrate in the direction of an increasing concentration of that ligand, that is, to undergo chemotaxis, are called chemoattractants. Among the most important are:

1. An activated complement component, C5a.
2. N-formyl-methionyl-oligopeptides derived from bacterial protein breakdown and from mitochondrial protein breakdown.
3. Leukotriene B_4, an oxidation product of arachidonic acid formed within the neutrophilic granulocyte itself.
4. Materials secreted from platelet alpha granules—platelet factor 4 and platelet-derived growth factor.

Chemoattractants also trigger other events of the phagocytic response. Whether a chemoattractant stimulates chemotaxis or, instead, stimulates granulocyte aggregation, activation of the "respiratory burst," and degranulation appears to depend upon several factors:

1. The concentration of the chemoattractant. In low concentration, a chemoattractant may stimulate chemotaxis. In high concentration, it may stimulate the other responses.
2. The affinity state of the chemoattractant's surface receptor. Receptors in a high-affinity state transduce chemotactic signals, whereas receptors in a low-affinity state transduce signals for

the other responses. (Guanine nucleotides can apparently convert high-affinity receptors into low-affinity receptors).
3. Changing properties of the surface membrane related to translocation of secondary granule contents to the membrane.

MEDIATORS GENERATED BY ACTIVATED GRANULOCYTES

Stimulated granulocytes generate at least two types of mediators important for phagocytosis and inflammation:

1. Toxic oxygen radicals.
2. Lipid mediators.

Toxic Oxygen Radicals. During phagocytosis, oxygen is consumed in a burst (respiratory burst). This increased oxygen uptake results from two linked biochemical events:

1. Reduction of molecular oxygen to form superoxide anion (O_2^-).
2. Consumption of glucose by way of the oxidative hexose monophosphate shunt pathway.

Activation of a membrane-associated oxidase by an unknown mechanism sets off these reactions. The oxidase catalyzes a reaction in which NADPH is used to reduce molecular oxygen to superoxide anion (O_2^-). Much of the superoxide anion is then rapidly transformed into H_2O_2 in a reaction catalyzed by the enzyme superoxide dismutase. The hexose monophosphate shunt (see Chapter 7) is activated to generate NADPH, which is consumed in the generation of O_2^- and in replenishing GSH (Fig. 14-1). The latter is depleted by one of the two mechanisms the granulocyte uses to detoxify excess H_2O_2, which might otherwise damage the granulocyte itself. (The second mechanism, which is independent of GSH, uses the enzyme catalase.)

The crucial importance of generating toxic oxygen radicals during phagocytosis was established when a fatal X-chromosome linked hereditary disorder—chronic granulomatous disease of childhood—was shown to stem from a deficiency of the membrane-bound oxidase catalyzing superoxide anion production. In this disorder, bacterial species possessing catalase which breaks down H_2O_2—and so makes H_2O_2 made by the bacteria themselves unavailable to the granulocyte—are not killed after phagocytosis but instead proliferate within neutrophilic granulocytes.

As mentioned earlier, neutrophilic granulocytes use H_2O_2, hal-

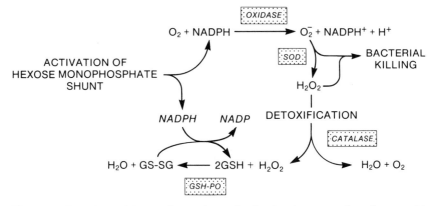

Fig. 14-1. Reactions of the respiratory burst that lead to the generation of superoxide anion and H_2O_2 in a stimulated granulocyte. The reactions by which the cell detoxifies H_2O_2 are also shown. Abbreviations: SOD, the enzyme superoxide dismutase; GSH-PO, the enzyme glutathione peroxidase; GSH and GS-SG, reduced and oxidized forms of glutathione.

ides, and the primary granule enzyme myeloperoxidase to form oxidized halogens with powerful microbicidal activity. In contrast to children with chronic granulomatous disease, individuals deficient in the enzyme myeloperoxidase do not have repeated and chronic bacterial infections. (Some have an increased susceptibility to infection with a particular fungus, *Candida albicans*, but many are asymptomatic.) This must mean that toxic oxygen radicals are required for an additional mechanism of bacterial killing that is independent of myeloperoxidase. This could be the Haber-Weiss reaction, a reaction in which O_2^- and H_2O_2 interact to generate a hydroxyl radical (OH·) with microbicidal activity.

Lipid Mediators. Stimulated granulocytes generate lipid mediators through complex reactions in which:

1. Phospholipases are activated—phospholipase C, which liberates diacyl glycerol from phosphatidyl inositol, and phospholipase A_2, which liberates arachidonic acid from membrane phospholipids.
2. Diacyl glycerol activates a c-AMP independent kinase, protein kinase C, which phosphorylates as yet unknown proteins important for the activation of cells.
3. Arachidonic acid is oxidized by way of the lipoxygenase pathway to generate leukotriene B_4. Leukotriene B_4 functions as a

powerful endogenous amplifier, attracting new granulocytes to a tissue site and activating them.

Pharmacologic doses of adrenal glucocorticoids suppress inflammation. This stems partly from their ability to stimulate synthesis if an intracellular material called lipocortin, which inhibits phospholipases and so inhibits important cellular events including the generation of lipid mediators.

INGESTION AND DEGRANULATION

Granulocytes have surface membrane recognition sites for:

1. The altered configuration of the Fc portion of an IgG molecule (see Chapter 20) formed when its antigen binding sites react with antigen.
2. C3b, an activated component of complement.

Coating of bacteria with IgG and C3b (opsonization) causes bacteria to adhere to the granulocyte at these surface recognition sites and so facilitates phagocytosis.

Binding to the Fc receptor site appears particularly important for initiating ingestion. (When particles not coated with IgG are ingested, it is assumed that they contain structural groups on their surface that substitute for IgG and react with the Fc recognition site on the granulocyte surface.) During ingestion, the granulocyte surface membrane invaginates and simultaneously extends pseudopods. The pseudopods come together to enclose the engulfed particle within a surface membrane-lined vacuole, which is called a *phagocytic vacuole*. Primary and secondary granules are attracted to the phagocytic vacuole. Their membranes fuse with the membrane of the phagocytic vacuole and their contents are discharged into the phagocytic vacuole. The pH of the vacuole falls. Conditions are thus achieved for an attack upon microorganisms by granule enzymes, many of which function best at an acid pH, and by toxic oxygen metabolites which diffuse into the phagocytic vacuole and initiate oxygen-dependent microbial killing.

Although secondary granules secrete materials into phagocytic vacuoles, their major function, as mentioned earlier, may be to translocate materials to the surface membrane during granulocyte adherence, chemotaxis, and activation. In contrast, the major function of the primary granule is to secrete its enzymes within the phagocytic vacuole to break down ingested material; however, some primary granule enzymes are discharged into the phagocytic vacuole before it closes and so the enzymes can escape extracellularly. As discussed earlier, these enzymes, such as the enzyme elastase, may then attack substrates in the surrounding tissues with resultant inflammatory tissue damage.

EOSINOPHILS

A separate progenitor cell and a specific colony stimulating factor (CSF) are thought to exist for eosinophils, which mature in the marrow through stages similar to those described for neutrophilic granulocytes. Eosinophils normally make up about 3% of circulating leukocytes.

Eosinophils often accumulate at sites of invasion of tissues by worms (helminths) and at sites of allergic tissue reaction. In both circumstances, this may reflect release of materials from activated tissue mast cells (see below) that are chemotactic for eosinophils. Eosinophilic granules contain large amounts of two materials—major basic protein and eosinophil myeloperoxidase—that are released when eosinophils are activated and degranulate. Upon their release, these materials can damage the larva-tissue stage of helminthic parasites, which are much too large to be ingested by phagocytic cells. Release of major basic protein and eosinophil myeloperoxidase can also induce tissue damage, and this contributes to the pathologic changes found in certain disorders in which eosinophils may accumulate in tissues in large numbers (see Chapter 21).

For unknown reasons, eosinopenia, associated with a diminished release of marrow eosinophils, is characteristic of acute bacterial infections. Adrenal glucocorticoids also cause eosinopenia, possibly by inducing margination of circulating cells.

BASOPHILS AND TISSUE MAST CELLS

Basophils, which are the least numerous of human leukocytes, also mature in the bone marrow through stages similar to those of neutrophilic granulocytes. Basophils remain in the blood for only hours; their tissue fate is unknown. Tissues contain abundant numbers of cells called mast cells, which resemble basophils in possessing granules that stain blue-black with Wright's stain but which differ in having a round, rather than a segmented, nucleus. Although blood basophils are not precursors of tissue mast cells, both apparently arise from a common marrow precursor cell.

Tissue mast cells may have evolved as specialized cells to combat tissue invasion by parasites and fungi. Antigens of these organisms often stimulate synthesis of antibodies of the IgE class (see Chapter 20). Tissue mast cells possess surface membrane receptors for the Fc fragment of IgE, and this provides a mechanism for concentrating IgE in the tissues on mast cell surfaces with the antigen binding sites of the immunoglobulin free to react with antigens of these organisms. One consequence of such antigen-antibody reactions is degranulation of the mast cells. The released granule contents include chemotactic materials that bring eosinophils to the tissue site, with resultant liberation from the eosinophils of major basic protein that can damage the invading organisms.

In allergic patients, other antigens (for example, pollens, food antigens) may also induce synthesis of IgE molecules that bind to basophils and tissue mast cells by their Fc fragment. The release of granule contents following combination of antigen with the antigen binding sites of such bound IgE may provoke an immediate hypersensitivity reaction (an acute asthmatic attack, generalized urticaria).

MONOCYTES–MACROPHAGES

The monocyte is the precursor of the macrophage and of related phagocytic cells with nonsegmented nuclei that make up what was formerly called the reticuloendothelial system and is now more appropriately called the *mononuclear phagocyte system*. As mentioned, the monocyte and the neutrophilic granulocyte arise from a common marrow progenitor cell. Within the marrow, the monocyte maturation sequence is progenitor to monoblast to promonocyte to monocyte. Monocytic elements make up from 1% to 3% of the nucleated cells of normal bone marrow; a bone marrow reserve of monocytes does not exist.

Components of the Mononuclear Phagocytic System

Like the neutrophilic granulocyte, the monocyte spends only a short time—perhaps up to 24 hours—in the circulation before entering the tissues. Unlike the neutrophilic granulocyte, which enters the tissues fully differentiated and survives only a short time, monocytes undergo further differentiation within the tissues to form a variety of mononuclear phagocytic cells, some of which survive for many days to months. The tissue pool of macrophages and related cells, which far exceeds the combined size of the marrow and blood monocyte pools, include the following:

1. Wandering macrophages (histiocytes) scattered in variable numbers throughout most of the tissues and within the pleural and peritoneal cavities.
2. Fixed macrophages that, together with endothelial cells, make up the cells lining the sinusoids of the liver, spleen, and bone marrow. (These macrophages are strategically placed to remove materials from the circulating blood.)
3. The macrophages lining the peripheral sinus of and distributed throughout lymph nodes.
4. The alveolar macrophages of the lung.
5. The osteoclasts of bone.
6. The microglial cells of the central nervous system.
7. The Langerhans cells of the skin.

In addition, macrophages that have accumulated at a site of chronic tissue inflammation often differentiate further to form epitheloid cells or may fuse to form multinucleated giant cells.

Functions of Monocytes–Macrophages

Monocytes–macrophages perform amazingly diverse and important functions in body defense and homeostatic reactions. These include:

1. The *phagocytosis of certain types of microorganisms* (for example, mycobacteria) and of the tissue debris of inflammation. Microorganisms ingested by macrophages either proliferate or are killed within the macrophages. What happens depends partly upon the function of T-lymphocytes. After exposure to antigens of the invading microorganism, T-lymphocytes can liberate soluble factors (lymphokines), particularly γ interferon, that activate or "arm" the macrophage. With its heightened ability to synthesize lysosomal enzymes and toxic oxygen radicals, the activated macrophage can then kill microorganisms attempting to multiply within it.
2. The clearance from blood—as its flows through the marcophage-lined sinusoids of the spleen, liver, and bone marrow—of senescent RBCs, of denatured plasma proteins, and of invading microorganisms.

3. The processing of antigen for presentation to lymphocytes in immune responses (see below).
4. The secretion of soluble materials (monokines) with important biologic activities. These include:
   a. Interleukin 1, a key agent for body defense and homeostasis. Its multiple activities include stimulation of:
      (1) T cells to secrete interleukin 2 (see below).
      (2) Hepatocytes to synthesize acute phase proteins (such as fibrinogen, haptoglobin).
      (3) Cells of the marrow microenvironment to make GM-CSF and probably other growth factors.
      (4) Fibroblasts to proliferate.
      Interleukin 1 also functions as an endogenous pyrogen, inducing fever as part of the body's response to infection.
   b. Cachexin, or tumor necrosis factor, which shares some of the functions of interleukin 1 and which may be important for host defense against tumor growth. Cachexin also exerts major deleterious effects through its ability to impede the function of mRNA for anabolic enzymes. It is responsible for the anorexia and wasting that develops in chronic infections and in advanced malignant disease. It is also thought responsible for the vascular dilitation leading to shock that characterizes acute, overwhelming infection with gram-negative organisms (endotoxic shock).

LYMPHOCYTES

Components of Lymphoid Tissue

Lymphocytes consist primarily of two functional classes of cells:

1. The T-lymphocyte, which is involved in cellular immune processes and in the regulation of antibody synthesis.
2. The B-lymphocyte, which participates only in humoral immune processes and is the precursor of the principal antibody-forming cell of the body—the plasma cell.

A third class of lymphocyte, the natural killer (NK) cell, has also been identified. It diverges from the T cell lineage at an early stage; does not require thymic conditioning; and differs functionally from the T cell in attacking certain types of target cells without prior sensitization by antigen on the target cell.

Lymphoid tissue in man consists of:

1. A marrow stem cell pool, which is a source of primitive precursors of T cells and B cells.
2. The central lymphoid tissue, which has two components:
   a. The thymus, where precursors are processed into immunologically competent T cells.
   b. The bone marrow, where precursors are processed into immunologically competent B cells.
3. The peripheral lymphoid tissues, which are the sites to which the immunologically competent T and B cells are distributed. These include:
   a. The lymph nodes.
   b. The spleen.
   c. The tonsillar tissues of the oropharynx (Waldeyer's ring).
   d. The submucosal accumulations of lymphocytes in the gut, respiratory, and urinary tracts.
   e. The bone marrow, which also contains immunologically competent lymphocytes, primarily B cells but also some T cells.

T and B cells are distributed differently in the peripheral lymphoid tissue. B cells are found as aggregates called follicles (Fig. 14-2) in the cortex of lymph nodes, the white pulp of the spleen, and the submucosa of the gut and respiratory tract. As mentioned, most of the small lymphocytes of the bone marrow are also B cells. T cells occupy the paracortical areas of the lymph nodes and the interfollicular areas of the lymphocyte accumulations in the submucosa of the gut, respiratory, and urinary tracts. T cells also form a dense sheath surrounding the central arterioles of the white pulp of the spleen.

T cells move back and forth between the tissues and the blood; this provides a mechanism for continuous T cell monitoring of antigens throughout the body. Normally, T cells make up about 70% of the lymphocytes in the blood. B cells, which make up 10% to 15% of circulating lymphocytes, also move back and forth between the blood and tissues but to a lesser extent than do T cells.

One should note that lymphocytes and granulocytes differ fundamentally in their life cycle. Granulocytes cannot divide, have a short life span in the tissues, and must be replaced continuously by new granulocytes from the bone marrow. Lymphocytes released from the central lymphoid tissue into the peripheral lymphoid tissue, particularly T cells, may survive as immunocompetent quiescent cells

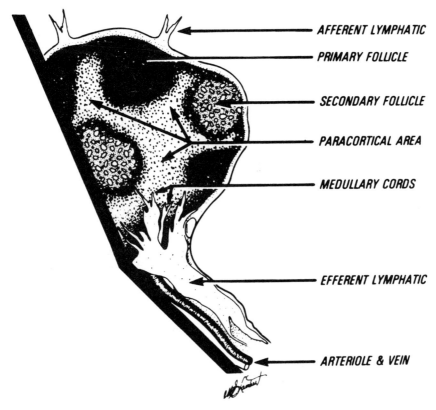

AFFERENT LYMPHATIC

PRIMARY FOLLICLE

SECONDARY FOLLICLE

PARACORTICAL AREA

MEDULLARY CORDS

EFFERENT LYMPHATIC

ARTERIOLE & VEIN

Fig. 14-2.   A schematic representation of the structure of a lymph node. B cells are found in the cortex in primary and secondary follicles. Primary follicles are uniform aggregates of small, quiescent B cells. Secondary follicles contain a central area of large, activated B cells with a surrounding mantle of small B cells. T cells are found in the paracortical areas. Plasma cells accumulate in the medullary cords. Lymphocytes, primarily T cells, leave the node via efferent lymphatic channels, eventually to enter the blood. (Reprinted by permission from Rapaport SI, Taetle R: Lymphocytes and immune responses. In West JB [ed]: Best and Taylor's Physiologic Basis of Medical Practice, 11th ed. Baltimore, Williams & Wilkins, 1984)

for long periods of time. However, when exposed to an immunologic determinant to which it is programmed to respond, a quiescent lymphocyte undergoes activation and divides. As the process continues, an expanded clone of lymphocytes responsive to that immunologic determinant is formed.

T Cells

THYMIC PROCESSING

T cells precursors migrate from the bone marrow to the thymic cortex. Here the cells divide rapidly and repeatedly, but most of the newly formed cells die. This cell wastage results from trial and error mechanisms, whereby T cells combine segments of germ-line DNA into functional genes for the polypeptide chains of a surface membrane receptor, the T cell antigen receptor. The structure of these polypeptide chains closely resembles the structure of the polypeptide chains of immunoglobulin molecules (see Chapter 20). Differences in how the germ-line DNA is rearranged results in differences in the amino acid sequences of segments of the polypeptide chains that confer selectivity of antigen recognition to the receptor.

Surviving lymphocytes in the cortex then migrate to the medulla of the gland where differentiation, but not cell division, continues. When processing is complete, the T-lymphocyte possesses a surface membrane antigen receptor that can:

1. Respond selectively to specific immunogenic sequences of foreign antigenic determinants.
2. Distinguish between self and non-self histocompatibility surface membrane determinants (see later).

Immunocompetent T cells are released from the medulla to the peripheral lymphoid tissues. They circulate freely throughout the peripheral lymphoid tissues but never return to the thymus. The thymus synthesizes soluble materials (for example, thymosin) that exert a supportive hormonal effect upon T cell function in the peripheral lymphoid tissues.

Processing of T cell precursors in the thymus begins in fetal life and continues through infancy and childhood. This gives rise to a repertoire of long-lived T-lymphocytes in the peripheral lymphoid tissues programmed to respond selectively to different antigens. Processing of new T cells then declines. The thymus, which weighs 70 g at the end of infancy, shrinks after puberty and in the elderly weighs only 3 g. Involution of the gland—with inability to process new T cells and a diminished thymic hormonal support for existing T cells—impairs the vigor of immune responses in older individuals.

T CELL SUBSETS

The immunocompetent T cells released from the thymus are programmed to perform different functions. Two major subpopulations have been recognized:

1. T-lymphocytes which, after exposure to foreign antigen on cells (for example, viral antigen on the surface of infected cells) in conjunction with histocompatability determinants, become *cytotoxic cells* that can lyse the target cells.
2. T cells which, after exposure to antigen in conjunction with histocompatability determinants, act as *immunoregulatory T cells* with helper functions. These helper functions support:
   a. The development of cytotoxic T cells.
   b. The acquisition by macrophages of microbicidal properties.
   c. The secretion of antibodies by B cells.

Other immunoregulatory cells have suppressor functions that dampen and so prevent excessive immune responses.

As discussed later, there are two types of histocompatibility determinants—Class I and Class II determinants. T cells are programmed to recognize one or the other of these determinants. T cells that recognize Class I determinants have a surface membrane antigen that reacts with a monoclonal antibody called CD8 (T8). T cells that recognize Class II determinants have a surface membrane antigen that reacts with a monoclonal antibody called CD4 (T4). CD8 cells are either cytotoxic cells or suppressor cells. Most, but not all, CD4 cells have helper functions.

PROLIFERATION OF T CELLS AFTER EXPOSURE TO ANTIGEN

Upon exposure to antigen, small quiescent T cells in the peripheral lymphoid tissue are transformed into large cells with a nucleus containing fine chromatin and nucleoli and with increased amounts of cytoplasm. The transformed cells then begin to divide. Proliferation results from two events:

1. The production by the T cell of a growth factor called interleukin 2 (Il 2).
2. The expression on the surface of the T cell of a receptor for Il 2.

The amount and duration of production of Il 2 and the density of its cell surface receptors determine the extent of T cell proliferation. As proliferation proceeds, the cells differentiate into the subsets of effector cells described above. These effector cells have finite life spans and, as stimulation by antigen ceases, diminish in number. A small number of T cells, "educated" by their exposure to the antigen, persist as immunologic memory cells capable of initiating more rapid and effective immunologic responses if the body is exposed again to that antigen. Memory T cells are very long-lived, apparently persisting for many years.

CLINICAL MANIFESTATIONS OF ALTERED T CELL FUNCTION

When T cell-mediated cellular immune mechanisms fail, a patient is subjected to repeated, serious infection by organisms that proliferate within cells. Many of these organisms are opportunistic organisms, that is, organisms that do not cause serious disease in normal individuals. Also, when T cell-mediated immune function is impaired, patients are at increased risk of developing a malignant proliferation of B cells (B cell lymphoma). In some instances, this reflects the need for T cells to curb proliferation of B cells infected with Epstein-Barr virus (see Chapter 21).

Responses mediated by T cells (and also possibly by natural killer cells) are responsible for rejection of bone marrow or other organ transplants and for the graft-versus-host reactions that may follow bone marrow transplantation. After an organ transplant, patients are frequently given adrenal cortical steroids and cyclosporine, both of which impair production of Il 2 and so dampen T cell responses.

B Cells

B CELL PROCESSING

B cells are processed in the bone marrow, which, like the thymic cortex, contains a fraction of lymphocytes undergoing rapid cell division and a high rate of cell death. During processing, each precursor of a B cell attempts to combine segments of germ-line DNA into rearranged functional genes supporting the synthesis of first the heavy chain and then the light chain of an immunoglobulin molecule unique for that cell in possessing but one of literally millions of possible antigenic specificities. As these gene rearrangements proceed, many cells are formed with aberrant DNA rearrangements or with DNA rearrangements coding for immunoglobulins reactive against antigens recognized as self. Such cells die and account for the large cell wastage.

The demonstration, by DNA analysis, of beginning rearrangement of the germ-line DNA for the heavy and light chains of IgM (see Chapter 20) provides the earliest evidence that a cell is committed to the B cell lineage. At the next stage, a pre-B cell is formed that contains μ chains in its cytoplasm as evidence of the cell's commitment to immunoglobulin synthesis. Then, μ chains disappear from the cytoplasm to be replaced by whole IgM molecules embedded in the surface membrane of the maturing B cell. This surface-bound IgM serves as the cell's initial antigen recognition site, that is, a surface recognition site for the specific haptenic determinant against which the cell, by its germ-line DNA rearrangements, has become committed to make antibody. At this stage, if the haptenic determinant is recognized as self, the cell is eliminated. As development proceeds, a second immunoglobin, IgD, also becomes embedded in the cell surface.

With these two classes of antigen recognition sites in place, the B cell is now programmed to function as an immunocompetent cell. It joins the pool of peripheral lymphoid tissue B cells ready to respond to the innumerable foreign antigens to which the body may be exposed. This pool of mature but "naive", that is, not yet exposed to antigen, B cells presumably turns over continuously throughout a person's life as new B cells are processed to replace senescent cells.

The mature B cell possesses cell surface components in addition to embedded immunoglobulin antigen receptors. These include Class II histocompatibility determinants (see below), receptors for the Fc site of immunoglobulins, and receptors for fragments (C3b and C3bi) of the complement component, C3. The physiologic functions of most of these surface components are not well understood.

RESPONSE OF B CELLS TO ANTIGEN

Upon exposure to an antigen it recognizes, the quiescent B cell is activated. This presumably results from cross-linking by antigen of the surface immunoglobulin antigen recognition sites. The activated B cell enlarges; its nucleus first becomes irregular and cleaved and then becomes "blast-like" in appearance, with fine chromatin and nucleoli.

The activated B cell expresses a cell surface receptor to a factor, the B cell growth factor (BCGF), which is made by T cells. Under the influence of BCGF, activated B cells begin to proliferate. At the same time, some B cells differentiate into a cell with properties intermediate between a lymphocyte and a plasma cell (plasmacytoid lymphocyte) that secretes IgM antibodies. These are the first antibodies the body makes to a new antigen.

The remainder of the activated B cells undergo further changes that include:

1. Replacement of their surface IgM and IgD by IgG, IgA, or IgE (rarely).
2. Expression of a second set of surface receptors, which are receptors for a second factor of T cell origin called B cell differentiation factor (BCDF).

The cells are now ready, upon exposure to BCDF, to differentiate into plasma cells secreting high-affinity IgG, IgA, or IgE antibodies.

How T cells are stimulated to release the factors necessary for B cells to proliferate and differentiate into plasma cells is incompletely understood. It involves an activation of helper T cells by exposure to the same antigen on macrophage surfaces and then an interaction of the activated T cells with B cells. These cell-cell interactions require that the T cell recognize Class II determinants, first on the macrophage and then on the B cell.

Plasma cells are short lived. Thus, as stimulation by antigen diminishes (and also as the result of other regulatory influences), antibody production declines. Some members of the activated B cell clone do not differentiate into plasma cells but persist as B memory cells with antigen-specific IgG (or IgA or IgE) embedded in their surface membrane. These cells can initiate an enhanced antibody response upon a second exposure to antigen. (Vaccination schedules in which a first dose of a vaccine is followed within several weeks to months by a second dose of the vaccine take advantage of this phenomenon.)

Antibodies are required for the body to combat infection by virulent bacteria (pneumococci, streptococci), since coating of bacteria by antibody is key to their phagocytosis by neutrophilic granulocytes. Patients with impaired antibody synthesis are, therefore at risk for recurrent pyogenic infections. Antibodies are also important in the control of viral infections since, by combining with antigens on shed virus from infected cells, antibodies may prevent the infection of new cells.

Natural Killer Cells

Natural killer cells differ from cytotoxic T cells in that they can lyse certain target cells without prior sensitization by antigen on the target cell surface. They may do so directly or by a mechanism known as antibody-dependent, cell-mediated cytotoxicity (ADCC). In the latter:

1. IgG binds by its antigen binding sites to antigen on a cell surface.
2. Natural killer cells, which have receptors for the Fc portion of IgG, bind to the Fc portion of the surface bound antibody, and this triggers the killing of the target cell.

The importance of natural killer cells for cell-mediated immune responses in humans is unclear.

RECOGNITION MECHANISMS FOR IMMUNE RESPONSES

Three types of surface recognition sites—related in evolution in that they are at least partly the products of genes arising from a common ancestral gene—are required for cells participating in immune responses to function normally. These are:

1. *The B cell antigen receptor.* As already discussed, the B cell uses the specificity of antigen binding sites of immunoglobulin molecules embedded in its surface membrane to recognize a specific immunogenic determinant of an antigen.
2. *The T cell antigen receptor.* This receptor, which allows a T cell to recognize a specific immunogenic determinant of an antigen in conjunction with histocompatibility determinants, has a complex structure. It consists of two polypeptide chains, called α and β and additional smaller subunits. The β chain has considerable homology with the heavy chain of immunoglobulin molecules. The structure of the α chain has yet to be determined. (The smaller subunits possess an antigen that reacts with a particular monoclonal antibody called OKT3. As discussed in Chapter 15, the T3 antigen is used as a surface marker for mature T cells.)
3. Two different surface recognition units, which have been named the *Class I and Class II determinants of the major his-*

tocompatibility complex. These surface recognition units are needed for cells participating in the immune response to identify and react with each other and with target cells. They also possess the major histocompatibility antigens that determine whether a tissue transplant "takes" or is rejected. These important surface membrane proteins and their genes are discussed in the next section.

THE MAJOR HISTOCOMPATIBILITY COMPLEX AND ITS PRODUCTS

A cluster of genes on human chromosome 6 code for polypeptide chains of the Class I and Class II determinants. This cluster is called the MHC (mixed histocompatibility complex) because, as already mentioned, antigens on these surface molecules determine whether a tissue transplant (for example, marrow transplant) is accepted as self or identified as foreign and rejected. In humans, the cluster is frequently referred to as the human leukocyte antigen (HLA) region, because the antigens were first characterized by incubating peripheral blood lymphocytes (as the source of antigens) with sera containing different antibodies to leukocytes (obtained from patients immunized to leukocytes by multiple transfusions or from multiparous women immunized transplacentally by fetal leukocytes).

Although the HLA region contains an increasing number of recognized genes, for simplicity, these may be thought of as making up four loci—HLA-A, HLA-B, HLA-C, and HLA-DR (D related). Multiple alleles exist for the genes at each locus. For example, an individual inherits from each parent one of at least 20 known alternative HLA-A genes and one of more than 40 known alternative HLA-B genes. This gives rise to the diversity of antigenic determinants on the Class I and Class II molecules needed by a sensing mechanism distinguishing self from non-self. Fortunately for transplantation purposes, the HLA genes are located so close to each other on chromosome 6 that cross-overs are uncommon. Therefore, the HLA genes are usually inherited from each parent as a unit or *haplotype.* (Since an individual inherits one of two possible haplotypes from each parent, a sibling of a patient needing a bone marrow transplant has a 25% chance of having the same haplotypes as the patient and so serving as a potential donor for the transplant.)

Class I determinants contain a heavy chain and a light chain. The HLA-A, B, and C loci, which are thought to have arisen by tandem gene duplication, each code for a polypeptide that can be used as the heavy chain of a Class I determinant. Therefore, the Class I determinants on a cell are a mixture of determinants whose heavy chains are products of HLA-A, B, or C genes. The light chain, which is coded for by a gene on chromosome 15, does not vary. It is a 12,000 dalton molecule, which the cell sheds, since it is also present in plasma and secreted in urine. Indeed, the light chain was first recognized as a serum protein and given the name β_2-microglobulin before its role as part of the Class I histocompatibility determinant was discovered. Homology exists between amino acid sequences in β_2-microglobulin and some constant region domains of immunoglobulins.

Class I molecules are present on the vast majority of all cells. As mentioned earlier, Class I determinants are involved in the sensitization of cytotoxic T cells to foreign antigens (for example, viral antigens) on cell surfaces and, subsequently, in the lysis by the sensitized cytotoxic T cells of target cells possessing both the foreign antigen and class I molecules on its surface.

Class II determinants (sometimes referred to as HLA-DR or Ia determinants) also contain two polypeptide chains. Both chains are coded for by genes at the HLA-DR locus. Class II determinants are restricted in their distribution and have so far been identified only on hemopoietic progenitor cells, endothelial cells, macrophages, B-lymphocytes, and activated but not quiescent T-lymphocytes. In immune responses involving immunoregulatory T cells with helper functions, antigens do not directly activate the T cells but are "presented" to the T cells by macrophages. To respond to the antigen on the macrophage surface, the T cell must also recognize the Class II determinant on the surface of the macrophage. The reasons for this dual recognition mechanism are not fully understood but are thought related to how vigorously the immune system can respond to a given immunogenic determinant. As mentioned earlier, Class II determinants on B cells are required for the interactions between helper T cells and B cells that result in B cell proliferation and differentiation during antibody production.

SELECTED READING

1. Acuto O, and Reinherz EL: The human T-cell receptor. Structure and function. N Engl J Med 312:1100, 1985.
2. Gabig TG, and Babior BM: The killing of pathogens by phagocytes. Ann Rev Med 32:313, 1981.

3. Goetzl EJ: Oxygen products of arachidonic acid as mediators of hypersensitivity and inflammation. Med Clin North Am 65:809, 1981.
4. Heberman RB: Natural killer cells. Hosp Prac 17:93, 1982.
5. Metcalf D: The granulocyte-macrophage colony-stimulating factors. Science 229:16, 1985.
6. Rosen FS, Cooper MD, and Wedgwood RJP: The primary immunodeficiencies. N Engl J Med 311:235 and 300, 1984.
7. Snyderman R, and Goetzl EJ: Molecular and cellular mechanisms of leukocyte chemotaxis. Science 212:830, 1981.

15

Hematologic Malignancies: General Concepts

CHARACTERISTICS OF HEMATOLOGIC MALIGNANCIES

The hematologic malignancies include the *leukemias*, the *lymphomas*, and two *monoclonal gammopathies*, multiple myeloma and Waldenström's macroglobulinemia. These diseases fulfill all of the criteria for a malignant proliferation of hematopoietic cells, which are:

1. *Monoclonality.* This key criterion was first recognized from studies of female patients heterozygous for the enzyme marker G6PD. In such heterozygotes, normal tissues are made up of a mixture of cells containing G6PD encoded by one allele and cells containing G6PD encoded by the other allele. In contrast, the cells of a hematologic malignancy contain G6PD encoded by one allele only, which means that all of the cells arose from a single clone.
2. *Clonal progression.* Once started, proliferation does not stop. Although sometimes only slowly, the malignant clone continues to expand.
3. *Clonal dominance.* Wherever it grows—the bone marrow, the lymphoid tissues, or both—a proliferative advantage allows the malignant clone to replace normal cell lines.
4. *Extinction of normal clones.* Early in the disease, normal clones are suppressed but still present. Later, they may die out, and only the progeny of the malignant clone are left.

5. *Genetic instability.* As the malignant clone proliferates, sub-clones arise with properties less and less like normal cells. A proliferation of differentiated cells frequently changes into a proliferation of less differentiated forms.

Sometimes one decides arbitrarily when to call a hematologic disorder malignant. For example, the *myelodysplastic syndromes* (see Chapter 11) are monoclonal disorders in which the progeny of an abnormal clone replace normal marrow elements but give rise to dysplastic hematopoiesis with bone marrow failure rather than to a progressive proliferative process. However, in a subset of patients, marrow blast cells become increasingly prominent; when they reach 30%, the diagnosis is changed to acute leukemia. A recently described syndrome involving expansion of a clone of large granular lympho-cytes (natural killer cells) affords another example. When the expan-sion of the clone is still minimal and recognizable only by molecular genetic analysis (see later), it can give rise to autoimmune phenomena such as persistent neutropenia. At this stage, the disorder is consid-ered an autoimmune disease; however, in some patients the clone expands to produce a moderate, persisting lymphocytosis. Some then consider the disorder a chronic form of T cell lymphocytic leukemia.

All of the non-lymphocytic proliferative disorders of bone marrow cells are often grouped together as the *myeloproliferative syndromes.* This includes disorders that are frank hematologic malignancies of myeloid cell lines (for example, chronic myelogenous leukemia) and monoclonal proliferative disorders not usually considered malignant (for example, polycythemia vera). The proliferative process in the latter advances slowly, often over years with active periods that may be followed by quiescent periods. However, such disorders have an enhanced risk of transformation into a hematologic malignancy, par-ticularly after treatment with agents that damage DNA (for example, after treatment of polycythemia vera with radioactive phosphorous or alkylating agents).

CATEGORIES OF HEMATOLOGIC MALIGNANCIES

Leukemias

The common feature of all leukemias is an *unregulated proliferation in the bone marrow of a cell of hematopoietic origin.* The leukemic cell overgrows and replaces normal elements in all areas of hemato-poietic marrow; consequently, marrow aspirated from any site will reveal the leukemic infiltrate (Fig. 15-1). The leukemic cell also proliferates in extramedullary sites of bygone fetal hematopoiesis, that is, the spleen and liver, and, in lymphocytic leukemias, in the lymph nodes. In addition, leukemic cells may invade and proliferate within nonhematologic organs and tissues, such as the central nervous system, testis, gastrointestinal tract, and skin.

The leukemias are classified by cell type. *Most often the cell is in the white blood cell series,* but occasionally it is of megakaryocytic lineage and rarely of erythroid lineage (erythroleukemia). Usually the leukemia involves only a single cell series, but surface marker studies with monoclonal antibodies (see later) have taught us that leukemic stem cells need not always follow a single program of cell differentiation. So-called mixed phenotype leukemias are now recognized in which one subclone of cells has surface markers characteristic of early myeloid cells and another subclone of cells has surface markers char-

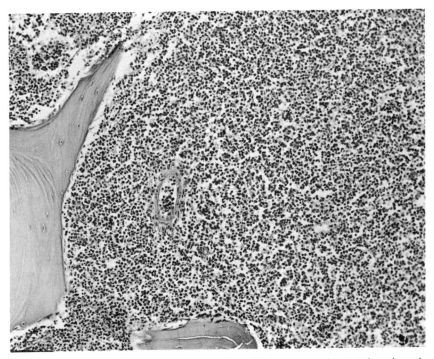

Fig. 15-1. Low-power view of histologic section of bone marrow in acute lymphocytic leukemia. Note hypercellularity of the marrow in leukemia, with replacement of normal marrow elements and of fat by proliferation of a single cell series.

acteristic of early lymphocytic forms. In rare instances, leukemic cells have been found to have a mixed pattern of cell surface antigens, indicating that the same cell is attempting to differentiate along more than one lineage.

The leukemias are divided on the basis of *degree of cell differentiation* into:

1. The *acute leukemias,* in which the marrow infiltrate consists predominantly of blasts or of cells with evidence of only early differentiation (for example, acute promyelocytic leukemia).
2. The *chronic leukemias,* in which the marrow infiltrate consists of a major proportion of differentiated cells.

In untreated acute leukemia, the peripheral blood WBC count may be high if many immature cells escape into the peripheral blood, or low (for example, a WBC count of 2000 per μL) if the leukemic proliferation depresses normal WBC production and only a few immature cells escape into the peripheral blood. In contrast, in untreated chronic leukemia, the peripheral blood WBC count is high, almost without exception, because mature WBC are less cohesive and can readily enter the peripheral blood.

The names acute and chronic leukemia were more appropriate in the past when patients whose leukemic cells were primarily undifferentiated used to die within a few weeks of diagnosis, whereas patients whose leukemic cells were differentiated could live for several years. Today, some patients with acute leukemia obtain complete remissions lasting many months to years, and many children with acute lymphocytic leukemia appear to be cured.

Lymphomas

Lymphomas are usually neoplasms of B- or T-lymphocytes of the peripheral lymphoid tissues (see Chapter 14). The malignant cell may have the morphologic features of normal, dormant, small lymphocytes but more often has morphologic and other phenotypic features of one of the different stages of activation or transformation that normal B or T cells go through after exposure to antigen. One form of lymphoma (lymphoblastic lymphoma) arises, not from cells of the peripheral lymphoid tissue, but as a neoplasm of thymic pre-T cells, that is, from cells of the central lymphoid tissue.

Lymphoma most often begins in a lymph node; however, it sometimes begins in an extranodal site, such as lymphoid tissue in the submucosa of the stomach or intestine. Certain T cell lymphomas characteristically first appear as lymphocytic infiltrates of the skin. Occasionally, lymphoma begins in unusual extranodal sites, for example, the brain, lung, ovary, or thyroid gland.

In some patients, lymphoma initially may appear confined to a single anatomic site, such as, a single lymph node or several adjacent lymph nodes. In other patients, multiple node sites are involved by the time the patient is first seen. Frequently, the spleen, liver, gastrointestinal tract, and bone marrow are also involved. In patients with advanced disease, lymphomatous infiltrates may be found at autopsy in many organs: the gastrointestinal tract, pancreas, liver, kidney, lung, endocrine glands, skeletal system, and skin.

Blurred Distinctions Between Leukemia and Lymphoma

A lymphoma beginning in lymph nodes or at an extranodal site may spread as lymphomatous masses analogous to other solid tumor metastases to many organs, including the bone marrow. If lymphomatous "metastases" in the bone marrow grow together to become a uniform marrow proliferation, then the appearance of the marrow is indistinguishable from that of a leukemia. The recognition of the neoplasm as a lymphoma may depend on knowledge of its initial pattern of distribution. For example, the acute lymphoblastic lymphoma of thymic pre-T cells mentioned earlier may present as a mediastinal lymphoma but often quickly moves into a leukemic phase with diffuse marrow infiltration and a high peripheral WBC count.

Lymphocytic neoplasms in which large numbers of lymphocytes from the peripheral lymphoid tissue enter the blood (yet the marrow remains only minimally involved) may also be labeled as leukemia. An example is a disorder called adult T cell leukemia in which one may find a high WBC count due to circulating T-lymphocytes; a rapidly progressive proliferation of T cells in the skin, peripheral lymph nodes, and other peripheral lymphoid tissue sites; but only minimal involvement of the bone marrow. A table listing related leukemias and lymphomas is found in Chapter 18.

Monoclonal Gammopathies

In monoclonal gammopathies, a single clone of activated B-lymphocytes or plasma cells secretes large amounts of a whole immunoglobulin molecule, of a light chain of an immunoglobulin molecule (see Chapter 20), or of both. The whole immunoglobulin molecule will be found in high concentration in the plasma, where, because all of its molecules have the sàme charge, it appears as a narrow protein band or "spike" in the gamma globulin region on serum protein electrophoresis (hence the name, monoclonal gammopathy). Light chain molecules are not retained in plasma, but are excreted into the urine as a protein with distinctive properties (Bence Jones protein, see Chapter 20).

Two of the monoclonal gammopathies fulfill the criteria for a hematologic malignancy. One is Waldenström's macroglobulinemia, a proliferative disorder of B cells secreting an immunoglobulin of the IgM class. Waldenström's macroglobulinemia, thus, represents one form of a lymphoma. The other, multiple myeloma, is a malignant proliferation of plasma cells primarily within the bone marrow. In its diffuse marrow distribution, multiple myeloma resembles a leukemia. Only in the unusual patient, in whom large numbers of plasma cells circulate in the peripheral blood, is the disorder referred to as plasma cell leukemia.

PATHOGENETIC AND ETIOLOGIC FACTORS

Abnormal Expression of Cellular Oncogenes

Certain RNA tumor viruses rapidly induce malignancies in laboratory animals through the action of transforming proteins produced by unique viral genes, which are therefore called viral oncogenes (v-onc). Studies of the origin of these genes revealed that some normal cellular genes share base sequences with viral oncogenes. These cellular genes were therefore given the name cellular oncogenes (c-onc) or proto-onc genes. They code for products that regulate normal cell differentiation and division—growth factors, receptors for growth factors, a G protein regulating adenylate cyclase activity, and proteins that affect the state of DNA in the cell nucleus. Accidental recombinations between viral genetic material and these normal cellular genes give rise to the v-onc genes. Fortunately, v-onc genes are not essential for replication of the virus and are therefore rapidly lost from the genome of the RNA virus. They do not appear to cause epidemics of cancer in animals in natural settings and have not been implicated in human malignant disease.

However, *abnormal expressions of cellular oncogenes* that trigger metabolic alterations increasing the ability of cells to divide are now thought key to the pathogenesis of malignant disease. Abnormal expression may be quantitative, reflecting escape from control of normal transcriptional promoter-enhancer regulators, or qualitative, resulting from a structural mutation affecting the function of an oncogene product.

Mechanisms inducing altered expression of oncogenes include:

1. *Chromosome breaks*, for example, a translocation of part of a chromosome that separates an oncogene from its promoter-enhancer regulator or a translocation that causes a portion of an oncogene and a partner gene in the translocation to combine to form an abnormal gene coding for an altered protein product. Cytogenetic studies (see later) in two hematologic malignancies have revealed translocations affecting oncogenes thought important for the development of each malignancy. These malignancies are:

   a. *Burkitt's lymphoma*, a rapidly growing lymphoma of transformed B-lymphocytes in which the terminal portion of chromosome 8 (location of the c *myc* oncogene) in cells of the malignant clone has exchanged with the terminal portion of chromosome 14 (location of the heavy chain genes of the immunoglobulin molecule) or with regions on chromosomes 2 or 22 (locations of the kappa and lambda light chains of immunoglobulins). The positioning of the *myc* gene next to the genes for immunoglobulin chains, a site that one might expect to favor transcription in cells programmed to produce immunoglobulins, apparently deregulates the *myc* gene and leads to overproduction of its product.

   b. *Chronic myelogenous leukemia*, in which an exchange between the terminal portion of chromosome 9 and chromosome 22 causes recombination between the *abl* oncogene from chromosome 9 and a partner gene on chromosome 22. The resultant *abl* protein has an altered amino terminal segment and presumably an altered function important for the sequence of events leading to the unrelenting proliferation of granulocytes characterizing that disease.

2. *Stimulation of transcription of cellular oncogenes by long terminal repeating sequences of viruses*. Certain RNA tumor viruses, unlike the rapidly transforming viruses mentioned earlier, cause tumors in animals only after a very long time. These viruses possess sequences from the ends of the viral genome called long terminal repeating sequences (LTRs), which possess promoter-enhancer activity. The virus can replicate within cells indefinitely without killing the cells, and so viral genes are integrated

randomly into the DNA of the cells. When, by chance, LTRs are inserted near cellular oncogenes, the oncogenes may be activated, and events are set in motion that eventually convert the cell into a tumor cell. Whether tumor viruses induce hematologic malignancies in humans by this mechanism is not yet known.
3. *Stimulation of transcription of cellular oncogenes by a stimulatory viral protein.* The human T cell leukemia viruses (HTLV) possess a gene coding for a viral protein that stimulates, not only its own long terminal repeats (and so propagation of the virus), but also the promoter-enhancer activity of cellular genes. This mechanism of activation, called *trans* activation, differs from the preceding in that the viral gene does not need to be inserted at a specific integration site next to a cellular oncogene in order to stimulate its transcription. The human T cell leukemia virus, HTLV-I, is thought to activate cellular oncogenes by this mechanism in the pathogenesis of a form of leukemia called adult T cell leukemia.

Viral Infection

As already described, three types of RNA tumor viruses have been identified: acute transforming tumor viruses containing viral oncogenes, nontransforming tumor viruses that produce tumors only after a very long period, and human T cell leukemia viruses. Only the last has as yet been proved to cause hematologic malignancy in humans.

As discussed in Chapter 21, a DNA virus called the Epstein-Barr (EB) virus can "immortalize" B lymphocytes in in vitro cultures. In vivo, cytotoxic T cells prevent uncontrolled proliferation of B cells infected with EB virus; however, in unusual hereditary immunodeficiency states and in certain acquired disorders in which T cell function is severely impaired, unchecked proliferation of B cells infected with EB virus can induce malignant lymphoma.

Aberrant Immune Function

An increased incidence of lymphocytic leukemia or lymphoma is found in patients with hereditary immunologic deficiency states, for example, hereditary X-linked immunodeficiency, common variable immunodeficiency, ataxia-telangiectasia. Similarly, patients with acquired causes for impaired immune function have an increased risk for developing lymphoma, for example, patients with acquired immune deficiency syndrome (AIDS) (see Chapter 21) or patients receiving chronic immunosuppressive therapy after organ transplantation. One mechanism for this has already been mentioned—unchecked proliferation of B-lymphocytes infected with EB virus. Other mechanisms are as yet unknown.

Chronic stimulation of immunoproliferative tissue may eventually lead to unregulated growth of a clone of cells, that is, to a lymphoproliferative malignancy. Thus, lymphoma arising in the wall of the small intestine may be a late complication of celiac disease, a chronic immunoinflammatory disorder resulting from hypersensitivity to a protein found in wheat products (gluten). A hypersensitivity reaction to a drug, for example, to phenytoin, may initate a continuing immunoproliferative disorder, angioblastic lymphadenopathy (see Chapter 18), that can progress to a frank immunoblastic sarcoma. Lymphoma of the thyroid gland may arise in the setting of chronic autoimmune thyroiditis (Hashimoto's thyroiditis).

Patients in whom chronic antigenic stimulation is combined with impaired immune function may be at particular risk for development of lymphoma, for example, a patient with a cardiac transplant in whom the host's immune system is simultaneously being stimulated by foreign antigens of the donor's heart and being suppressed by drugs given to suppress its rejection.

Environmental Agents Damaging DNA

Individuals exposed to agents that can damage the DNA of bone marrow cells have an increased incidence of acute myelogenous leukemia or other forms of acute non-lymphocytic leukemia. The increase in acute myelogenous leukemia found in the Japanese population exposed to radiation from the atomic bomb established that *radiation* is leukemogenic in man. *Chemical agents* that damage bone marrow may also be leukemogenic. Workers chronically exposed to *benzene* have been shown to have an increased risk for developing acute myelogenous leukemia. Patients with malignant or immunoinflammatory disorders treated with alkylating agents (for example, cyclophosphamide, melphalan, chlorambucil), which cross-link DNA strands, have an increased late incidence of acute non-lymphocytic leukemia.

Karyotypic analysis (the characterization of the morphology of the chromosomes of cells in mitosis) has revealed a strikingly high frequency of abnormalities of chromosomes 5 and 7 in the leukemic cells of patients developing acute non-lymphocytic leukemia after known exposure to radiation or alkylating agents. Similar karyotypic abnormalities have been observed in some patients with acute non-lymphocytic leukemia and no known exposure to a leukemogenic agent. One suspects that such patients have been exposed to an unrecognized agent damaging the DNA of bone marrow stem cells.

PATHOGENESIS OF CLINICAL MANIFESTATIONS

The major clinical manifestations of hematologic malignancies stem from the following pathologic processes:

1. *Bone marrow failure.* Bone marrow function fails early in acute leukemia and eventually in all forms of leukemia. Bone marrow function also fails in lymphomas that extensively infiltrate the bone marrow and in multiple myeloma in its advanced stage. As a result, patients become anemic, thrombocytopenic, and (except in chronic myelogenous and chronic myelomonocytic leukemias) granulocytopenic.

2. *Organ and tissue infiltration.* This varies in the different leukemias and lymphomas (as described in later chapters) but often results in lymphadenopathy, splenomegaly, or both. It may lead to obstructive findings (for example, hydronephrosis from large retroperitoneal nodes obstructing the ureters); to pain from compression of nerve roots, stretching of the capsule of organs, or an expanding proliferation of cells in the marrow cavity; and to symptoms and signs of central nervous system involvement (severe headaches, cranial nerve palsies).

3. *Immunologic abnormalities.* These develop primarily in patients with the chronic forms of lymphocytic leukemia, lymphoma, or multiple myeloma and may result in:
   a. Disturbed antibody synthesis, leading to an increased susceptibility to infection or to the synthesis of autoantibodies that may cause anemia or thrombocytopenia.
   b. Disturbed cellular immune function that may:
      (1) Increase susceptibility to infection with opportunistic microorganisms.
      (2) Impair erythropoiesis, granulopoiesis, or both due to excessive activity of suppressor T cells or natural killer cells.

4. *Effects of tumor cell products,* such as hyperviscosity secondary to formation of large amounts of a high molecular weight IgM in Waldenström's macroglobulinemia, osteoporosis and pathologic fractures due to formation of osteoclast activating factor in multi-

ple myeloma, and renal failure due to precipitation of uric acid within renal tubules in patients in whom a rapid turnover of malignant cells liberates large amounts of uric acid.

NEWER INVESTIGATIVE AND DIAGNOSTIC APPROACHES

Conventional morphologic techniques may not permit one:

1. To recognize a clonal proliferation in its early stages or when it persists as minimal residual disease after treatment.
2. To establish the cell lineage of immature-appearing blasts that are found in some acute leukemias.
3. To determine whether malignant lymphocytes are of T or B cell origin.

New techniques for analyses of gene rearrangements, structural alterations of chromosomes, and patterns of cell surface antigens now allow one to obtain such information. Diagnostic ability has been raised to a new level of sensitivity and specificity, and therapy can be modified for different disorders previously not distinguishable from each other.

Molecular Genetic Analysis

The genes for the polypeptide chains of an immunoglobulin molecule and for the polypeptide chains of the T cell antigen receptor exist in germ-line DNA as multiple, discontinuous pieces of genetic material. Very early in B cell processing, the germ-line DNA of a heavy chain and then a light chain are rearranged to bring selected discontinuous portions of each gene together to form functional genes. A similar rearrangement of the genes for the chains of the T cell antigen receptor occurs during T cell processing.

The different combinations of genetic segments possible during gene rearrangement, plus reading frame shifts that occur when certain of the segments come together, allow a limited amount of germ-line genetic material to code for literally millions of different variable regions of T cell surface antigen receptors and immunoglobulin molecules. Since the gene rearrangements of each processed T cell and B cell are uniquely designed to code for a specific antigenic determinant, a polyclonal population of T or B cells consists of myriad cells differing from each other in their gene rearrangements. Thus, not enough DNA of a particular rearrangement is present to permit its recognition. If a lymphocyte population contains an expanded number of cells from a single clone, then enough DNA will be present with the same gene rearrangement to identify the rearrangement by molecular hybridization techniques. This involves cleaving the DNA with enzymes called restriction endonucleases, separating segments into different sizes by gel electrophoresis, and identifying rearranged genetic segments by their hybridization with commercially available radiolabeled probes for regions of antigen receptor and immunoglobulin genes.

Analysis of immunoglobulin gene and of T cell receptor gene rearrangements has provided a way to recognize:

1. *Very early B or T cell differentiation in lymphoblasts of acute lymphocytic leukemia.* (A suprise has been the discovery of some leukemic lymphoblasts in which both a gene for the heavy polypeptide chain of an immunoglobin molecule and the gene for a polypeptide chain of the T cell antigen receptor have undergone rearrangement.)

2. *A monoclonal proliferation of differentiated T cells.* Whereas staining for the light chain type of surface immunoglobulin provides a relatively simple way to establish B cell monoclonality (see below), identifying a rearrangement of T cell antigen receptor genes by molecular hybridization assay is the only generally applicable way to establish T cell monoclonality.

3. *A limited clonal expansion of lymphocytes,* such as that found in some patients with the large granular lymphocyte syndrome mentioned earlier.

Surface Marker Analysis

As hematopoietic cells differentiate and mature, they express surface membrane and cytoplasmic proteins recognizable with commercially available monoclonal antibodies. The monoclonal antibodies, which are of murine origin, react with specific epitopes on these proteins and so are bound to the cell. Bound monoclonal antibody is then identified by use of a second antibody—a peroxidase- or fluorescein-labeled, anti-mouse immunoglobulin antibody.

Surface antigens identifiable by this technique are of two general types:

1. *Lineage specific*, that is, antigens present only on cells of a single cell line. Some lineage-specific antigens persist throughout

cell differentiation, whereas others appear or disappear from the surface membrane at different stages of cell differentiation.
2. *Lineage nonspecific.* Such antigens are often activation antigens, for example, antigens present on growth factor receptors, such as the transferrin receptor, that become expressed on the surface of cells of a number of lineages when they are stimulated to grow and divide.

Thus, to characterize a cell population fully, one must determine its pattern of reaction to a panel of monoclonal antibodies directed against a number of different cell surface antigens. This is referred to as surface marker analysis.

In many hematologic malignancies, the cells bear surface markers resembling those found on normal cells at a particular stage of differentiation. Therefore, surface marker analysis often allows one to relate a neoplastic proliferation to cell lineage and to a stage of cell differentiation. Surface marker studies have proved particularly useful:

1. In acute leukemias when conventional staining of blood smears or marrow aspirates reveals only primitive-appearing blasts without morphologic evidence of differentiation. Surface marker analysis can establish whether the cells are lymphoblasts, myeloblasts, or megakaryoblasts, which is essential for selecting treatment.
2. In distinguishing between reactive hyperplasia of B cells and B cell lymphoma. B cells contain immunoglobulin on their cell membrane. Reactive proliferations are polyclonal, and so the B cells will be a mixture of cells reacting with an antiserum against kappa-type light chains and cells reacting with an antiserum against lambda-type light chains (see Chapter 20). Neoplastic proliferations are monoclonal and therefore will be made up of B cells reacting exclusively with antiserum against only one type of light chain.
3. In determining whether a lymphoma or lymphocytic leukemia is of B cell or T cell origin. Although sometimes possible from clinical and conventional morphologic findings, surface marker analysis is frequently necessary to establish this. The distinction is important because B cell and T cell malignancies often have different prognoses and therapy.
4. To relate lymphocytic leukemias and lymphomas to stages in the differentiation or transformation of B lymphocytes and to different categories of T cells (see Chapter 14). This has led to a growing understanding of the differing biologic behavior of these neoplasms.

A confusing nomenclature of surface marker analysis developed after commercial monoclonal antibodies, which reacted with different epitopes on the same surface molecule or molecular complex and so identified the expression of the same surface phenomenon, became available. An international workshop group has recently proposed a Cluster Designation, or CD, nomenclature that assigns to such monoclonal antibodies the same CD number. (The CD nomenclature for lymphocyte surface markers is summarized in Table 17-2).

Cytogenetic Studies

Techniques have been developed to separate and stain the individual chromosomes of dividing cells. Photographs are taken of single dividing cells, and from such photographs, the 46 chromosomes of a human cell are arranged in 22 pairs of autosomal chromosomes and a sex chromosome pair, either XX or XY. This yields what is referred to as a karyotype.

Each chromosome, after being stained, usually with Giemsa, has its own characteristic pattern of banding. This provides a morphologic map of the chromosome and makes possible the localization of an abnormality to a particular segment of a chromosome (Fig. 15-2).

NOMENCLATURE

A human cell with 46 chromosomes is called a *diploid* cell, whereas a cell with greater or fewer than 46 chromosomes is referred to as an *aneuploid* cell. If the cell has fewer than 46 chromosomes, it

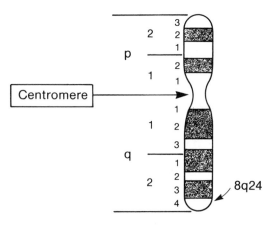

Fig. 15-2. A schematic representation of chromosome 8 illustrates the nomenclature used to identify the arms, regions, and bands of a chromosome. An arrow points to 8q24, which is the site of the c-myc gene.

is *hypodiploid*; if it has more than 46 chromosomes, it is *hyperdiploid*. If a cell has 46 chromosomes but there have been structural rearrangements of the chromosomes, then it is called a *pseudodiploid* cell.

The chromosomes are numbered from 1 to 22 in order of decreasing size. Each chromosome has two arms that meet at a segment called the centromere. The short arm is referred to by the letter p and the long arm by the letter q (see Fig. 15-2). Each arm is divided into regions, with region 1 being the region closest to the centromere. Each region is divided into numbered bands and a band may, in turn, be further divided into sub-bands. The terminology is "read backwards." For example, 8q24 (which is the site of the c-myc oncogene (see Fig. 15-2)) denotes a site in the fourth band of the second region of the q arm of chromosome 8. When localizing a site to a sub-band, one places a decimal point before the sub-band, for example, 1p34.3 would indicate the third sub-band of the fourth band of the third region of the p arm of chromosome 1.

A terminology also exists for chromosomal abnormalities. When a whole chromosome is gained or lost, a plus or minus sign is placed in front of the chromosome number. When part of a chromosome is gained or lost, a plus or minus sign is placed after the chromosome number. For example, −5 means that the cell contains only one chromosome 5; 14q+ means that extra material has been identified on the q arm of chromosome 14. Translocation of a segment of one chromosome to another is denoted by the letter t, followed in brackets by the chromosomes involved, with the lesser chromosome number coming first. The chromosome bands in which the breaks have occurred are indicated in a second set of brackets. For example, a translocation designated as t(8;14) (q24;q32) means a translocation between chromosomes 8 and 14 that involves the fourth band of the second region of the q arm of chromosome 8 and the second band of the third region of the q arm of chromosome 14. Symbols for other chromosomal alterations include "inv" for inversion, "i" for isochromosome (a daughter chromosome formed when a chromosome divides not longitudinally, as is normal, but transversely at its centromere), and "r" for ring chromosome.

KARYOTYPIC ANALYSIS IN HEMATOLOGIC MALIGNANCIES

The cells of most hematologic malignancies will have chromosomal abnormalities. In some disorders, consistent chromosomal defects have been identified (Table 15-1), either as a single defect or in combination with other apparently random defects. At times, a chro-

Table 15-1. Consistent Chromosomal Alterations in Leukemias and Lymphomas*

DISORDER	ABNORMALITY	APPROXIMATE FREQUENCY (%)
Chronic myelogenous leukemia	t(9;22) (q34;q11)	> 90
Acute non-lymphocytic leukemias		
Acute myeloid leukemia with some differen-tiation	t(8;21) (q22;q22)	18
Acute promyelocytic	t(15;17) (q22;q21)	100
Acute myelomonocytic with eosinophilia	Abnormalities of 16q22	—
Secondary to cytotoxic agents	−5, 5q−, −7, +8	—
Lymphomas		
Burkitt's lymphoma	t(8;14) (q24;q32) or t(8;22) (q24;q11) or t(2;8) (q12;q24)	100
Follicular lymphoma	t(14;18) (q32;q21)	85
Diffuse B cell lymphoma	t(11;14) (q13;32)	—
Chronic lymphocytic leukemia	t(11;14) (q13;q32) +12	—

*See text for explanations of nomenclature.

mosomal spread may reveal a mixture of cells containing only the consistent abnormality and cells containing the consistent abnormality plus other abnormalities. The latter cells are thought to arise as subclones of the original clone.

Karyotypic analysis has provided information at two levels of understanding:

1. Certain specific chromosomal abnormalities have been identified with a substantial frequency in a particular type or subtype of hematologic malignancy, but the meaning of the association for the pathogenesis of either the malignancy itself or one of its manifestations is not clear. Nevertheless, identifying the chromosomal abnormality may provide diagnostic or prognostic information (for example, in acute non-lymphocytic leukemia, an inversion of chromosome 16 appears to be associated with complete remissions after chemotherapy that are sustained for long periods).

2. Chromosomal breaks in several translocations are now known to occur at a cellular oncogene site on one chromosome and a site of a gene involved in an essential function of the cell on the other chromosome. Several translocations found consistently in different types of B cell lymphoma or leukemia involve a site on chromosome 14 that normally breaks to allow the separate V, J, and D segments of the germ-line heavy chain gene to come together in the formation of a functional heavy chain gene. Translocations apparently result from the mistaken incorporation into the normal breaking point of genetic material with a similar signal sequence from another chromosome. As mentioned, in Burkitt's lymphoma, the partner gene in the translocation is chromosome 8, which breaks at the site of the c-myc gene. The translocation deregulates the c-myc gene and a rapidly growing tumor results. Such cytogenetic observations are leading to major advances in the understanding of disturbed cellular oncogene expression in the hematologic malignancies.

THERAPEUTIC CONSIDERATIONS

In planning treatment for a patient with a hematologic malignancy, one must first decide whether its goal is cure or palliation. *Cure* is possible:

1. When tumoricidal doses of radiation therapy can be delivered to disease confined to a circumscribed anatomic site or sites as, for example, in stage I or II Hodgkin's disease (see Chapter 19). In such patients, one must establish by thorough clinical and laboratory studies that the planned field of radiation encompasses all known disease.
2. In some types of rapidly growing disseminated lymphoma with a high proportion of cells in growth cycle if intensive courses of combination chemotherapy can kill all of the malignant cells before a drug-resistant cell line emerges.
3. In some patients with acute leukemia, particularly children with the most common type of acute lymphocytic leukemia (see Chapter 17). A combination of drugs is given that produces essentially total marrow hypoplasia. Previously suppressed normal stem cells may then repopulate the marrow with normal hematopoietic cells. Residual leukemic cells are still present, and further therapy is given over many months to destroy these

residual cells. (In some centers, bone marrow transplantation is recommended for young patients with acute *non-lymphocytic* leukemia who have been brought into remission and who have a compatible sibling donor. This strategy assumes that the very large dose of alkylating agent given to prepare the patient for transplant, plus a second effect related to a degree of graft-versus-host reaction after transplantation, kills all residual leukemic cells.)

Paradoxically, cure is not yet achievable for lymphomas that grow more slowly and whose natural history, therefore, may be compatible with survival for a number of years. Nor is cure achievable in the chronic leukemias or multiple myeloma, in which the predominant forms are not blasts but differentiated WBCs. (A possible exception may be some patients with chronic myelogenous leukemia subjected to intensive chemotherapy followed by bone marrow transplantation).

Palliative therapy for hematologic malignancies serves the following purposes:

1. To treat existing complications of advanced disease, for example, pain secondary to organ enlargement, anemia secondary to marrow infiltration, hyperviscosity secondary to an elevated plasma IgM level.
2. In some patients with less advanced disease, to slow the rate of tumor growth and so forestall the development of complications. Before treating for this purpose, one often watches the patient for a time to determine how fast the disease is moving on its own.

Types of Chemotherapeutic Agents

Drugs presently used to treat hematologic malignancies fall into these classes:

1. *Alkylating agents.* Alkylating agents can substitute an alkyl group for a hydrogen atom on organic molecules, including the bases of DNA. This results in a cross-linking of the strands of DNA that interferes with its replication and the transcription of RNA. Alkylating agents act on cells in cycle and on resting cells. Therefore, they are particularly useful as chemotherapeutic agents for slow-growing hematologic malignancies (for example, chronic lymphocytic leukemia) in which a high proportion of cells are in a resting phase. The alkylating agents in common use

today include: nitrogen mustard, cyclophosphamide (Cytoxan), chlorambucil (Leukeran), melphalan (Alkeran), and busulfan (Myleran). In addition, a group of drugs called the nitrosoureas (CCNU, BCNU) are lipid-soluble alkylating agents with a different tissue distribution and longer duration of action.

2. *Antimetabolites* are compounds that can block DNA synthesis by inhibiting the function of enzymes required for normal purine or pyrimidine metabolism. Thus, they are mostly used in disorders with a high proliferative rate in which many cells are in the DNA synthetic phase (S phase) of the growth cycle. The antimetabolites include:

   a. Folic acid antagonists. The most important is methotrexate, a compound that competes with dihydrofolate for the enzyme dihydrofolate reductase. This enzyme catalyzes formation of tetrahydrofolate, which is an essential reaction for DNA synthesis (see Chapter 4).

   b. Pyrimidine analogues, of which cytosine arabinoside (Ara-C, cytarabine) is the most important. This agent inhibits DNA synthesis by inhibiting the enzyme DNA polymerase.

   c. Purine analogues (6-mercaptopurine, 6-thioguanine), which inhibit de novo purine synthesis and purine nucleotide interconversions.

   d. Hydroxyurea, which inhibits the enzyme ribonucleoside reductase, and so prevents the conversion of ribonucleotides to deoxyribonucleotides.

3. *Mitotic inhibitors.* These include two closely related derivatives of the periwinkle plant, vincristine and vinblastine. These cycle-specific drugs cause metaphase arrest, thus interfering with cell generation at a step just preceding mitosis. They have proved useful in acute lymphocytic leukemia, the lymphocytic lymphomas, and Hodgkin's disease. Etoposide (VP 16) is another agent that appears to act as a mitotic inhibitor and to be useful in the treatment of lymphoma.

4. *Antibiotics.* Daunorubicin (daunomycin) and doxorubicin (Adriamycin), which are antitumor antibiotics isolated from a *Streptomyces* species, interfere with DNA synthesis by their ability to intercalate between DNA base pairs. Daunorubicin has proved particularly valuable for the induction of remission in acute leukemia, and doxorubicin has proved particularly valuable for treatment of rapidly growing lymphoma. Another antitumor antibiotic, bleomycin, has had a limited usefulness in the treatment of Hodgkin's disease and other lymphomas.

5. *Hormones.* Adrenal steroids can lyse some types of lymphocytes and can also interfere with the production of interleukin 2. They have proved valuable in inducing remissions in acute lymphocytic leukemia and also in the treatment of chronic lymphocytic leukemia and lymphocytic lymphomas.

6. *Biologic enhancers.* These agents, which are materials that can enhance immune function through actions upon lymphocytes and macrophages, are still experimental drugs at this writing. One agent, interferon alpha 2, a leukocyte product now available from recombinant DNA technology, has proved effective in treatment of patients with a form of lymphocytic leukemia known as hairy cell leukemia (see Chapter 17) and in some patients with cutaneous T cell lymphomas.

7. *Miscellaneous.* L-Asparaginase, an enzyme from bacteria that deaminates arginine and so makes this amino acid unavailable to tumor cells, has been found useful in treatment regimens for acute lymphocytic leukemia. *Deoxycoformycin,* an inhibitor of the enzyme adenosine deaminase, causes toxic levels of deoxyATP to accumulate in lymphocytes. Deoxycoformycin has induced disease remissions in patients with hairy cell leukemia, with acute T cell lymphocytic leukemia, and in occasional patients with chronic lymphocytic leukemia through mechanisms that are not yet clear.

Toxic Effects of Chemotherapeutic Agents

All of the chemotherapeutic agents except vincristine, bleomycin, L-asparaginase, and adrenal steroid hormones depress bone marrow function. This is the toxic effect that often limits optimal use, particularly when the disease itself has already encroached upon bone marrow function. When pushed to toxicity, the alkylating agents can produce long-standing marrow hypoplasia. The antimetabolites can also severely depress marrow function, but it usually recovers within days after the agent is discontinued.

Alkylating agents may permanently damage the DNA of stem cells, and the prolonged use of alkylating agents is associated with a risk for the development of secondary acute non-lymphocytic leukemia. Alkylating agents may also induce sterility in men and a premature menopause in women.

Many of the chemotherapeutic agents cause nausea and vomiting for a number of hours after they are given. Many also cause a temporary loss of hair. A number of drugs have unique side effects, the most important of which are listed in Table 15-2.

Complications of Therapy

As mentioned, severe granulocytopenia following intensive chemotherapy enhances the risk for infection. The onset of fever in a granulocytopenic patient signifies infection until proved otherwise. One must act promptly to identify the site and organism and to begin broad-spectrum antibiotic coverage while awaiting culture results. If fever continues, the antifungal agent, amphotericin, is often added. Platelet concentrates (see Chapter 30) are given when infected patients are also severely thrombocytopenic (platelet counts below about 15,000 per μL) as prophylaxis against life-threatening bleeding.

Patients with large masses of leukemic or lymphomatous tissue sensitive to radiation or chemotherapy must be protected against developing uric acid nephropathy after therapy. The drug, allopurinol, a xanthine oxidase inhibitor, is given to block the oxidation of hypoxanthine and xanthine to uric acid. Since hypoxanthine and xanthine are more soluble than uric acid, they do not precipitate in the kidney. A patient with large tumor masses extremely sensitive to chemotherapy, for example, a patient with Burkitt's lymphoma, may

Table 15-2. Unique Side Effects of Chemotherapeutic Agents

AGENT	SIDE EFFECTS
Busulfan	Pulmonary fibrosis,* Asthenia-hyperpigmentation syndrome*
Cyclophosphamide	Hemorrhagic cystitis
Bleomycin	Pneumonitis, skin hyperpigmentation and keratosis
Daunorubicin, doxorubicin	Cardiomyopathy
Methotrexate	Hepatic fibrosis,* mucositis
6-Mercaptopurine, 6-thioguanine	Hepatotoxicity, jaundice
Vincristine	Nervous system toxicity (peripheral neuritis, autonomic nervous system dysfunction with obstipation)
L-Asparaginase	Pancreatitis, diabetes mellitus, decreased synthesis of coagulation factors
Adrenal steroids	Diabetes mellitus, masking of signs of infection, osteoporosis*

*Develops after prolonged use.

also develop hyperkalemia, hypocalcemia, and hyperphosphatemia as a consequence of tumor lysis.

SELECTED READING

1. Foon KF, Todd RF III: Immunologic classification of leukemia and lymphoma. Blood 68:1, 1986.
2. Knopf MKT, Fischer DS, and Welch-McCaffrey D: Cancer Chemotherapy. Treatment and Care, 2nd ed. Boston, G K Hall, 1984.
3. Rowley JD: Chromosome abnormalities in leukemia and lymphoma. Ann Clin Lab Sci 13:87, 1983.
4. Weinberg RA: The action of oncogenes in the cytoplasm and nucleus. Science 230:770, 1985.
5. Yunis JJ: The chromosomal basis of human neoplasia. Science 221:227, 1983.

16

Myeloproliferative Disorders

The myeloproliferative disorders are clonal proliferative diseases affecting granulocytic, monocytic, erythroid, and megakaryocytic cell lines. They include very different diseases that can be divided into two major subgroups:

1. Frank hematologic malignancies.
   a. The acute non-lymphocytic (myeloid) leukemias.
   b. Chronic myelogenous leukemia.
   c. Chronic myelomonocytic leukemia.
2. A group of disorders usually viewed as non-malignant because the proliferative process advances slowly, often only over years. Three findings are characteristic of these disorders:
   a. The proliferative process involves more than one cell series. The disorders are classified largely by which cell series exhibits the most prominent proliferation. Since this may change with time, one disorder may shift into another.
   b. Proliferation of megakaryocytes occurs so consistently that in its absence one hesitates to make a diagnosis of a disorder in this group.
   c. The proliferative process prominently involves extramedullary sites as well as the bone marrow. Consequently, the spleen is usually enlarged.

The myeloproliferative disorders that fall within this subgroup include:

a. Polycythemia vera (see Chapter 13), in which erythroid, granulocytic, and megakaryocytic proliferation occurs but in which, for many years, erythroid proliferation predominates.
b. Myelofibrosis with myeloid metaplasia, in which proliferation of megakaryocytes is combined with a secondary, reactive proliferation of fibroblasts with resultant fibrosis of the bone marrow. In some patients, considerable granulocytic proliferation may also be observed.
c. Essential thrombocythemia, in which extreme megakaryocytic proliferation may give rise to a platelet count in the 1 to 2 million per μL range.
d. Myeloid metaplasia without myelofibrosis, in which proliferation of neutrophilic granulocytes predominates, but in a much less aggressive pattern than in chronic myelogenous leukemia (see later).

THE ACUTE NON-LYMPHOCYTIC (MYELOID) LEUKEMIAS

In the acute non-lymphocytic leukemias, a mutant hematologic stem cell gives rise to a monoclonal population of myeloid cells whose ability to differentiate beyond early forms is markedly impaired. In addition, the cells possess a proliferative advantage and, therefore, blasts and other early forms increasingly replace the normal hematopoietic marrow elements. Often, leukemic forms will have almost totally replaced normal elements before the patient is seen, and the diagnosis is unequivocal. Sometimes, however, blasts and other early forms are increased but are still a minority of the nucleated marrow cells. Then, one must arbitrarily decide whether the diagnosis is acute leukemia or a preleukemic myelodysplastic syndrome (see Chapter 11). For the acute myeloblastic and monoblastic leukemias, many hematologists use a criterion proposed by the French-American-British (FAB) group that blasts make up 30% or more of nucleated marrow cells.

Types of Acute Non-Lymphocytic (Myeloid) Leukemia

Current FAB criteria for classifying the acute myeloid leukemias into seven types are summarized in Table 16-1. This classification is based largely, although not entirely (see criteria for megakaryoblastic leu-

Table 16-1. The French-American-British (FAB) Classification of Acute Myeloid Leukemias

CATEGORY	CRITERIA
M1-Myeloblastic leukemia without maturation	90% or more of nonerythroid marrow cells are myeloblasts; 3% or more of blasts stain for myeloperoxidase or for granule phospholipid (Sudan black).
M2-Myeloblastic leukemia with maturation	30% to 80% of nonerythroid marrow cells are myeloblasts, >10% are promyelocytes to mature neutrophils, and <20% are monocytic elements.
M3-Promyelocytic leukemia	Most marrow cells are abnormal hypergranular promyelocytes, some may contain bundles of Auer rods.
M4-Myelomonocytic leukemia	30% or more of all nucleated marrow cells are blasts. Granulocytic elements make up >20% of nonerythroid marrow cells. A monocytic component is identified by: a. 5000 per μL or more monocytic elements in the peripheral blood and either (1) 20% or more cells of monocytic lineage in the bone marrow, or (2) A serum lysozyme level > three times normal. b. If monocytic elements in the peripheral blood are <5000 per μL, recognition of 20% or more cells of monocytic lineage in the bone marrow with conformation by cytochemical stains showing fluoride-inhibited nonspecific esterase activity or by elevated serum or urine lysozyme.
M5-Monocytic leukemia	80% or more of nonerythroid marrow cells are monoblasts, promonocytes, or monocytes. In subtype $M5_a$, 80% or more of all monocytic cells are monoblasts; in subtype $M5_b$, less than 80% of monocytic cells are monoblasts.
M6-Erythroleukemia	50% or more of nucleated marrow cells are erythroid precursors and 30% or more of the remaining nonerythroid cells are blasts.

(continued)

Table 16-1. The French-American-British (FAB) Classificatin of Acute Myeloid Leukemias (continued)

CATEGORY	CRITERIA
M7-Megakaryoblastic leukemia	30% or more of cells of megakaryocytic lineage in a bone marrow aspirate. If aspirate unobtainable because of marrow fibrosis, then: a. A bone marrow biopsy showing excess blasts and, often, increased numbers of maturing megakaryocytes plus, b. Circulating megakaryoblasts. Megakaryocytic lineage of blasts should be confirmed by platelet peroxidase reaction on electron microscopy or immunologic identification with antibodies to platelet glycoproteins or von Willebrand factor.

kemia), upon the morphology of the leukemic cells on light microscopy. Cytochemical stains are used to confirm the identification of:

1. *Myeloblasts*, by the demonstration of cytoplasmic myeloperoxidase, phospholipid (Sudan black), or a specific esterase (chloroacetate esterase).
2. *Monoblasts*, by the demonstration of a nonspecific cytoplasmic esterase (for example, alpha-naphthyl acetate esterase) inhibitable with sodium fluoride.

The recognition of different types of acute myeloid leukemia is evolving further through cytogenetic observations. One can now identify:

1. A subgroup within the M2 (myeloblastic leukemia with maturation) category characterized cytogenetically by a translocation involving chromosomes 8 and 21 and morphologically by large blasts with prominent azurophilic granules and Auer rods.
2. Acute promyelocytic leukemia by a translocation involving chromosomes 15 and 17. This has led to recognition of a variant form also causing hypofibrinogenemia (see later) but containing fine granules seen only by electron microscopy rather than the

heavy azurophilic granules and bundles of Auer rods characteristic of the form first recognized.

3. A subgroup within the M4 (myelomonocytic leukemia) category characterized cytogenetically by abnormalities of chromosome 16 and morphologically by increased numbers of marrow eosinophils. (Prolonged remissions after chemotherapy have been described in patients with this subtype.)

4. Loss of all or part of chromosome 5, chromosome 7, or both in acute leukemia secondary to exposure to cytotoxic agents. Such chromosomal changes may also be a marker for acute leukemia secondary to exposure to unrecognized toxic environmental agents.

Surface marker analysis is also now widely used to characterize cell types in acute leukemias. Immunofluoresence with monoclonal antibodies for myeloid cell surface antigens (for example, My4, My7, My8, My9) or with monoclonal antibodies for lymphoid cell antigens (see Chapter 17) may permit one to decide whether primitive blasts are myeloblasts or lymphoblasts. The My antibodies also yield surface marker patterns useful in distinguishing leukemic cells with early granulocytic differentiation from leukemic cells with early monocytic differentiation.

Clinical Manifestations

The acute non-lymphocytic leukemias are adult diseases. Although exceptions occur, childhood acute leukemia is acute lymphocytic leukemia (see Chapter 17). Patients usually seek medical help because of manifestations of failure of normal bone marrow function, for example,

1. Fatigue and weakness secondary to anemia.
2. Abnormal bleeding or bruising due to thrombocytopenia.
3. Fever and systemic toxicity from an infection reflecting impaired phagocytic function of granulocytes.

Sometimes findings develop abruptly in a previously apparently healthy person. In other patients, an anemia worsening over months, often associated with neutropenia and moderate thrombocytopenia, may precede the appearance of overt acute leukemia. Such a preleukemic prodrome is frequently seen in older patients and in patients who develop acute leukemia after treatment with a cytotoxic agent.

MYELOBLASTIC LEUKEMIA

Myeloblastic leukemia, with or without maturation and with or without a monocytic component (types M1, M2, and M4 of Table 16-1), makes up about 75% of all acute non-lymphocytic leukemia.

Physical Findings. The patient may appear well nourished and need not look seriously ill. Unless infected, he or she will not have fever. Lymphadenophathy is rare; the spleen tip is occasionally palpable. With severe anemia, hemorrhages and exudates may be seen in the eye grounds. Sometimes, pressure on the sternum or other bones causes pain. In many patients, the only abnormal findings are pallor, petechiae, and an occasional small ecchymosis.

Laboratory Findings.

1. *Peripheral blood count.* A normochromic and normocytic anemia is usually present and sometimes severe. The reticulocyte count is low. The total WBC count may be high but is more often normal or low. If high, most of the cells on the blood smear are blasts. If normal or low, blasts are still usually recognized without difficulty. Most patients have a very low platelet count, but an occasional patient, discovered early, may still have a normal platelet count.
2. *Bone marrow.* The marrow is usually markedly hypercellular. The normal elements are largely replaced by immature cells, which are myeloblasts plus varying proportions of more differentiated forms in the different subtypes (see Table 16-1 and Figs. 16-1 and 16-2). In a few patients, usually older males, the marrow may appear hypocellular and thus resemble marrow aplasia. However, most of the cells present are blasts and other early myeloid forms rather than the plasma cells, small lymphocytes, macrophages, and fibroblasts that make up the residual marrow population in aplasia.

PROMYELOCYTIC LEUKEMIA

The cytogenetic and morphologic features of promyelocytic leukemia have already been described. The important clinical feature is an unusually severe bleeding tendency. In addition to the thrombocytopenia found in all types of acute leukemia, the patient with promyelocytic leukemia has clotting factor deficiencies: *hypofibrinogenemia and low levels of factors V and VIII.* These probably stem

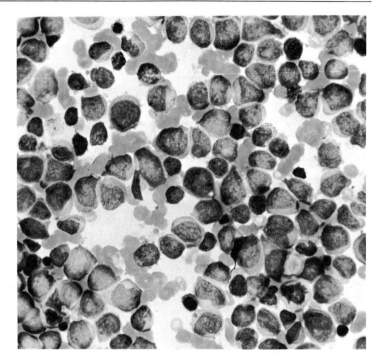

Fig. 16-1. Bone marrow smear in acute myeloblastic leukemia. Note marked proliferation of early myeloid forms.

from diffuse intravascular clotting triggered by release of material with tissue factor activity from the leukemic promyelocyte. The recent finding of lower plasma levels of alpha$_2$ antiplasmin, the primary inhibitor of plasmin, than of antithrombin III, the primary inhibitor of thrombin, in these patients suggests that excessive fibrinolytic activity also contributes significantly to the development of the clotting factor deficiencies.

MONOCYTIC LEUKEMIA

Monocytic leukemia differs clinically from myeloblastic leukemia in that:

1. The gums may hypertrophy, and oral ulcers are frequently noted.
2. Skin infiltrates are common.
3. The spleen is often palpable.

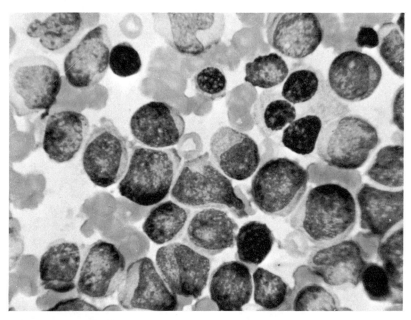

Fig. 16-2. Higher-power view of bone marrow smear in acute myeloblastic leukemia (M2 type; see Table 16-1). Note morphologic features of leukemic myeloblasts and the dysplastic, more differentiated myeloid elements.

4. Anorectal ulcerations frequently occur.

5. The central nervous system is frequently involved.

The peripheral WBC count is usually high, with large numbers of monoblasts and immature monocytes on the peripheral blood smear. Monoblasts and other monocytic elements virtually replace the other elements of the bone marrow. Serum lysozyme (also called muramidase) levels are elevated and large amounts of lysozyme are excreted in the urine. This may injure the renal tubules, with resultant excessive urinary potassium loss and hypokalemia.

MEGAKARYOBLASTIC LEUKEMIA

Megakaryoblastic leukemia (acute megakaryocytic leukemia, acute myelofibrosis), once considered rare, is now recognized to make up 5% to 10% of acute non-lymphocytic leukemia. Its increased rec-

ognition stems from the use of newer techniques for identifying megakaryoblasts, for example, demonstrating that the blasts:

1. React with antibodies to platelet surface antigens or to von Willebrand factor (which is made in megakaryocytes and endothelial cells).
2. Contain platelet peroxidase in a characteristic distribution on
   electron microscopy.

Patients with megakaryoblastic leukemia may present with fever
not attributable to infection and with hemorrhagic phenomena. The
spleen may or may not be palpable. The usual patient is both anemic
and leukopenic with few circulating blasts. Platelet counts may be
low, normal, or elevated, and dysplastic, giant platelets are often
noted on the blood smear.

Occasional patients have elevated WBC counts and many circulating blasts that vary in size and other morphologic features. Some
blasts may have a deeply basophilic cytoplasm and exhibit cytoplasmic budding or have cytoplasmic vacuoles. Cytochemical stains
are negative for myeloperoxidase and chloroacetate esterase but
weakly positive for fluoride inhibitable alpha-napthyl acetate esterase. A few patients may also have a prolonged prothrombin time
associated with a reduced plasma factor V level.

One often cannot aspirate bone marrow because of marrow fibrosis, a probable consequence of stimulation of fibroblasts by growth
factors released from proliferating cells of megakaryocytic lineage.
When obtainable, aspirates may be either hypocellular or hypercellular with increased numbers of blasts. Marrow biopsy sections are
hypercellular and contain a mixture, in varying proportions, of blasts,
abnormal appearing megakaryocytes, mononuclear cells, and fibroblasts in a background of increased diffuse reticulin fibrosis. The
combination of megakaryocytic proliferation and fibrosis resembles
the bone marrow findings of myelofibrosis with myeloid metaplasia
(see later), which is why one earlier name for the disease was acute
myelofibrosis.

Megakaryoblasts are often resistant to current chemotherapeutic
regimens for acute non-lymphocytic leukemia. Therefore, it may
prove important to use immunochemical techniques, not only to identify megakaryoblastic leukemia, but to recognize myeloblastic leukemias that may have a megakaryoblastic component.

Treatment

INITIAL THERAPY TO INDUCE A REMISSION

A common approach is to begin treatment with a combination of:

1. Cytarabine, 100 mg per square meter of body surface area (m^2) per day by continuous intravenous infusion for 7 days.
2. Daunorubicin, 45 mg per m^2 for patients under 60 years or 30 mg per m^2 for patients over 60 years, on 3 successive days.

This regimen will induce an initial remission in over 60% of persons with acute non-lymphocytic leukemia. It causes severe marrow aplasia, following which, in the patient who obtains a remission, previously suppressed normal stem cells repopulate the marrow with normal hematopoietic cells. Patients with leukemia secondary to earlier treatment with cytotoxic agents (for example, cyclophosphamide, melphalan, busulfan, nitrosourea compound) are less likely to obtain a remission, possibly because they have fewer residual normal stem cells that can repopulate the marrow. As mentioned, patients with megakaryoblastic leukemia are also less responsive to this chemotherapeutic regimen.

During the aplastic period, some patients—usually older patients—will die from infection or hemorrhage. Virtually all patients develop fever, which is treated with combinations of antibiotics effective against a wide spectrum of bacteria. If fever persists despite antibiotics, the antifungal agent, amphotericin, is added. Platelet transfusions are given as prophylaxis against hemorrhage when platelet counts fall below 20,000 per μL.

In some older patients, acute non-lymphocytic leukemia may smoulder. For weeks to several months, the circulating blast count remains low, and enough residual normal hematopoietic function persists to maintain granulocyte levels above 1000 per μL and platelet counts above 20,000 per μL. One withholds chemotherapy from such patients, particularly if the bone marrow is hypocellular rather than hypercellular. When the leukemia eventually worsens, less intensive chemotherapy—a 21-day course of low-dose cytarabine, 10 mg per m^2 given twice daily either subcutaneously or intravenously—has been tried. The effectiveness of this regimen, which has also been used in patients with myelodysplastic syndromes with excess marrow blasts (see Chapter 11), is not yet clear.

SPECIAL THERAPEUTIC PROBLEMS

The Patient Who Presents with Infection. If a patient presents with infection but still has reasonable numbers of circulating granulocytes, one attempts to bring the infection under control with several days of antibiotic treatment before beginning chemotherapy that will wipe out the remaining granulocytes. However, if a patient presents with infection and severe granulocytopenia (for example, less than 500 granulocytes per µL), then one should begin chemotherapy with little delay, since antibiotics in the absence of granulocytes will not bring infection under control.

High Blast Counts. In patients with blast counts exceeding 50,000 per µL, masses of adherent blasts may plug cerebral vessels and fatal cerebral bleeding will result. Adherent blasts may also impede flow through the pulmonary microcirculation, causing pulmonary infiltrates and hypoxia. Therefore, one attempts to reduce the number of circulating blasts in such patients without delay, often by combining leukapheresis with administration of large doses of hydroxyurea.

Bleeding Due to Depleted Coagulation Factors. Prothrombin times and fibrinogen levels should be measured before and during induction chemotherapy in patients with promyelocytic leukemia and also in patients with other types of acute non-lymphocytic leukemia and high WBC counts. If the fibrinogen level is less than 150 mg per dL or falls below this level during chemotherapy, some hematologists will give heparin in a reduced dosage (for example, 500 U per hour by continuous intravenous drip) to combat disseminated intravascular coagulation and cryoprecipitate (see Chapter 30) to raise the fibrinogen level.

MANAGEMENT AFTER INDUCTION OF REMISSION

What to do after a patient with acute non-lymphocytic leukemia obtains a remission is not yet clear. At some centers, bone marrow transplantation is recommended for patients under the age of 35 years who have an HLA compatible sibling. The intensive chemotherapy given to prepare the patient for transplant may destroy all remaining leukemic cells, and relapse rates after transplantation are below 20%. However, a number of patients will die of interstitial pneumonitis or of graft-versus-host disease during the first year after transplantation.

Patients who are not subjected to transplantation should be given post-remission chemotherapy whenever possible on protocol in a clinical study. Non-cross-resistant drugs different from those used to induce remission are usually added in such protocols. Nevertheless, 50% of patients will relapse within 18 to 24 months. Between 20% and 30% of patients will have extended disease-free survival.

CHRONIC MYELOGENOUS LEUKEMIA

Pathogenesis

Cytogenetic studies and studies using G6PD as a marker (see Chapter 7) have established that chronic myelogenous leukemia (CML) is a clonal disorder resulting from malignant transformation of a pluripotent hematopoietic stem cell. A specific chromosomal abnormality, the Ph[1] chromosome, and monoclonality of G6PD have been demonstrated in granulocytic cell lines (neutrophilic, eosinophilic, basophilic), in monocytes, erythroid precursors, megakaryocytes, and also in B-lymphocytes. Abnormalities have only rarely been demonstrated in peripheral blood T-lymphocytes, probably because the precursors of these long-lived cells have left the bone marrow long before its take over by the transformed pluripotent stem cell of CML.

The chromosomal abnormality of CML was recognized first as a small chromosome 22, which was named the Philadelphia chromosome (Ph[1]) after the city of its discovery. We know now that the chromosome is small because of a specific translocation in which much of its long arm is translocated to chromosome 9, t(9;22) (q34;q11). The break points for the translocation occur in a small region of 22q called the "break point cluster region," or bcr, and in a region on chromosome 9 where the oncogene c-abl is located. (C-abl is the cellular homologue of the transforming oncogene of the Abelson murine leukemia virus.) The remaining bcr sequences on chromosome 22 act as an accepter for the c-abl gene, and a new fusion gene is formed. This chimeric gene is active, giving rise to a chimeric bcr/c-abl messenger RNA and a resultant abnormal chimeric protein. The abnormal protein, unlike the normal protein product of the c-abl gene but like the protein coded for by the viral abl oncogene, has tyrosine kinase activity and, therefore, the potential to activate cells.

The Ph[1] chromosome defect is found in about 95% of patients with CML. It appears very early in the disease, and in rare patients has been discovered before any other manifestation of CML. Although possibly not the first event of a multistep process causing malignant transformation of a hematopoietic stem cell in CML, the Ph[1] translocation, with resultant deregulation of the kinase activity of the protein product of the chimeric *bcr/c-abl* gene, is thought to represent a key pathogenetic event for the disease. (The 5% of patients with Ph[1] negative CML are a heterogenous group. Some patients probably have mutations of c-*abl* that are occult and do not produce a readily recognizable cytogenetic abnormality; other patients probably do not have true CML but a variant myeloproliferative disorder with features resembling CML.)

The transformed hematopoietic stem cell of CML gives rise to an increasingly expanded pool of committed stem cells of granulocytic and, at least initially, megakaryocytic cell lines. As a consequence, an abnormal granulocytic series overgrows the marrow, crowding out the normal granulocytic and erythroid elements and spilling over in ever-increasing numbers into the peripheral blood. The abnormal cells retain their capacity for maturation, giving rise to mature polymophonuclear neutrophils that have a normal functional activity, yet are not totally normal in that they have low levels of some of the enzymes of normal mature granulocytes, for example, alkaline phosphatase (see later). Since the proliferation involves all granulocytic cell series, the number of eosinophils and basophils in the peripheral blood also increases. Early in the disease, megakaryocytes are increased in the bone marrow and the peripheral blood platelet count is usually elevated.

The expanded committed progenitor pool spreads from the marrow to extramedullary sites. Granulocytes proliferate profusely in the spleen, growing out from the red pulp to replace the normal lymphoid elements of that organ. Granulocytes also proliferate within the sinusoids of the liver.

CML is an unstable disease. In its initial phase, it is a disorder of increasing overproduction of relatively normal granulocytes readily responsive to chemotherapeutic control; however, over months to several years, the malignant clone undergoes further mutations that cause the disease to enter into an accelerated phase. Then, increased numbers of basophils and of dysplastic-appearing mature neutrophilic granulocytes may be noted on the peripheral blood smear. The proportion of early myeloid elements—blasts, promyelocytes, and early myelocytes—increases in the bone marrow and, often, also in the peripheral blood. The disease becomes increasingly resistant to chemotherapy. A cytogenetic study at this time reveals added chromosomal abnormalities; these often include a Ph[1] abnormality of the second chromosome 22, along with one or more abnormalities of other chromosomes, for example, trisomy of chromosome 8.

Finally, many patients enter a "blast crisis" in which blasts and other early forms virtually replace all other nucleated marrow cells. The disease is now acute leukemia. Although usually myeloblastic leukemia or another of the subtypes of acute non-lymphocytic leukemia, in about 30% of patients, the leukemia is acute lymphoblastic leukemia of B cell lineage. This conversion from a granulocytic to a lymphocytic neoplasm provides further evidence that CML originates in a primitive hematopoietic cell that can give rise to cells of both myeloid and lymphocytic lineages.

Manifestations

CLINICAL FINDINGS

Chronic myelogenous leukemia occurs primarily in middle-aged adults, occasionally in patients in their 20s and in elderly patients, and only very rarely in infants and children. Early disease is asymptomatic and often discovered accidentally. A patient with more advanced disease may seek medical attention because of an abdominal mass, which is an enlarged spleen, or because of weakness, fatigue, and weight loss.

The patient with early disease is afebrile and does not look ill. The only positive physical finding is a palpable spleen, which is found in virtually all patients by the time the peripheral blood count has risen to 50,000 per μL. As the disease progresses further, the patient may begin to lose weight because of hypermetabolism secondary to the increased production of granulocytes. The spleen grows bigger and the liver also enlarges. Peripheral lymph nodes do not enlarge.

The patient with far-advanced disease appears wasted. He or she often has an evening fever because of hypermetabolism. (However, high fever should also arouse suspicion of splenic infarction or a complicating infection.) The spleen is now very large. Ecchymoses and petechiae may be noted, and bone tenderness may be a troublesome complaint.

LABORATORY FINDINGS

1. *Peripheral blood count.*
   a. WBCs. The WBC count is high: in the 20,000 to 50,000 range in early disease, above 100,000 and even up to 400,000 per

μL in patients with advanced untreated disease. *Chronic granulocytic leukemia with a normal or low WBC count before treatment is so rare that it may be considered nonexistent.* Segmented neutrophils predominate on the blood smear, but frequent band forms and late metamyelocytes are also usually present, as are increased numbers of eosinophils and basophils. Scattered, more immature granulocytic elements—myelocytes, promyelocytes, and even an infrequent myeloblast—are also found. A modest increase in monocytes and in cells that have morphologic features resembling both monocytes and granulocytes may sometimes be noted.

  b. RBCs. Anemia secondary to failure of RBC production becomes progressively more severe as the disease advances. Reticulocyte counts may be in the normal range or depressed. Paradoxically, early in the disease or as a harbinger of relapse in a patient in remission, the hematocrit may rise briefly to levels slightly above normal. The RBCs are normochromic and normocytic. Occasional normoblasts may be noted, but frequent normoblasts in the peripheral blood arouse suspicion of myelofibrosis with myeloid metaplasia (see Table 16-3).

  c. Platelets. A mild to moderate thrombocytosis is a characteristic early manifestation of CML; however, late in the disease, most patients become thrombocytopenic because of a combination of:

    (1) Diminished megakaryocytic proliferation as granulocytic proliferation becomes more aggressive.

    (2) Suppressed megakaryopoiesis from chemotherapy.

    (3) Sequestration of platelets in a massively enlarged spleen.

2. *Bone marrow.* Histologic sections of aspirated particles or a marrow biopsy reveal a marked hypercellularity due to intense granulocytic hyperplasia (Fig. 16-3). As already mentioned, megakaryocytes are increased in number in early disease and usually reduced in number in patients with advanced, heavily treated disease. On the aspirate smear, granulocytic elements at different stages of development are seen in overwhelming numbers (Fig. 16-4). Segmented neutrophils, bands, and late metamyelocytes predominate, but myeloblasts, promyelocytes, and early myelocytes are also prominent. Cells of the eosinophilic series, basophils, and cells containing both eosinophilic and basophilic granules are frequently noted. Erythroid precursors are proportionately greatly reduced in number.

    Occasionally, one cannot aspirate marrow. Needle biopsy reveals an organized granulocytic proliferation along an underlying

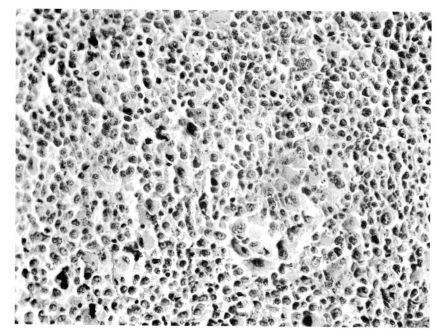

Fig. 16-3. Histologic section of a marrow particle in chronic myelogenous leukemia. Note intense hypercellularity caused by myeloid hyperplasia with loss of marrow fat.

network of reticulin fibers. In unusual patients with long-standing disease, the marrow is markedly fibrotic and resembles the marrow of myelofibrosis with myeloid metaplasia (see later).

3. *WBC alkaline phosphatase.* The cytoplasm of normal mature neutrophilic granulocytes contains alkaline phosphatase activity, which increases during infection or other stress. In contrast, the segmented neutrophil in CML contains little or no alkaline phosphatase activity. Therefore, an alkaline phosphatase stain can help to distinguish CML from other causes of marked leukocytosis.

4. *Cytogenetic studies.* When CML is suspected, marrow aspirate should be subjected to cytogenetic study. As already mentioned, a Ph[1] chromosome will be found in 95% of patients. Some patients will also have additional chromosomal abnormalities when first seen and, therefore, a greater likelihood of an aggressive course of the disease.

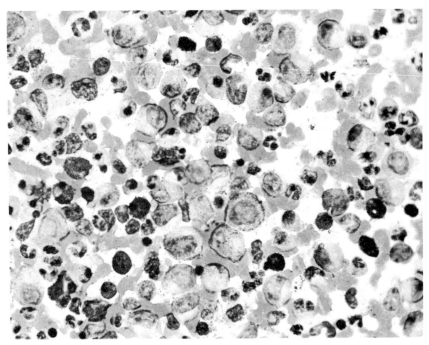

Fig. 16-4. Bone marrow smear in chronic myelogenous leukemia. Note not only the abundance of mature granulocytic forms, but also the increased numbers of early myeloid elements.

Differential Diagnosis

When a leukocytosis of segmented neutrophils in the 15,000 to 25,000 per μL range persists for several weeks in an otherwise clinically well person, one must consider the possibility of early chronic myelogenous leukemia. Finding a low WBC alkaline phosphatase activity heightens concern and signals the need for a cytogenetic study of a marrow aspirate to look for a Ph^1 chromosome.

A marked granulocytosis with a WBC count above 50,000 per μL may be found, not only in CML, but in occasional patients with:

1. A leukemoid reaction to an infection or malignancy.
2. Myelofibrosis with myeloid metaplasia.
3. Late polycythemia vera.

The differences between CML and a leukemoid reaction are summarized in Table 16-2. The differences between CML and mye-

Table 16-2. Differences Between Chronic Myelogenous Leukemia and a Leukemoid Reaction

PARAMETER	CHRONIC MYELOGENOUS LEUKEMIA	LEUKEMOID REACTION
Spleen	Palpable	Rarely palpable
Myeloblasts and promyelocytes	Present in significant numbers on blood smear	Rarely found on blood smear
Eosinophils and basophils	Increased on blood smear	Decreased on blood smear
RBC morphology	Occasional nucleated RBC sometimes seen	RBC abnormalities normally not seen
WBC alkaline phosphatase	Low	High

lofibrosis with myeloid metaplasia are listed in Table 16-3. The distinction between CML and late polycythemia vera has been discussed in Chapter 13.

Course, Complications, and Treatment

Chronic myelogenous leukemia steadily worsens in the untreated patient; therefore, unless the disease is discovered very early, the patient is treated as soon as the diagnosis is made. Either busulfan (Myleran), an oral alkylating agent, or hydroxyurea, an antimetabolite inhibiting ribonucleotide reductase activity, can be given. With few exceptions, patients initially respond to either drug with a return of a sense of well-being, shrinkage of the spleen, correction of anemia, and a fall of the WBC count to a normal or near normal level. Busulfan is easier to use because, once these initial effects have been obtained, the drug may be discontinued or given in a minimal maintenance dose, and the patient may remain in remission without disease progression for many months. In contrast, hydroxyurea, being an enzyme inhibitor, requires continuous full-dosage, suppressive therapy and frequent patient visits to monitor drug effect. Nevertheless, some physicians prefer to use hydroxyurea because of concern that DNA damage induced by an alkylating agent could hasten the additional mutations of the CML clone that increase its aggressiveness. Moreover, busulfan given for many months may produce serious side effects—diffuse pulmonary fibrosis and a peculiar syndrome of hyperpigmentation, weakness, weight loss, and gastrointestinal symptoms.

Despite initial ready control of disease with these agents, treatment has not lengthened survival substantially. In 1924, untreated chronic myelogenous leukemia had a median survival time of 31 months. In a recent report of over 600 patients with CML under the age of 45 years, the actuarial death rate was 5% for the first year after diagnosis, 12% for the second year, and 22.5% for each year thereafter. This reflects the inability of present agents to prevent the further intraclonal mutations that convert CML into a disease refractory to treatment.

In unusual patients, CML suddenly transforms into acute leukemia. A patient under apparent good control appears at the next visit with many blasts on the peripheral blood smear and a marrow fully occupied by blasts and other early forms. If the acute leukemia is acute myeloblastic leukemia or another of the acute non-lymphocytic types, it rarely responds to standard induction chemotherapy for these leukemias with cytarabine and daunorubicin. If the acute leukemia is acute lymphoblastic leukemia, a brief remission is often obtained with vincristine and prednisone.

In the usual patient, the disease worsens more gradually as subclones of cells increasingly resistant to chemotherapy emerge. Busulfan or hydroxyurea may still depress the total WBC count—only now immature WBCs persist on the blood smear, the enlarged spleen fails to shrink, anemia and thrombocytopenia worsen, and repeated transfusions become necessary. Splenic infarcts may occur and pro-

Table 16-3. Differences Between Myelofibrosis and Chronic Myelogenous Leukemia

PARAMETER	MYELOFIBROSIS	CHRONIC MYELOGENOUS LEUKEMIA
Relation of spleen size to WBC count	Massive splenomegaly out of proportion to WBC count, which rarely exceeds 50,000 per μL	When spleen is massively enlarged, WBC count usually exceeds 100,000 per μL
Peripheral blood smear	Many nucleated RBCs	Nucleated RBCs present but not numerous
Bone marrow	Fibrosis and megakaryocytic hyperplasia	Hypercellular with marked myeloid hyperplasia; megakaryocytes sometimes but not always prominent
WBC alkaline phosphatase	May be elevated or low	Low
Chromosome studies	Ph[1] chromosome absent	Ph[1] chromosome present in about 95% of cases

duce fever, pain in the left upper abdomen that may radiate to the left shoulder, and a friction rub over the spleen. The patient grows weaker and more wasted because of the combination of anemia and hypermetabolism. After reaching this stage, the patient usually succumbs within weeks to some complication of the disease, usually infection or bleeding.

Because most patients with CML treated as described above will die within 3 to 5 years of diagnosis, better approaches to therapy are needed. Recently, alfa interferon has been reported to induce remissions different from those obtained with busulfan or hydroxyurea in that normal cells without the Ph^1 abnormality reappear in the bone marrow. Whether this hopeful observation means that therapy with alfa interferon can prolong survival in CML is not yet known.

In many centers, high-dose chemoradiotherapy, followed by marrow transplantation, is now recommended for the patient under 40 years of age who has an HLA compatible sibling marrow donor. The high-dose chemoradiotherapy offers the possibility of eradicating the leukemic clone and actual cure. Transplantation as soon as a patient has been brought into initial remission with standard therapy provides the best chance of eradicating the leukemic clone. However, 30% of patients die of some complication within the first few months of marrow transplantation, so early marrow transplantation could shorten survival. As yet, criteria are not clear for deciding when to proceed with marrow transplantation in a young patient whose disease is under good control with standard chemotherapy.

CHRONIC MYELOMONOCYTIC LEUKEMIA

Chronic myelomonocytic leukemia is a disease of insidious onset of older persons. In some patients, it is discovered during examination for unrelated disease. Other patients seek attention because of bruising or symptoms of anemia.

Manifestations

Physical findings may be limited to pallor and, in about one half of patients, an enlarged spleen. *Laboratory examination* reveals the following:

1. *Peripheral blood count.*
   a. A moderate anemia (for example, Hgb of 10 g per dL) with disturbed RBC morphology that includes a population of ma-

crocytic RBCs and often cells with coarse basophilic stippling. In some patients, rare nucleated RBC may be found on the blood smear.

b. A WBC count that is usually elevated but, in some patients, may be normal or depressed. A monocytosis is characteristically present. Abnormal monocytic forms with a horseshoe-shaped nucleus or with convolution or attempted lobulation of the nucleus are often although not invariably seen (Fig. 16-5). Scattered, more immature-appearing monocytic forms, with a round nucleus and finer chromatin, may also be noted. Segmented neutrophils are often increased in number and may have abnormal features, such as hypersegmentation or absence of neutrophilic granules. Varying numbers of metamyelocytes, myelocytes, and cells with morphologic features in-

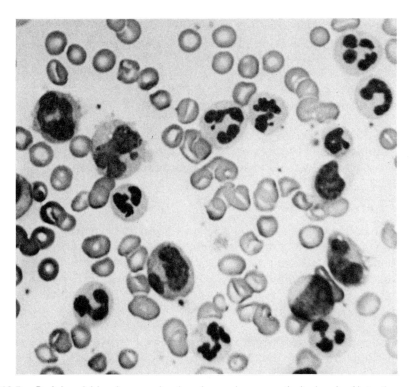

Fig. 16-5. Peripheral blood smear in chronic myelomonocytic leukemia. Note the mixture of segmented neutrophils and dysplastic monocytes with a horseshoe-shaped, convoluted, or even lobulated nucleus. A single early form with a prominent nucleolus is also present.

termediate between myelocytes and monocytes are noted. An occasional blast may also be seen but, by definition, blasts make up less than 5% of circulating WBC.

    c. Moderately reduced numbers of platelets, which usually look normal but in occasional patients are large and deficient in granules.

3. A *bone marrow* that is usually strikingly hypercellular, exceeding the degree expected from the peripheral blood count, and characterized by:

    a. Greater numbers of early forms than the appearance of the peripheral blood WBC would lead one to suspect. By definition, however, blasts make up less than 30% of nucleated marrow cells.

    b. Increased cells of both granulocytic and monocytic lineage, but the former usually predominate. Cells are also seen that appear intermediate between granulocytic and monocytic forms. Cytochemical stains for esterase activity often show a greater degree of monocytic proliferation than is apparent with routine stains.

    c. Depressed erythropoiesis with dysplastic nucleated RBCs which may have some features resembling megaloblasts.

    d. Normal numbers of megakaryocytes without dysplastic morphology.

4. *Abnormal blood chemistries* that include an increased serum lysozyme level in all patients and hyperuricemia and an unexpected polyclonal hypergammaglobulinemia in some patients.

Course and Treatment

The disease may be indolent or slowly progressive over many months to several years. (For this reason, as discussed in Chapter 11, some hematologists have considered chronic myelomonocytic leukemia a myelodysplastic, rather than a frankly malignant, disorder.) Anemia often gradually worsens to a degree that requires treatment with transfusions. Platelet counts usually remain adequate to prevent serious bleeding. Despite seemingly adequate numbers of circulating neutrophils, susceptibility to infection is increased, and a number of patients die from infection while the disease is still in its chronic phase. Aggressive chemotherapy should be avoided; the risk of death from infection during the resultant pancytopenia exceeds the likelihood of obtaining a long-lasting remission.

    If patients survive long enough, the disease will eventually transform into subacute or acute myelomonocytic leukemia. The WBC count and number of blasts in the peripheral blood then rise progressively, and blasts and other early forms crowd out the other marrow elements. Temporary remissions have been reported in a few patients at this stage following administration of vincristine and prednisone or of low doses of cytarabine.

MYELOFIBROSIS WITH MYELOID METAPLASIA

In this disorder, fibrosis occurs in the bone marrow and myeloid metaplasia (proliferation of granulocytic elements, normoblasts, and megakaryocytes) occurs in the spleen, liver, and, to a lesser extent, lymph nodes. It is characterized by the following triad:

1. Splenomegaly, which is frequently massive.
2. Leukoerythroblastic peripheral blood (described below).
3. Fibrotic bone marrow containing clusters of megakaryocytes.

Studies using G6PD as a marker have established that the disorder arises in a hematopoietic stem cell. Its monoclonal daughter cells and their progeny:

1. Take over what persists of hematopoiesis in a bone marrow that becomes increasingly fibrotic.
2. Colonize extramedullary sites, with resultant extensive proliferation of hematopoietic cells within the sinusoids of the red pulp of the spleen and of the liver.

Proliferation of megakaryocytes both within the marrow and in extramedullary sites is a characteristic feature of the disorder.

G6PD marker studies have also established that the marrow fibrosis stems from activation and proliferation of polyclonal fibroblasts. Thus, the fibrosis is secondary—a probable consequence of the release of PGDF (platelet derived growth factor) from proliferating megakaryocytes. Osteoclasts are also stimulated in many patients to lay down new bone in the marrow cavity with resultant osteosclerosis.

Manifestations

CLINICAL FINDINGS

The patient is almost always over 40 and is usually over 50 years of age. Most patients with early disease are asymptomatic; the disease is discovered during an examination for an unrelated complaint. The patient with more advanced disease may complain of fatigue, weight loss, and night sweats, of pressure symptoms stemming from a large spleen, of abnormal bruising or bleeding, or, less commonly, of bone pain.

The usual patient is afebrile, but occasional patients develop fever late in the disease. Wasting of muscles may also be noted in a patient with advanced disease. Splenomegaly is the striking finding; sometimes the spleen fills the left side of the abdomen. Some degree of hepatomegaly is also found. Ascites may be a late finding. Lymphadenopathy is rare.

LABORATORY FINDINGS

1. *Peripheral blood.* With rare exceptions, the patient is anemic, and frequently severely anemic. The reticulocyte count may be depressed (for example, less than 0.5%) but often is slightly elevated (for example, 4%, uncorrected) because of the escape of many immature RBCs into the peripheral blood. The WBC count may vary from leukopenic levels to counts of over 50,000 per μL. The platelet count may be low, normal, or elevated. Distinctive morphologic findings are seen on the peripheral blood smear:
   a. *Oval and teardrop shaped RBCs* (Fig. 16-6); "shift cells," that is, RBCs that stain more blue than red; and nucleated RBCs. (The nucleated RBCs are a reflection of intrasinusoidal hematopoiesis in the liver and spleen, which allows nucleated RBCs to be swept away easily into the circulating blood.)
   b. *Immature WBCs,* extending back as far as the blast stage. Eosinophils and basophils are often increased.
   c. *Large, bizarre platelets.* Occasionally a single-lobed megakaryocyte nucleus surrounded by platelets may be discovered in the feather edge of the smear.
   The term "leukoerythroblastic reaction" is used for this combination of immature RBCs, immature WBCs, and abnormal platelets on a peripheral blood smear.
2. *Bone marrow.* Attempts to aspirate marrow fail or yield only scanty, nondiagnostic material. Needle biopsy yields a core of marrow (Fig. 16-7) with the following characteristics:
   a. Fibrosis, with increased fibrillar reticulin (Fig. 16-8), collagen, and fibroblasts.
   b. Clusters of megakaryocytes (Fig. 16-9), with many atypical megakaryocytes.
   Dilated bone marrow sinusoids are also usually noted. Scattered residual islands of cellular marrow may be found.

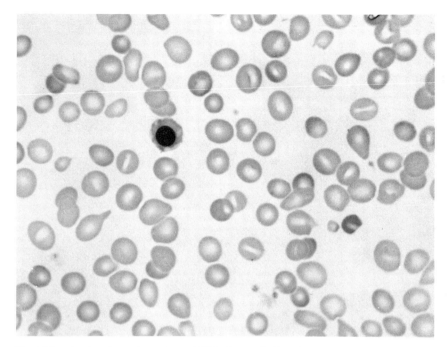

Fig. 16-6. Oval and teardrop-shaped RBCs in myelofibrosis with myeloid metaplasia. Note also the circulating normoblast.

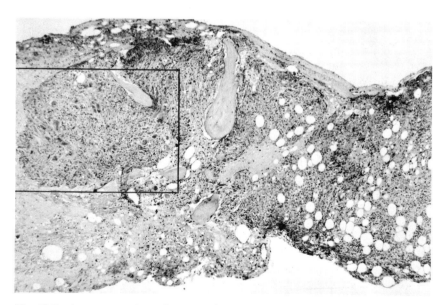

Fig. 16-7. Low-power view of a core of marrow obtained by needle biopsy from a patient with myelofibrosis with myeloid metaplasia. Extensive fibrosis and clusters of megakaryocytes are recognizable even at this magnification.

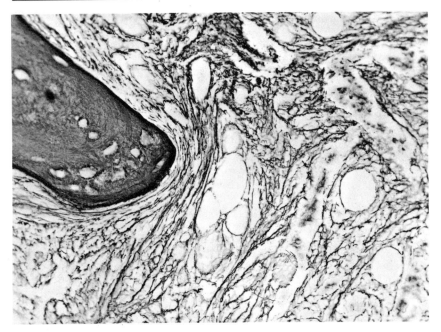

Fig. 16-8. Silver stain of a bone marrow biopsy specimen to demonstrate the marked increase in reticulin fibers found in the marrow in myelofibrosis with myeloid metaplasia.

3. *Other findings.*
   a. The serum uric acid is usually elevated.
   b. The WBC alkaline phosphatase test results vary. In some patients, the WBCs are strongly positive and resemble the WBCs of polycythemia vera; in other patients, the WBCs are negative and resemble the WBCs of chronic myelogenous leukemia.
   c. An increased density of the bones on bone films and an elevated serum alkaline phosphatase in the patient with osteosclerosis.

Disorders Confused with Myelofibrosis

CIRRHOSIS

A patient with early myelofibrosis who presents with moderate splenomegaly, anemia, and leukopenia may superficially resemble a patient with cirrhosis, congestive splenomegaly, and hypersplenism.

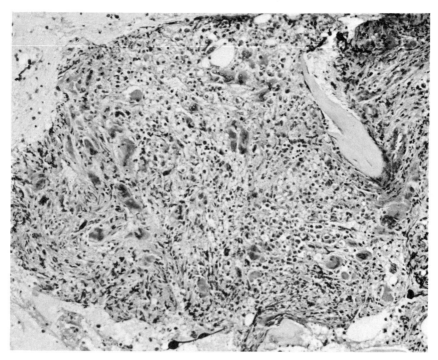

Fig. 16-9. High-power view of that portion of the biopsy specimen shown in the inset of Figure 16-7. Note increased numbers and atypical appearance of the megakaryocytes in myelofibrosis with myeloid metaplasia.

The teardrop-shaped RBCs and immature cells of myelofibrosis on the blood smear point the way to the correct diagnosis.

METASTATIC CARCINOMA IN BONE MARROW

Metastatic carcinoma to marrow may induce a reaction mimicking myelofibrosis, with a leukoerythroblastic peripheral blood and marked fibrosis of a marrow biopsy. The discovery of nests of tumor cells on the biopsy section establishes the diagnosis.

HAIRY CELL LEUKEMIA

In this disorder (see Chapter 17), a patient often presents with pancytopenia and massive splenomegaly. One may be unable to aspirate marrow because of increased marrow reticulin. Before marrow biopsy with a Jamshidi needle became standard practice, this combination of findings could be confused with myelofibrosis. Marrow biopsy, however, should reveal the distinctive histologic appearance of hairy cells growing in the marrow (see Fig. 17-9).

POLYCYTHEMIA VERA

The findings in a patient with late stage polycythemia (see Chapter 13)—anemia, spenomegaly, leukocytosis, increased marrow megakaryocytes, and marrow fibrosis—may resemble closely the findings of myelofibrosis.

CHRONIC MYELOGENOUS LEUKEMIA

The differences listed in Table 16-3 usually allow one to distinguish readily between myelofibrosis with myeloid metaplasia and chronic myelogenous leukemia. However, late in the course of chronic myelogenous leukemia, after a patient has received large amounts of busulfan and no longer responds to the drug, the marrow may be fibrotic, the anemia severe, the WBC count not greatly elevated, and the spleen massively enlarged. Then the findings of the two diseases may closely resemble each other.

Course and Complications

In a recent review of 56 patients, median survival was 5 years from the date of the first bone marrow biopsy demonstrating the fibrosis and 8 years from the date of the first symptoms or other signs attributable to the disease. The range of survival was very wide—from a few months to over 30 years. Prognosis for an individual patient was unpredictable. When patients developed unexplained fever, body wasting, severe thrombocytopenia, or severe anemia, they usually succumbed to the disease within the next 24 months.

Major complications of the disease are:

1. *Anemia,* which may become so severe that the patient can survive only with repeated transfusions. Although the anemia stems primarily from failure of production of RBCs, in some patients splenic sequestration of RBCs contributes significantly to its severity.

2. *Abnormal bleeding.* Some patients are thrombocytopenic, but even patients who are not thrombocytopenic may bleed abnormally because of qualitative defects of platelet function. If surgery must be done (for example, a prostatectomy to relieve uri-

nary retention), platelet concentrates should be given to control postoperative bleeding.

3. *Inanition and intercurrent infection.* The massive splenomegaly and, sometimes, massive hepatomegaly interfere with the patient's ability to eat. This, plus the hypermetabolism that accompanies extensive myeloid metaplasia, leads to muscle wasting and a decreased resistance to infection.

4. *Portal hypertension.* Myeloid metaplasia in the sinusoids of the liver may interfere with flow from the portal to the hepatic venous system, with resultant portal hypertension. This may lead to ascites and even bleeding from esophageal varices.

5. *Acute leukemia.* Although not itself considered a hematologic malignancy, myelofibrosis transforms into acute non-lymphocytic leukemia in 5% to 10% of patients.

Treatment

Large doses of androgens have been given to patients in an attempt to increase effective erythropoiesis but are of questionable value and may cause further splenic enlargement and fluid retention. Myelosuppressive agents in small doses or small doses of radiation are sometimes used to shrink temporarily a massively enlarged spleen. Such measures must be used cautiously to avoid making anemia or thrombocytopenia worse. Allopurinol is usually given to reduce serum uric acid levels as prophylaxis against attacks of secondary gout.

Splenectomy should be considered for the patient with:

1. Persistent pain from massive splenomegaly.
2. Severe thrombocytopenia.
3. Anemia so severe that transfusions are required every 2 to 4 weeks.

The operation is associated with a substantial risk for postoperative bleeding or infection. After splenectomy, the liver may enlarge rapidly in about 10% of patients.

ESSENTIAL THROMBOCYTHEMIA

This disorder, also known as primary thrombocythemia, is characterized by:

1. A persistently elevated platelet count in the 1,000,000 per μL or higher range.

2. Bone marrow findings of:
   a. Megakaryocytic hyperplasia.
   b. Absence of a Ph^1 chromosome.
   c. Absence of marrow fibrosis.
   d. Normal iron stores.
3. No evidence of an increased erythroid mass.

The disease is seen primarily in older adults, but occasionally appears in a young individual, usually a woman. Mild splenomegaly is found in some patients but less frequently than in other myeloproliferative disorders with thrombocytosis (for example, myelofibrosis, polycythemia vera). In an unusual patient, the spleen may atrophy after a splenic vein thrombosis. Mild granulocytic proliferation, with WBC counts in the 10,000 to 15,000 per μL range, is usually present.

All patients are thought to have an increased risk of excessive bleeding from mucous membranes, particularly bleeding from the gastrointestinal tract. Older patients also have a high incidence of neurologic manifestations attributable to cerebrovascular vasomotor or thromboembolic events—headache and paresthesias, transient ischemic episodes, and even strokes. Platelet emboli in small peripheral vessels may give rise to a syndrome of burning of the fingers or toes that small doses of aspirin dramatically relieves. In older patients, chemotherapy with hydroxyurea or small doses of busulfan is frequently used to reduce the platelet count. Asymptomatic younger individuals have been watched for long periods without giving drugs to reduce the platelet count. Splenectomy should never be performed in a patient with essential thrombocythemia, for it results in extreme thrombocytosis and a high risk for death from thrombosis.

MYELOID METAPLASIA WITHOUT MYELOFIBROSIS

This rare disorder, which clearly differs from chronic myelogenous leukemia, is characterized by:

1. A modestly increased proliferation of granulocytes with a strongly positive alkaline phosphatase test.
2. Splenomegaly.
3. Mild megakaryocytic proliferation and thrombocytosis.
4. Absence of marrow fibrosis.
5. Absence of a Ph^1 chromosome.

It differs from polycythemia vera in the absence of an elevated erythroid mass and from essential thrombocythemia in the lesser degree of megakaryocytic hyperplasia.

SELECTED READING

Acute Non-Lymphocytic Leukemia

1. Bennett JM, Catovsky D, Daniel MT, Flandrin G, Galton DAG, Gralnick HR, and Sultan C: Proposed revised criteria for the classificaton of acute myeloid leukemia. A report of the French-American-British Cooperative Group. Ann Intern Med 103:626, 1985.
2. Champlin RE, Ho WG, Gale RP, Winston D, Selch M, Mitsuyasu R, Lenarky C, Elashoff R, Zighelboim J, and Feig SA: Treatment of acute myelogenous leukemia. A prospective controlled trial of bone marrow transplantation versus consolidation chemotherapy. Ann Intern Med 102:285, 1985.
3. Drabkin HA: The molecular biology of chromosome alterations in myelogenous leukemia. West J Med 143:825, 1985.
4. Huang M-J, Li C-Y, Nichols WL, Young J-H, and Katzmann JA: Acute leukemia with megakaryocytic differentiation: a study of 12 cases identified immunocytochemically. Blood 64:427, 1984.

Chronic Myelogenous Leukemia

1. Gale RP: The molecular biology of chronic myelogenous leukemia. Br. J. Haematol 60:395, 1985.
2. Sokal JE, Baccarani M, Tura S, Fiacchini M, Cervantes F, Rozman C, Gomez GA, Galton DAG, Canellos GP, Braun TJ, Clarkson BD, Carbonell F, Heimpel H, Extra JM, Fiere D, Nissen NI, Robertson JE, and Cox EB: Prognostic discrimination among younger patients with chronic granulocytic leukemia: relevance to bone marrow transplantation. Blood 66:1352, 1985.

Chronic Myelomonocytic Leukemia

1. Solal-Celigny P, Desaint B, Herrera A, Chastang C, Amar M, Vroclans M, Brousse N, Mancilla F, Renoux M, Bernard J-F, and Boivin P: Chronic myelomonocytic leukemia according to FAB classification: analysis of 35 cases. Blood 63:634, 1984.

Myelofibrosis with Extramedullary Myeloid Metaplasia

1. Silverstein MN, and ReMine WH: Splenectomy in myeloid metaplasia. Blood 53:515, 1979.
2. Varki A, Lottenberg R, Griffith R, and Reinhard E: The syndrome of idiopathic myelofibrosis. A clinicopathologic review with emphasis on the prognostic variables predicting survival. Medicine 62:353, 1983.

Essential Thrombocythemia

1. Hoagland HC, and Silverstein MN: Primary thrombocythemia in the young patient. Mayo Clin Proc 53:578, 1978.
2. Jabaily J, Iland HJ, Laszlo J, Massey EW, Faguet GB, Briere J, Landaw SA, and Pisciotta AV: Neurologic manifestations of essential thrombocythemia. Ann Intern Med 99:518, 1983.

17

The Lymphocytic Leukemias

The lymphocytic leukemias consist of the acute lymphoblastic leukemias and the leukemias of differentiated lymphocytes (Table 17-1). With a rare exception (described later), the former are malignant proliferations of cells that are at early stages of processing into B or T cells. The latter are malignant proliferations of cells with properties of differentiated B or T cells in either a quiescent or activated state (see Chapter 14). The acute lymphoblastic leukemias are usually childhood illnesses, whereas the leukemias of differentiated lymphocytes rarely become evident before middle or late adult life.

As first discussed in Chapter 15, immune marker analysis has been crucial in relating the lymphocytic leukemias, not only to T or B cell lineage, but to stages of differentiation or activation of lymphocytes. A partial list of antibodies used for this purpose is given in Table 17-2.

ACUTE LYMPHOBLASTIC LEUKEMIA

Childhood Disease

Acute lymphocytic leukemia is the most frequent malignancy of childhood. In the United States, it occurs much more frequently in white children than in black children. Its incidence peaks between 3 to 5 years of age, but it is not unusual to find the disease in infants under the age of 1 year and in older children and adolescents.

Table 17-1. The Lymphocytic Leukemias

I. Acute lymphoblastic leukemias
  a. B cell lineage
    1. Leukemias of cells with increasing evidence of B cell processing (see Fig. 17-2)
        (a) Early B cell-committed leukemia
        (b) Common acute lymphoblastic leukemia (common ALL)
        (c) Pre-B cell leukemia
    2. Unusual other B cell lineage acute leukemias
        (a) Transformed B cell (Burkitt cell) leukemia
        (b) Lymphoblastic crisis of chronic myelogenous leukemia*
  b. Acute T-lymphoblastic leukemia. (Immune marker profiles may correspond to those found in early or later stages of thymic T cell processing; see Table 17-2.)
II. Leukemias of differentiated lymphocytes
  a. B cell leukemias
    1. Chronic lymphocytic leukemia. (The cell has properties of a dormant, differentiated B cell.)
    2. Less common leukemias of lymphocytes with properties of different stages of activation or transformation of normal B cells.
        (a) Leukemic phase of small, cleaved cell lymphoma (lymphosarcoma cell leukemia)
        (b) Prolymphocytic leukemia*
        (c) Hairy cell leukemia*
        (d) Plasmacytoid lymphocytic leukemia
  b. T cell leukemias
    1. Adult T cell leukemia (associated with HTLV-I infection).
    2. Cutaneous T cell lymphoma with circulating T lymphocytes (Sézary syndrome).
    3. Tγ cell lymphocytosis/leukemia

* In rare patients, the leukemia may be of T cell lineage.

In this disorder, an immature lymphocyte overgrows the bone marrow (see Figs. 15-1 and 17-1). This is a cell committed to B cell ontogeny (Fig. 17-2) in about 85% of children and to T cell ontogeny in about 15% of children. In about 1% of children, the cell has the phenotypic properties of the transformed blast-like cell (Burkitt cell) that develops after differentiated B cells are incubated with an activating agent in vitro.

MANIFESTATIONS

Clinical Findings. The child may be first seen because of nonspecific complaints such as malaise, loss of appetite, and low-grade fever or because of complaints arising from bone marrow failure, for example,

Table 17-2. Antibodies Commonly Used in Immune Marker Studies*

I. T cell markers
  A. For antigens appearing early in thymic T cell processing

CD2(T11)	Marks for the sheep cell receptor now known to function physiologically as an antigen-independent receptor needed for initiating activation and division of cells during early thymic processing.
CD1(T6)	Marks for a surface molecule appearing a little later during thymic processing as gene rearrangements for T cell antigen receptor chains begin. Not present on mature T cells.

  B. For components of the T cell antigen receptor complex

CD3 (T3)	Marks for a component of the T cell antigen receptor formed later in thymic processing and present on all mature T cells.
CD4 (T4)	Marks for a component on the T cell antigen receptor allowing T cells to recognize Class II MHC determinants. Usually found on T helper cells.
CD8 (T8)	Marks for a component on the T cell antigen receptor allowing T cells to recognize Class I MHC determinants. Found on cytotoxic T cells.

  C. Other useful antibodies

CD5 (T1, T101)	Marks for a surface molecule present on both immature and mature T cells and also on the B cells of chronic lymphocytic leukemia.
Tac	Marks for the Il-2 receptor and thus for activated T cells (Also reacts with the abnormal B cells of hairy cell leukemia).
HNK-1	Marks for a surface molecule present on T-related cells with natural killer cell function.

II. B Cell Markers
  A. For identifying cells in different stages of B cell differentiation

CD10 (CALLA)	Recognizes a surface antigen found on the common form of acute lymphocytic leukemia.
CD24 (BA-1)	Recognizes a second surface antigen found on the common form of acute lymphocytic leukemia.
CD19 (B4)	Recognizes an antigen found on both early and differentiated B cells.
CD20 (B1)	Recognizes a second antigen found on both early and differentiated B cells.

(continued)

Table 17-2. Antibodies Commonly Used in Immune Marker Studies*
(continued)

B. For identifying the presence of immunoglobulin in or on B cells

Anti-SIg	An antibody recognizing polyclonal surface immunoglobulin and so staining all cells of a B cell suspension, regardless of chain type of a surface immunoglobulin.
Anti-k chain	An antibody recognizing only kappa immunoglobulin light chains and therefore useful in recognizing a monoclonal proliferation.
Anti-λ chain	An antibody recognizing only lambda immunoglobulin light chains and therefore useful in recognizing a monoclonal proliferation.
Anti-μ chain	An antibody recognizing the heavy chain of IgM. Useful in recognizing beginning immunoglobulin formation in the cytoplasm of differentiating B cells.
III. Anti-TdT.	A marker for a nuclear enzyme found in cells at an early stage of processing into either T or B cells. (Distinguishes these immature cells, which are TdT positive, from immature-appearing cells that represent transformed, differentiated B or T cells, for example, the transformed cell of Burkitt cell leukemia, which is TdT negative.)

*CD nomenclature is used with older names given in parenthesis.

pallor and lethargy stemming from anemia or abnormal bruising caused by thrombocytopenia. Occasionally, fever and bone and joint pain mimic the findings of juvenile rheumatoid arthritis.

Pallor, purpura, and petechiae may or may not be prominent on the initial examination. Peripheral lymphadenopathy and splenomegaly are often but not always found. In most children, results of the initial neurologic examination are normal.

Laboratory Findings

1. *Peripheral blood count.* Normochromic, normocytic anemia and a thrombocytopenia are usually discovered on the initial blood count and are often severe. The WBC count may be low, normal, or high. When low, the peripheral blood findings resemble those of marrow hypoplasia. When high, the differential count will re-

veal a preponderance of immature-appearing lymphocytes. The morphologic features of these cells may vary and a FAB group has described three cytologic types:

a. L1 (most common type). The cell is small with regular homogenous chromatin, inconspicuous nucleoli, and very scanty cytoplasm. Often the nucleus appears to occupy the entire cell, and only a thin rim of cytoplasm can be seen in a limited portion of the cell.

b. L2. The cell is larger. The nucleus may be irregular and its chromatin is clumped. Nucleoli are prominent and cytoplasm is moderately abundant.

c. L3 (rare). The cell is large. Nuclear chromatin is fine and homogenous. Nucleoli are prominent. The cytoplasm is abundant, deeply basophilic, and frequently contains multiple vacuoles. This morphology is diagnostic of the transformed B cell (Burkitt cell) variant.

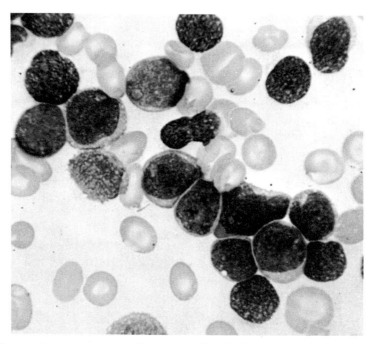

Fig. 17-1. Smear of a bone marrow aspirate in acute lymphoblastic leukemia. Contrast the dispersed appearance of the nuclear chromatin in these minimally differentiated cells with the condensed "smuggy" look of the chromatin in the small, mature lymphocytes of chronic lymphocytic leukemia as shown in Figure 17-3.

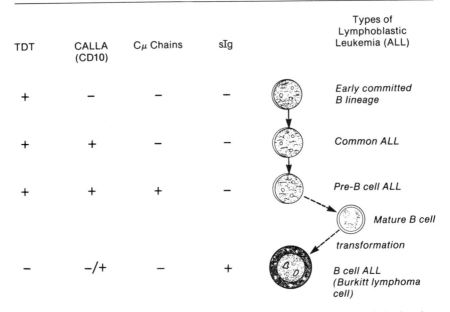

TDT	CALLA (CD10)	Cμ Chains	sIg		Types of Lymphoblastic Leukemia (ALL)
+	–	–	–		*Early committed B lineage*
+	+	–	–		*Common ALL*
+	+	+	–		*Pre-B cell ALL*
					Mature B cell
					transformation
–	–/+	–	+		*B cell ALL (Burkitt lymphoma cell)*

Fig. 17-2. The immune marker phenotypes of acute B cell lymphoblastic leukemias of cells at different stages of B cell evolution. Heading abbreviations: TDT, terminal deoxynucleotidyl transferase; Cμ chains, cytoplasmic μ chains; sIg, surface immunoglobulin.

2. *Chest radiography.* This film is taken to look for a mediastinal mass, which will be found in some of the patients with acute T-lymphoblastic leukemia.

3. *Bone marrow.* In most patients, normal bone marrow elements will be essentially totally replaced by sheets of lymphoblasts (see Fig. 15-1). In an unusual patient, the initial marrow may be hypoplastic, but many of the cells that are present will be identified as lymphoblasts.

4. *Spinal fluid examination.* This is done to rule out meningeal involvement at the time of diagnosis, which alters the type of central nervous system treatment given. (If the patient is severely thrombocytopenic, platelet concentrates are given before doing the spinal tap.)

DIAGNOSIS

Problems in diagnosis arise when:

1. The patient presents with pancytopenia, the marrow is hypoplastic, and the possibility of aplastic anemia must be considered.

2. The type of acute leukemia—lymphocytic or non-lymphocytic—
   is difficult to determine from the morphologic appearance of
   the cells. This is less of a problem now that immune marker
   techniques are available. Lymphoblasts (with the exception of
   the rare L3 cell) will contain the nuclear enzyme terminal
   deoxynucleotidyl transferase (TdT), whereas blasts of the non-
   lymphocytic leukemias will not. (This enzyme, which can add
   deoxynucleoside triphosphates onto the single-strand, free end
   of DNA in the absence of a template, is thought to be involved
   in the gene rearrangements that take place during beginning B
   and T cell differentiation.) Moreover, surface membrane antigens on lymphoblasts will usually react with B or T lineage-
   specific monoclonal antibodies, whereas surface membrane
   antigens on the blasts of acute non-lymphocytic leukemias
   will usually react with granulocytic- or monocytic-specific
   monoclonal antibodies. Nevertheless, diagnostic problems
   occasionally persist, as when leukemic blasts mark with both
   lymphocytic and myeloid cell markers (so-called lineage
   infidelity).

Making a complete diagnosis of acute lymphoblastic leukemia
requires determining its subtype. T cell lymphoblastic leukemia is
more aggressive and requires more intensive treatment than does the
common form of B cell lymphoblastic leukemia. Measuring TdT does
not distinguish T cell from B cell disease, since this enzyme is present
in the early cells of both lineages. Monoclonal antibodies reacting
with surface antigens specific for early B or T cells (Table 17-2) are
used to identify cell lineage.

It also appears important to establish into which subgroup of B-
related disease, an acute leukemia falls (see Fig. 17-2). Both the
leukemia of very early B-committed lymphocytes (which do not yet
possess a surface membrane antigen reacting with an antibody called
CD 10 or CALLA) and the so-called pre-B cell leukemia (which reacts
with this antibody but has progressed in differentiation far enough to
have heavy chains of IgM in its cytoplasm that react with an anti-μ
chain antibody) have a higher relapse rate with current therapy than
a more frequent, in-between group. This in-between group, referred
to as common acute lymphocytic leukemia, reacts with the CD 10
(CALLA) antibody but does not yet have cytoplasmic μ chains. The
rare transformed B cell lymphoblastic leukemia, which is readily
recognizable by its distinctive L3 morphology, the absence of TdT,
and the presence of surface membrane IgM, has the highest relapse
rate of all of the acute lymphoblastic leukemias.

FACTORS INFLUENCING PROGNOSIS

Chemotherapy induces a remission in almost all children; unfortunately, many will relapse despite continuing chemotherapy for a prolonged period. Factors affecting the risk for relapse include:

1. *Cell type.* As already mentioned CD 10 (CALLA) positive, μ chain negative, early B cell leukemia has the best prognosis for cure. T cell and pre-B cell leukemias have a somewhat poorer prognosis, and the rare transformed B cell variant has the poorest prognosis of all. Patients with L2 morphology have also been reported to have a higher risk of relapse than patients with L1 morphology.
2. *Age and sex.* Infants under the age of 1.5 years and children over the age of 10 years have a higher frequency of relapse than do children in whom the disease begins between the ages of 1.5 and 10 years. This partly reflects a higher prevalence of very early B lineage leukemia in infants and of T-lymphoblastic leukemia in older children. For an unknown reason, girls have a better prognosis for disease-free survival than boys.
3. *Extent and distribution of disease at the time of diagnosis.* Children with extensive disease, as evidenced by massively enlarged lymph nodes, prominent hepatosplenomegaly, WBC counts above 50,000 per μL, or evidence of central nervous system (CNS) involvement have a high risk for relapse. So do children who have a mediastinal mass, because this means that they have T cell disease.

COURSE AND TREATMENT

The use of only two drugs, vincristine and prednisone, will induce a remission in almost all children. The marrow will then appear normal, but many leukemic cells still remain. Consolidation therapy is therefore given with L-asparaginase plus other agents used in different treatment protocols. Since chemotherapeutic agents fail to cross the blood-brain barrier, a course of intrathecal chemotherapy with methotrexate is also begun shortly after the patient enters remission. If such prophylactic CNS therapy is not given, 75% of children will relapse with CNS involvement within 2 years, despite a negative initial spinal fluid examination. Maintenance therapy, for example, continuous methotrexate and 6-mercaptopurine plus intermittent bolus therapy with vincristine and prednisone, is then continued for 3 years. With such management, about 50% of children may be expected to survive without further evidence of disease after the drugs are stopped.

Despite CNS prophylaxis, relapse often occurs first in the CNS with manifestations such as ocular disturbances (diplopia, strabismus, blindness), cranial or peripheral nerve palsies, or symptoms of increased intracranial pressure. The spinal fluid examination will frequently show an increased pressure, presence of lymphoblasts in the spinal fluid, decreased sugar, and normal protein. Rarely, the spinal fluid may be normal despite clear clinical evidence of CNS involvement.

In boys, relapse may first appear as a painless enlargement of the testis due to leukemic infiltration. A bone marrow relapse usually quickly follows. Patients with relapse can often be brought into a second remission, but their chances for prolonged survival are markedly diminished.

Because T cell lymphoblastic leukemia and transformed B cell leukemia are more aggressive disorders, they are treated more intensively. Daunorubicin is added during the induction phase, and both daunorubicin and cytosine arabinoside are frequently added to the other drugs mentioned earlier for maintenance. Children with T cell disease are given prophylactic CNS therapy with cranial radiation as well as intrathecal methotrexate despite a risk for late impaired mental performance after cranial radiation.

Acute Lymphoblastic Leukemia in Adults

About 10% of acute lymphoblastic leukemia occurs in adults. Although about one half of patients will have CD10 (CALLA) positive, early B lineage leukemia, the proportion of patients with very early (CD10 negative) B-committed disease or with T cell disease is higher than in children. Lymphoblast morphology is more often of the L2 type.

Adults do less well than children. A remission can be induced in about 85% of adults but requires using daunorubicin in addition to vincristine and prednisone. L-asparaginase is given for consolidation. Cranial radiation and intrathecal methotrexate are combined for CNS prophylaxis. Intensive continuing chemotherapy regimens are currently being tried to reduce the frequency of relapse. These often include daunorubicin, cyclophosphamide, and cytosine arabinoside in addition to the 6-mercaptopurine, methotrexate, vincristine, prednisone combinations used in children.

LEUKEMIAS OF DIFFERENTIATED B CELLS

Chronic Lymphocytic Leukemia

In chronic lymphocytic leukemia, lymphocytes morphologically indistinguishable from normal small lymphocytes infiltrate the bone marrow and circulate in large numbers in the peripheral blood (Fig. 17-3). In early disease, lymphocytic infiltrates are non-diffuse, that is, are separated by areas of uninvolved marrow (Fig. 17-4). Later, a diffuse, uniform infiltrate of lymphocytes usually fills the entire marrow space. Lymphocytes also proliferate within other organs, particularly the lymph nodes, spleen, and liver. Although rarely performed, a biopsy of an involved lymph node reveals a diffuse proliferation of small lymphocytes replacing the normal histologic pattern of the node. The lymph node histopathologic pattern is that of a diffuse lymphocytic lymphoma of small lymphocytes (see Fig. 18-1 and Table 18-1).

Lymphocytes gradually accumulate in chronic lymphocytic leukemia at a rate that varies in different patients. Nevertheless, except

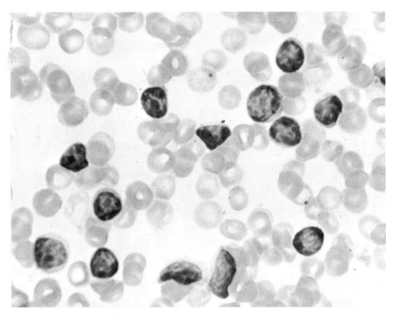

Fig. 17-3. Peripheral blood smear in chronic lymphocytic leukemia showing increased numbers of ordinary-appearing small lymphocytes.

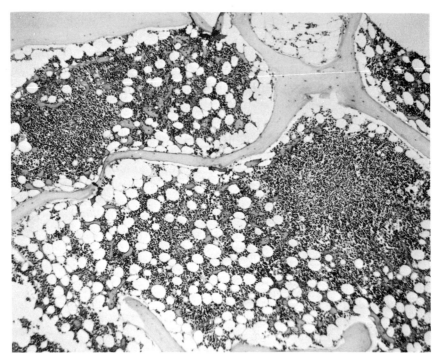

Fig. 17-4. Low-power view of a histologic section of bone marrow in early chronic lymphocytic leukemia. Note nodular areas of lymphocytic infiltration separated by areas of normal marrow.

for a few patients in whom the disease stabilizes, the malignant clone inexorably expands and an untreated patient eventually accumulates an extensive tumor cell burden.

PROPERTIES OF THE MALIGNANT CELL

Like normal circulating B-lymphocytes, the lymphocytes of chronic lymphocytic leukemia exhibit immunofluorescent staining for surface immunoglobulin (SIg), which may be IgM alone or IgM plus IgD (see Chapter 14). However, immune marker studies differ from those of normal circulating B cells in that:

1. The cells stain only weakly for SIg.
2. The SIg of all cells is of the same light chain type. Because the proliferation is clonal, a mixture of cells staining for kappa chains and of cells staining for lambda chains is never found.

3. The cells react with CD5 (T1, T101), an antibody thought originally to react with a surface membrane antigen found only on T cells.

Although absent from normal peripheral blood, a careful search may uncover a few cells with a similar surface marker phenotype in a normal lymph node. Many such cells can be demonstrated in the B areas of fetal lymph nodes at an early gestational age. They have also been described in the peripheral blood of patients during reconstitution of the immune system after bone marrow transplantation. Thus, the proliferating cell of chronic lymphocytic leukemia may represent a cell of normal B cell ontogeny that is "hidden" wthin B cell areas of peripheral lymphoid tissue after they develop beyond a certain stage. The cell has been described as a "virgin", early differentiated B cell unaltered by exposure to antigen.

DISEASE MANIFESTATIONS

Clinical Findings. Chronic lymphocytic leukemia is a disease of older adults. Ninety percent of patients will be over 50 years of age. Men outnumber women about two to one.

The disorder is often discovered accidentally during an examination for an unrelated complaint. Other patients seek medical attention because of enlarged lymph nodes or because of increasing fatigue and weakness.

The patient is afebrile and may not look ill. Enlarged lymph nodes are usually found but may be absent in early disease. The spleen will be palpable in about one half of patients. Massive splenomegaly is rare.

Laboratory Findings

1. *Peripheral blood count.* The total WBC count ranges from about 20,000 to over 200,000 per μL with from about 70% to over 95% small, mature-appearing lymphocytes (see Fig. 17-3). In early stages of the disease, the Hgb level and the platelet count are normal or only minimally depressed. Later in the disease, severe anemia and thrombocytopenia may develop.
2. *Bone Marrow.* As already noted, the marrow will be infiltrated with small, well-differentiated lymphocytes (Fig. 17-5) in a diffuse or non diffuse pattern. Erythroid and myeloid elements are correspondingly reduced. However, if an autoimmune hemolytic anemia develops, erythropoiesis may become surprisingly

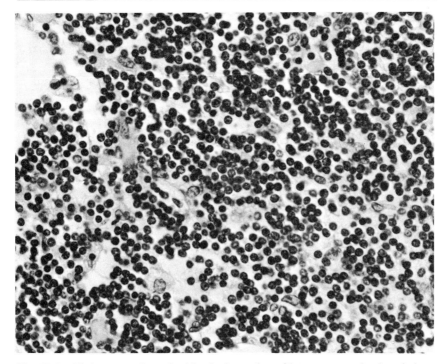

Fig. 17-5. High-power view of a histologic section of bone marrow in chronic lymphocytic leukemia. Note uniform infiltrate of small, well-differentiated lymphocytes.

prominent. Megakaryocytes are present but often diminished in number in advanced disease.

3. *Surface marker studies*. These are indicated whenever physical findings, for example, massive splenomegaly, or morphology of the lymphocytes in the peripheral blood (see Figs. 17-6, 17-7, 17-10) or bone marrow (Fig. 17-9) are atypical for chronic lymphocytic leukemia. The pattern of marker studies already described should be found.

4. *Other findings*. The *serum proteins* are normal early in the disease but many patients later develop *hypogammaglobulinemia* associated with impaired antibody synthesis. Uric acid levels are not elevated.

DIFFERENTIAL DIAGNOSIS

A persisting lymphocytosis of over 15,000 per μL of normal-appearing small lymphocytes in an adult permits a presumptive diagnosis of chronic lymphocytic leukemia. The possibility of one of the other, less common leukemias of differentiated B or T cells must be kept in mind, as well as the knowledge that an inexperienced technologist can occasionally confuse the small, immature-appearing lymphocytes of acute lymphoblastic leukemia of L1 type with the small, mature-appearing lymphocytes of chronic lymphocytic leukemia.

DISEASE EXTENT

A simple system—based on the number of areas of lymphoid enlargement and the degree of bone marrow failure—is frequently used to stage the extent of disease at the time of diagnosis. For this purpose the following are considered separate lymphoid areas: cervical, axillary, and inguinal lymph nodes (unilateral or bilateral), liver, and spleen. The stages are:

Stage A. No anemia or thrombocytopenia and two or less areas of lymphoid enlargement.
Stage B. No anemia or thrombocytopenia and three or more involved areas.
Stage C. Anemia of less than 10g per dL, thrombocytopenia of less than 100,000 per μL, or both, regardless of the number of areas of lymphoid enlargement.

PROGNOSIS AND MANAGEMENT

The median survival time for patients with newly diagnosed chronic lymphocytic leukemia is between 4 and 5 years, but survival varies widely from a few months to over 10 to 15 years in individual patients. Important determinants of prognosis are:

1. *The extent of disease at the time of diagnosis*, that is, into which of the above stages the patient fits. Patients presenting with Stage A disease have a median survival of 7 years, whereas patients who present with Stage C disease have a median survival of less than 3 years.
2. *The rate at which the malignant clone expands.* In some patients in Stage A or B, the disease may remain indolent over years. In other patients, a period of observation attests to a progressively rising WBC count (for example, a doubling of the lymphocyte count within 12 months), a falling hematocrit, and an increasing lymphadenopathy. Initial findings that lead one to suspect that a patient will follow this latter course are:
   a. A presenting lymphocyte count of greater than 50,000 per μL.
   b. Diffuse lymphocytic infiltration of the bone marrow with little if any intervening normal hematopoietic tissue or fat.

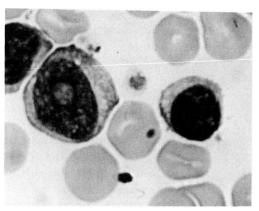

Fig. 17-6 The different morphology on a peripheral blood smear of a prolymphocyte and of the small, dormant-appearing lymphocyte of chronic lymphocytic leukemia. The prolymphocyte is large, contains more cytoplasm, and has a prominent nucleolus.

c. The presence on the blood smear of frequent larger lymphocytes with less condensed nuclear chromatin and a nucleolus (prolymphocytes) (Fig. 17-6).

Patients with Stage A or B disease are usually not treated initially to determine the pace of the disease. When treatment is started (for example, after noting that the WBC count has doubled within 12 months), it is often with pulse doses of an alkylating agent and prednisone. One regimen employs a single dose of chlorambucil of 0.4 to 0.6 mg per kg plus 5 days of prednisone, 60 mg per m² body surface area, every 2 weeks. Patients with severe anemia or thrombocytopenia may be treated for several weeks with prednisone alone, 40 to 60 mg daily, before adding an alkylating agent.

COMPLICATIONS

As the disease advances, the chances increase of a patient's developing one or more of the following complications:

1. *Severe anemia.* This may be one of two types:
   a. Anemia characterized by depressed, unresponsive erythropoiesis. It now appears that this results, not from a crowding out of erythroid precursors by the leukemic B cells, but from an excessive activity of T suppressor cells in the marrow. (Why this abnormality of T cell function occurs in a B cell proliferative disease is unknown.) The characteristics of this anemia are:
      (1) Normochromic, normocytic RBCs *without spherocytosis.*

(2) A low reticulocyte count and decreased numbers of erythroid precursors in the marrow.

(3) A negative Coombs' test.

b. Anemia secondary to autoimmune hemolysis. This may develop suddenly and produce severe anemia. Its characteristics are:

(1) Numerous spherocytes and polychromatophilic macrocytes on the blood smear.

(2) Elevated reticulocyte count and prominent numbers of erythroid precursors in the bone marrow.

(3) Positive direct Coombs' test.

(4) Slight elevation of the serum bilirubin level.

The hemolysis will frequently subside after treatment with large doses of adrenal steroids (for example, 60 to 80 mg of prednisone daily).

2. *Bleeding due to thrombocytopenia.* Severe thrombocytopenia (for example, a platelet count of 10,000 per μL) may develop despite the presence of adequate to moderately diminished numbers of megakaryocytes in the bone marrow. Although this presumably represents another autoimmune complication—the result of an antiplatelet autoantibody—the thrombocytopenia may not respond to adrenal steroid therapy.

3. *A second malignancy.* The incidence of a second primary neoplasm—skin cancer, colorectal cancer, lung cancer—is substantially higher in patients with chronic lymphocytic leukemia than in control normal populations.

4. *Infection.* Because of markedly impaired synthesis of humoral antibody and impaired cell-mediated immune responses, patients with advanced disease have a marked susceptibility to infections. Patients given adrenal steroids must be watched especially carefully for infection, since steroids further depress resistance to infection and also may mask its manifestations. Infection is the most frequent immediate cause of death in chronic lymphocytic leukemia.

TRANSFORMATION INTO MORE AGGRESSIVE DISEASE

"Prolymphocytoid transformation." In some patients, chronic lymphocytic leukemia increases in clinical aggressiveness in association with the appearance on the blood smear of a number of larger lymphocytes. Many of these larger lymphocytes have morphologic features of prolymphocytes (see Fig. 17-6). When prolymphocytes exceed an arbitrarily selected value of 15% of the lymphocyte count,

the disease is considered to have undergone "prolymphocytoid transformation." Biopsy of a lymph node shows a pseudofollicular pattern made up of many foci of larger, transformed cells dispersed within a background of small lymphocytes. (The histopathology can be confused with that of a follicular mixed small and large cell lymphoma). After prolymphocytoid transformation, the disease usually becomes refractory to further control with an alkylating agent and prednisone and many patients die within a few months.

Richter's Syndrome. A second pattern of increased aggressiveness may be seen in which the appearance of the circulating lymphocytes does not change but in which tumor growth accelerates in one or more groups of nodes and often also in other organs or tissues such as the gastrointestinal tract, liver, skin, or bone. The patient usually develops fever and sometimes complains of abdominal pain. Biopsy of an involved area reveals a diffuse proliferation of large cells. The histopathologic pattern (referred to in former terminology as "diffuse histiocytic lymphoma") is usually that of an immunoblastic sarcoma of B cells.

This combination of findings, which has been referred to as *Richter's syndrome*, may develop terminally in about 5% of patients with chronic lymphocytic leukemia. Although one assumes that it evolves from transformation of the original leukemic clone, this need not be true. In one recently reported patient, the small lymphocytes of the original leukemia and the large cells of the second lesion differed both in the rearrangements of their heavy chain genes and in the light chain type of their surface immunoglobulin. In this patient, Richter's syndrome clearly arose as a malignant proliferation of a second, independent B cell clone.

Other Leukemias of Differentiated B Cells

These less common disorders have distinctive clinical and laboratory findings (Table 17-3) that distinguish each from chronic lymphocytic leukemia.

LEUKEMIC PHASE OF SMALL CLEAVED FOLLICULAR CENTER CELL LYMPHOMA

In this disorder, which has also been referred to as lymphosarcoma cell or notched cell leukemia, the circulating lymphocytes have irregular nuclei and amitotic cleavage planes (see Fig. 17-7). In con-

Table 17-3. Properties Distinguishing Various Leukemias of Differentiated B Cells

LEUKEMIA	CELL MORPHOLOGY	sIg* STAINING	IMMUNE MARKERS
Chronic lymphocytic	Small, mature lympho-cyte	Weak	CD5 positive
Leukemic phase of cleaved cell lym-phoma (lymphosar-coma cell leukemia)	Cleaved nucleus	Bright	CD5 negative, CD10 (CALLA), positive
Prolymphocytic	Prominent nucleolus	Bright	CD5 positive or nega-tive
Hairy cell	Cytoplasmic projec-tions	Bright	CD5 negative, Tac pos-itive

* Abbreviation for surface immunoglobulin.

trast to chronic lymphocytic leukemia, the lymphocytes stain brightly for surface immunoglobulin (see Fig. 17-8) and show capping of surface immunoglobulin (a concentration of stained immunoglobulin at one pole of the cell). The cells also are CD 5 (Tl, T101) negative.

Patients with this disorder may have large, bulky lymphadenopathy. A lymph node biopsy shows a small cleaved follicular center cell lymphoma (see Fig. 18-2).

PROLYMPHOCYTIC LEUKEMIA

Patients with prolymphocytic leukemia have the following findings:

1. A very large spleen.
2. Minimal or no lymphadenopathy.
3. A very high WBC count, for example, greater than 100,000 per μL.
4. Lymphocytes of characteristic morphology. The cell is usually larger, with more cytoplasm and less condensed nuclear chromatin than the small, dormant lymphocyte. Its distinctive feature is a single, prominent nucleolus (see Fig. 17-6).

Typically, prolymphocytes stain brightly for SIg and so are clearly of B cell lineage. They may or may not react with a CD5 antibody (T1, T101). In a rare patient whose findings are otherwise not distinctive, immune markers will reveal that the prolymphocyte is of T cell lineage.

HAIRY CELL LEUKEMIA

Hairy cell leukemia is a chronic malignant disorder that requires for its diagnosis the demonstration on bone marrow biopsy of a lymphocytic proliferation with a distinctive histologic appearance (see Fig. 17-9). Noting lymphocytes with striking cytoplasmic projections, so-called hairy cells (see Fig. 17-10), on a peripheral blood smear may provide the first clue to the diagnosis. On cytochemical staining, these lymphocytes have a second distinctive feature, namely, they are positive for tartrate-resistant acid phosphatase. Although circulating hairy cells have given the disease its name, they may not be prominent on the blood smear of some patients.

In the vast majority of patients, hairy cell leukemia is a B cell disorder. The cells stain brightly for surface immunoglobulin and have rearranged genes for immunoglobulin chains on molecular ge-

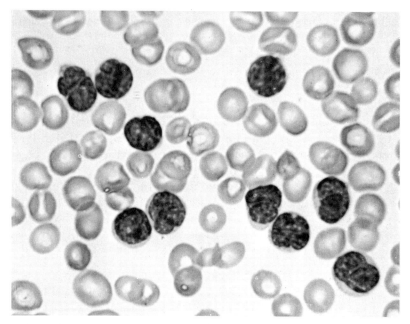

Fig. 17-7. Peripheral blood smear in the leukemic phase of small cleaved cell lymphoma showing lymphocytes with characteristic amitotic nuclear cleavage planes. Cells with this morphology are sometimes called "lymphosarcoma cells."

A Chronic Lymphocytic Leukemia   B Lymphosarcoma Cell Leukemia

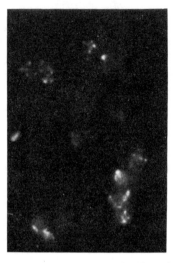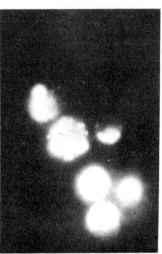

Fig. 17-8. Fluoresence of cells stained with fluorescein-conjugated polyvalent anti-human IgG to detect surface immunoglobulin (sIg). Contrast the weak staining for sIg of lymphocytes of chronic lymphocytic leukemia *(A)* with the bright staining for sIg of circulating lymphocytes in the leukemic phase of small cleaved cell lymphoma *(B)*.

netic analysis. The cells also react with a monoclonal antibody named Tac, which is directed against a determinant on the Il-2 receptor. (Initially thought specific for T cells, it now appears that at least the determinant of the Il-2 receptor recognizing Tac may also be found on activated cells of other lineages).

Rare patients have also been discovered with hairy cell leukemia of T cell origin and infection with an uncommon strain of human T cell leukemia virus called HTLV-II. Why this disorder of apparently different causation and cell lineage has the same clinical features as the common type of hairy cell leukemia is unknown.

Manifestations. Hairy cell leukemia is usually of insidious onset. The typical patient is a middle-aged male (4:1 male-to-female ratio). The characteristic finding on physical examination is an enlarged spleen (about 90% of patients) without associated peripheral lymphadeno-pathy. Sometimes splenomegaly is massive. Although peripheral lymphadenopathy is uncommon (less than 5% of patients), retroperi-

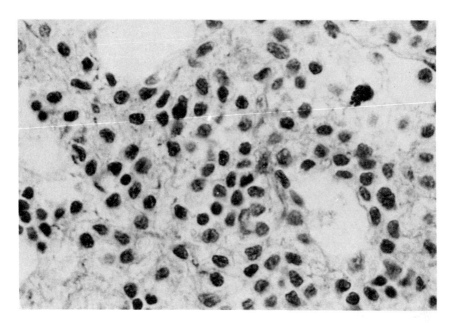

Fig. 17-9. High-power view of a histologic section of bone marrow in hairy cell leukemia showing the loose appearance of the infiltrate created by the abundant clear cytoplasm of the cells. Note also the uniform nuclear configuration of the cells.

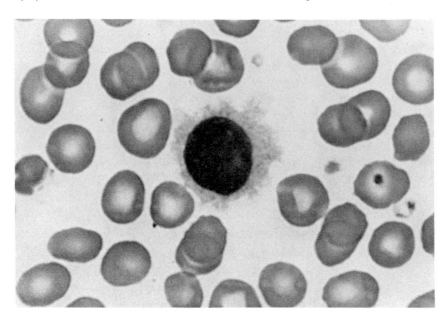

Fig. 17-10. Peripheral blood smear in hairy cell leukemia. The nucleus of the hairy cell is typically round and centrally placed, and the cytoplasm has numerous hair-like projections.

toneal lymphadenopathy is noted on CT scans in some patients.
The disease exists in two forms as defined by the peripheral blood count:

1. A common *pancytopenic form* characterized by moderate to severe anemia, leukopenia, and thrombocytopenia. Differential counts reveal a reduced percentage of both granulocytes and monocytes. Granulocyte levels may fall to the 500 μL range and platelet counts to less than 25,000 per μL. Hairy cells are readily seen in modest numbers on the blood smear of most patients, but in a rare patient, they are hard to find.
2. A *leukemic form* in which the WBC count exceeds 10,000 and greater than 50% of the WBC are hairy cells. An unusual patient may have a WBC count in the 50,000 per μL range. The leukemic form is found in about 15% of patients.

The bone marrow often cannot be aspirated. Biopsy reveals a monotonous infiltrate of mononuclear cells that has an illusory loose appearance due to a halo of clear cytoplasm surrounding the nucleus of the cell (see Fig. 17-9). A reticulin stain discloses that the cells grow in a stroma of reticular fibers, which explains why the cells are difficult to aspirate.

Course and Management. Patients who become severely granulocytopenic (less than 500 granulocytes per μL) are at high risk for infection, which is a major cause of death in hairy cell leukemia. A number of patients have developed atypical mycobacterial infection, and this possibility should be strongly considered in a patient who develops persistent fever and a pulmonary infiltrate. For reasons not yet clear, patients are also prone to develop manifestations of autoimmune disease, for example, nodular skin lesions that show an inflammatory vasculitis on biopsy.

The pancytopenia of hairy cell leukemia reflects two processes:

1. Underproduction of blood cells by an infiltrated marrow.
2. Splenic sequestration of blood cells.

Newly recognized patients with hairy cell disease who are not severely pancytopenic may be observed for a time to determine the rate of progress of the disease. As pancytopenia worsens, at some point splenectomy is performed. The resultant relief of splenic sequestration often allows the blood count to return to normal or near normal values for a long period. In most patients, RBC, granulocyte, and platelet counts eventually fall again as the proliferative process in the bone marrow slowly expands. One then treats the patient with one of two new agents, interferon or deoxycoformycin (pentastatin), which, although still in clinical trials, clearly appear to be effective in hairy cell leukemia. The initial experience with deoxycoformycin is particularly encouraging. Indeed, deoxycoformycin may possibly replace splenectomy as the initial therapy for hairy cell leukemia.

PLASMACYTOID LYMPHOCYTIC LEUKEMIA

Whereas the usual patient with chronic lymphocytic leukemia eventually becomes hypogammaglobulinemic, an occasional patient is found to have an elevated level of a monoclonal plasma immunoglobulin. The monoclonal protein may be IgG or IgM. Although the lymphocytes on the peripheral blood smear of such a patient may be difficult to distinguish from those of the usual patient with chronic lymphocytic leukemia, immune marker studies will reveal a difference. The cells do not react with CD5 (T1, T101). Thus, they differ from the "virgin" B cell of CLL and appear, instead, to resemble B cells activated by exposure to antigen to acquire properties of immunoglobulin secreting cells. Indeed, some of the lymphocytes in the bone marrow from such a patient will have a plasmacytoid look due to an increased amount of basophilic cytoplasm. Increased numbers of plasma cells may also be noted in the marrow. Many of the features of plasmacytoid lymphocytic leukemia resemble those of macroglobulinemia of Waldenström (see Chapter 20).

LEUKEMIAS OF DIFFERENTIATED T CELLS

Except for an unusual patient with hairy cell leukemia or prolymphocytic leukemia who will have T cell disease, the leukemias of differentiated T cells fall into the groups discussed below.

Adult T Cell Leukemia/Lymphoma

After an incubation period that may last for several years, infection with a human acute leukemia/lymphoma virus (HTLV-I) can give rise to an acute, rapidly fatal lymphoproliferative disorder. The disease may present as a lymphoma or in a leukemic phase; if the former occurs, a leukemic phase often develops during its course. Circulating lymphocytes vary both in size and in degree of nuclear irregularity. One type of cell is characteristic—a large cell with a polylobated, "knobby-looking" nucleus (Fig. 17-11). It can be found in variable numbers on the blood smear of most patients. Immune marker studies

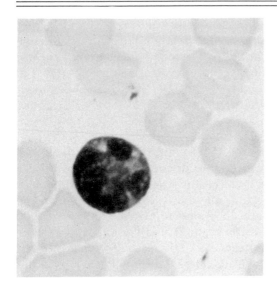

Fig. 17-11. Peripheral blood smear showing a highly poly-lobated lymphocyte. Such cells are seen on the peripheral blood smear of patients with adult T cell leukemia/lymphoma secondary to HTLV-I infection.

(Table 17-4) show that the malignant cell is a differentiated T cell, that is, is CD3 positive, and is of the CD4 subset. CD4 positive cells usually have helper immunoregulatory functions, but the CD4 positive cells from patients with this disease suppress immunoglobulin synthesis when they are cocultured in vitro with B cells. The cells characteristically have a high number of surface membrane receptors for Il-2 and so react strongly with the monoclonal antibody Tac.

EPIDEMIOLOGIC STUDIES

Adult T cell leukemia/lymphoma is endemic in southwest Japan, the Caribbean, and, to a lesser extent, in the southeastern United States. A cluster of cases has recently been discovered in Brooklyn, New York, and this raises the possibility that other geographic pockets may be found in the United States. All patients in the United States to date have been black.

Serologic studies have revealed a prevalence of antibodies to HTLV-I in normal persons in certain Caribbean areas of from 2% to 5% and in areas in southern Japan of from 10% to 15%. Prevalence of HTLV seropositivity and of clinical adult T cell leukemia/lymphoma are correlated. Family members of patients have a frequency of seropositivity approaching 50%, and occurrence of disease in more than one member of a family has been reported.

Although the majority of seropositive patients have remained well, instances of asymptomatic seropositive patients developing adult T cell leukemia/lymphoma several years later have been documented. Moreover, studies from Japan suggest that a "preleukemic" form of the disease exists in which small numbers of circulating abnormal cells can be repeatedly demonstrated in the peripheral blood of seropositive individuals. These individuals may be totally asymptomatic or may have transient fever, skin eruptions, and mild lymphadenopathy.

The relation between seropositivity and clinical disease resembles that seen with another HTLV type, HTLV-III. Exposure to this retrovirus causes a certain number of individuals to develop full blown AIDS, a larger group to develop evidence of smoldering AIDS-related clinical findings, and a much larger group to become seropositive yet remain asymptomatic and at unknown risk for developing later disease (see Chapter 21).

MANIFESTATIONS

The onset of disease is usually sudden in an adult between 30 and 60 years of age. Characteristic clinical findings include:

Table 17-4. Different Laboratory Findings in Adult T Cell Leukemia, Sézary Syndrome, and Tγ Cell Leukemia/Lymphocytosis

FINDING	ADULT T CELL LEUKEMIA	SÉZARY SYNDROME	Tγ CELL LEUKEMIA/ LYMPHOCYTOSIS
HTLV-I Serology	+	−	−
Lymphocyte morphology	Pleomorphic, polylobated nucleus	Cerebriform cell	Cytoplasmic cell with prominent azurophillic granules
Immune functional behavior	Suppressor	Helper	K cell, NK cell*
Immune markers			
CD3	+	+	− or +
CD4	+	+	−
CD8	−	−	+
Other	Tac +[†]		Fc receptor for IgG, HNK-1 +

* Abbreviations for killer cell and natural killer cell, see text.
[†] Indicates presence of Il-2 receptors on surface membrane.

1. Skin lesions, for example, nodules, erythematous patches, erythroderma. Biopsy of skin lesions may be indistinguishable from mycosis fungoides (see Chapter 18).
2. Hypercalcemia. Apparently, the malignant cells secrete a lymphokine that activates osteoclasts.
3. Lytic bone lesions on radiographs in about 50% of cases. These lytic areas are not areas of T cell proliferation but result from bone lysis secondary to osteoclast activation.
4. Lymphadenopathy, which may be peripheral, retroperitoneal, or hilar. However, a mediastinal mass is not found.
5. Enlargement of the spleen, liver, or both in about 50% of patients.

The *peripheral blood count* reveals no or minimal anemia. The total WBC count may be normal or, if large numbers of the malignant T cells are circulating, very high. If the WBC count is normal, the characteristic polylobated lymphocyte (see Fig. 17-11) may or may not be found on search of the blood smear.

Even when the WBC count is high, a *bone marrow examination* may be normal or show only scattered areas of lymphocytic infiltration. Thus, most of the circulating cells represent T cells entering the blood from other areas of proliferation. Histopathologic examination of a lymph node biopsy shows a diffuse lymphoma either of large cells or of mixed small and large cells.

COURSE

Intensive chemotherapy may induce a transient remission, but most patients die of some complication of the disease within 12 months of diagnosis. As with HTLV-III infection, patients with acute HTLV-I related disease have a decreased resistance to infection, particularly with opportunistic organisms. A number of patients develop bilateral interstitial pulmonary infiltrates, which may result from *Pneumocystis carinii* infection, from lymphomatous proliferation in the lungs, or from both. Patients also frequently develop CNS findings, usually as a consequence of lymphomatous leptomeningitis.

Leukemic Phase of Cutaneous T Cell Lymphoma

Malignant proliferations of T cells are seen in which the initial clinical manifestations appear primarily confined to the skin. The clinical course is more indolent than that of adult T cell leukemia/lymphoma. Patients are usually older and male patients predominate. The disease is not found in geographic clusters or in particular racial groups, and the patients do not have serum antibodies to HTLV-I.

A spectrum of skin lesions are seen. At one end is mycosis fungoides, a disorder in which the skin lesions take the form of indurated plaques that progress, sometimes over years, to nodules and fungating lesions. At the other end is Sézary's syndrome, a disorder characterized by a diffuse, progressive, intensely itching, erythematous, exfoliative erythroderma.

In many patients, occasional abnormal-appearing T cells can be found on the peripheral blood smear. The nucleus of the cell is less polyploid than that of the characterstic cell of adult T cell leukemia/ lymphoma and has a folded, "cerebriform" look (Fig. 17-12). As disease progresses, visceral disease becomes increasingly overt (for example, peripheral lymphadenopathy, hepatosplenomegaly). Visceral involvement tends to appear earlier in patients with Sézary's syndrome, some of whom develop a leukemic phase of the disease with a lymphocytosis in which a substantial proportion of the lymphocytes have an abnormal cerebriform appearance. These abnormal cells have, therefore, been given the name Sézary cells.

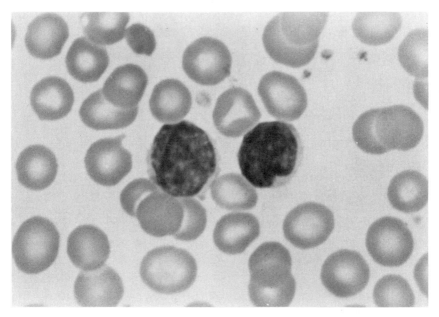

Fig. 17-12. Peripheral blood smear from a patient with a cutaneous T cell lymphoma showing the cerebriform appearance of the nucleus of the lymphocyte that characterizes the Sézary cell.

Tγ Cell Leukemia/Lymphocytosis

PROPERTIES OF Tγ CELLS

Tγ cells are cells that possess the following two surface membrane receptors:

1. A receptor allowing the cells to form rosettes with sheep erythrocytes and also causing the cell to react with the monoclonal antibody CD2 (T11). (This receptor, which is found on all T cells and which first appears on the surface membrane very early in T cell processing, establishes that the cells are related to the T lineage.)

2. A receptor allowing the cells to form rosettes with human RBCs coated with anti-D (Rh) antibody of the IgG class. Rosettes are formed because the receptor on the lymphocytes reacts with the Fc segment of the IgG antibody bound to the red cells. Since IgG is also called γ-globulin, T-related cells possessing this receptor are referred to as Tγ cells.

Some Tγ cells react with CD3, which means that they possess a determinant of the T cell antigen receptor that does not appear on the cell surface until a later stage of thymic T cell processing. Other Tγ cells do not react with CD3, which means that, although T-related, they have not been subjected to full thymic T cell processing. All Tγ cells react with CD8, which means that they can recognize Class I histocompatibility determinants.

Tγ cells function as K cells (killer cells), that is, they can kill tissue cells that have been coated by IgG antibody. Some T cells, particularly in the presence of gamma interferon, also function as NK cells (natural killer cells), that is, they can kill certain cells (for example, a myeloid cell line called K562) even though the cells have not been coated with antibody. Tγ cells also react with monoclonal antibodies thought to identify natural killer cells (HNK-1, Leu 7).

Tγ cells have a characteristic morphologic feature of prominent azurophilic cytoplasmic granules. Many are also large cells with increased amounts of cytoplasm. Such cells have been referred to as *large granular lymphocytes* (LGL).

MANIFESTATIONS OF PROLIFERATIVE Tγ CELL DISORDERS

A chronic, often indolent proliferative disorder of Tγ cells has been identified with the following characteristics:

1. Moderate splenomegaly without peripheral lymphadenopathy.
2. Lymphocytosis with lymphocyte counts in the 5000 to 40,000 per μL range. Most of the lymphocytes will have the morphologic appearance of LGL. (Their surface marker profile will be as discussed above: IgG Fc receptor positive; CD2, CD8, and HNK-1 positive; and CD3 positive or negative.)
3. Neutropenia, which is found in most patients and which may be severe and associated with recurrent skin infections.
4. Other cytopenias in a few patients, such as anemia secondary to red cell aplasia or thrombocytopenia.
5. Minimal to moderate lymphocytic infiltration of the bone marrow. Granulopoiesis is also abnormal in many patients in that cells beyond the myelocyte stage are not found. In the occasional patient with red cell aplasia, erythroid precursors are absent.
6. Evidence of abnormal B cell immunoregulation which may take the form of:
   a. Either polyclonal hypergammaglobulinemia or hypogammaglobulinemia.
   b. Elevated titers for rheumatoid factor or antinuclear antibody (ANA).
   c. Autoantibodies against granulocytes or RBCs.

Despite the chronic, nonaggressive nature of the lymphocytic proliferation, DNA analysis of polypeptide chain genes of the T cell antigen receptor reveals evidence of an expanded monoclonal population of T cells. Therefore, many view the disorder as a form of chronic T cell lymphocytic leukemia; however, because in most patients the proliferating clone does not continue to expand and because of the prominence of the neutropenia, others refer to the disorder as chronic T cell lymphocytosis with neutropenia.

Felty's syndrome (see Chapter 21) is a disorder characterized by rheumatoid arthritis (often advanced), splenomegaly, and severe persistent neutropenia. Although lymphocytosis is not present, DNA analysis has revealed the presence of an expanded clone of T lymphocytes in some patients. In these patients, Felty's syndrome appears to represent a variant of Tγ cell leukemia/lymphocytosis with only a minimal, subclinical clonal expansion.

Rare patients have also been described with an aggressive lymphoma characterized by an extensive proliferation of T-lymphocytes, particularly in the sinusoids of the liver and in the spleen. Immune marker profiles of the proliferating cells do not differ from those found in patients with nonaggressive Tγ cell leukemia/lymphocytosis. In striking contrast to the patient with Felty's syndrome, the patient with this aggressive, rapidly fatal lymphoma represents the other end of a wide spectrum of Tγ cell proliferative disease.

SELECTED READING

Acute Lymphoblastic Leukemia

1. Gottlieb AJ, Weinberg V, Ellison RR, Henderson ES, et al.: Efficacy of daunorubicin in the therapy of adult acute lymphocytic leukemia: a prospective randomized trial by cancer and leukemia group B. Blood 64:267, 1984.
2. Murphy S, and Jaffe ES: Editorial retrospective. Terminal transferase activity and lymphoblastic neoplasms. N Engl J Med 311:1373, 1984.
3. Smithson WA, Gilchrist GS, and Burgert EO, Jr: Childhood acute lymphocytic leukemia. CA 30:158, 1980.

Differentiated B Cell Leukemias

1. Gale RP, and Foon KA: Chronic lymphocytic leukemia: recent advances in biology and treatment. Ann Intern Med 103:101, 1985.
2. Galton DAG, Goldman JM, Wiltshaw E, Catovsky D, Henry K, and Goldenberg GJ: Prolymphocytic leukaemia. Br J Haematol 27:7, 1974.
3. Kjeldsberg CR, and Marty J: Prolymphocytic transformation of chronic lymphocytic leukemia. Cancer 48:2447, 1981.
4. Mangan KF, and D'Allesandro L: Hypoplastic anemia in B cell chronic lymphocytic leukemia: evolution of T cell-mediated suppression of erythropoiesis in early-stage and late-stage disease. Blood 66:533, 1985.
5. van Dongen JJM, Hooijkaas H, Michiels JJ, Grosveld G, de Klein A, van der Kwast ThH, Prins MEF, Abels J, and Hagemeijer A: Richter's syndrome with different immunoglobulin light chains and different heavy chain gene rearrangements. Blood 64:571, 1984.

Leukemias of Differentiated T Cells

1. Broder S, (moderator) Bunn PA Jr, Jaffe ES, Blattner W, Gallo RC, Wong-Staal F, Waldman TA, and Devita VT Jr (discussants): T-cell lymphoproliferative syndrome associated with human T-cell leukemia/lymphoma virus. Ann Intern Med 100:543, 1984
2. Harden EA, and Haynes BF: Phenotypic and functional characterization of human malignant T cells. Semin Hematol 22:13, 1985.
3. Newland AC, Catovsky D, Linch D, Cawley JC, Beverley P, San Miguel JF, Gordon-Smith EC, Blecher TE, Shahriari S, and Varadi S: Chronic T cell lymphocytosis: a review of 21 cases. Br J Haematol 58:433, 1984.

18

Non-Hodgkin's Lymphomas

As discussed in Chapter 15, lymphomas are neoplasms of cells of the immune system involving the lymph nodes, the lymphoid tissue of extranodal sites, or both. Lymphomas may be divided into:

1. The non-Hodgkin's lymphomas, which are (except for a disorder of pre-T cells, lymphoblastic lymphoma, and very rare instances of histiocytic lymphoma) *proliferative disorders of B- or T-lymphocytes of the peripheral lymphoid tissues* with different degrees of lymphocyte transformation (see Chapter 14).
2. Hodgkin's disease, a disorder whose histopathology differs fundamentally from other lymphomas and which is the topic of Chapter 19.

As also discussed in Chapter 15, the distinction between a non-Hodgkin's lymphoma and lymphocytic leukemia may become blurred when lymphoma also:

1. Diffusely infiltrates the bone marrow, or
2. Results in large numbers of lymphocytes entering the blood from tissues other than the bone marrow, for example, from the subcutaneous tissues and lymph nodes in a cutaneous T cell lymphoma.

Lymphomas and leukemias that represent proliferations of the same cell type are summarized in Table 18-1.

Table 18-1. Lymphocytic Neoplasms That May Present as Lymphoma or Leukemia

PROLIFERATIVE GRADE	CELL TYPE	LYMPHOMA	LEUKEMIA
Low	B	Small lymphocytic (B)	Chronic lymphocytic leukemia
	B	Small lymphocytic, plasmacytoid (Waldenström's macroglobulinemia)	Plasmacytoid lymphocytic leukemia
	B	Small cleaved cell, follicular	Lymphosarcoma cell leukemia
	T	Small lymphocytic (T)	T cell leukemia (T cell chronic lymphocytic leukemia)
High	B	Small non-cleaved cell diffuse (Burkitt's or Burkitt-like)	Acute B cell lymphoblastic leukemia (L3 morphology)
	T	Lymphoblastic lymphoma (convoluted T cell)*	Acute T cell lymphoblastic leukemia
	T	Cutaneous T cell lymphomas (mycosis fungoides, Sézary syndrome)	Sézary cell leukemia
	T	Adult T cell lymphoma+	Adult T cell leukemia

*Often presents with mediastinal mass
+Rapidly fatal disease related to HTLV-I infection

PATHOLOGIC DIAGNOSIS

Histologic Features

In lymphoma, proliferating cells of lymphoid tissue origin obliterate the normal architecture of a lymph node (see Fig. 14-2). The neoplastic cell may proliferate in either a diffuse (Fig. 18-1) or a follicular (nodular) pattern (Fig. 18-2). Lymphomatous follicular proliferations may sometimes be difficult to distinguish morphologically from benign follicular hyperplasias, for example, from the hyperplastic follicles found in an enlarged axillary node reacting to antigens in a vaccine injected subcutaneously into the arm. However, immunocytochemical staining for light chains of surface immunoglobulin usually allows one to distinguish the two processes. Follicular hyperplasias are polyclonal, and therefore the B cells of the follicles will be a mixture of cells staining for kappa light chains and cells staining for lambda light chains. Lymphomatous follicles are monoclonal; therefore, all of the cells in all of the follicles will stain for the same light chain type.

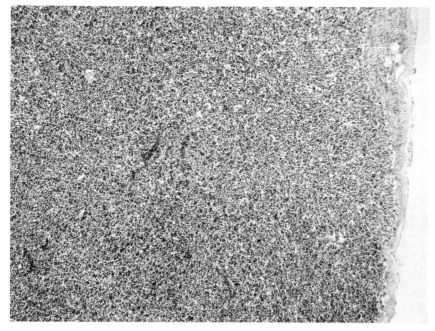

Fig. 18-1. Low-power view of a lymph node. Note diffuse proliferation of cells, which at higher magnification (see Fig. 18-6) are seen to be dormant-appearing small lymphocytes. Diagnosis: small lymphocytic lymphoma (chronic lymphocytic leukemia related).

Cytologic Types

RELATION OF CELL TYPE TO CELL SIZE

Non-Hodgkin's lymphomas can be divided into lymphomas of small cells, of large cells, or of a mixture of small and large cells. It was once thought that the small cells were lymphocytes and the large cells were histiocytes; now it is known that virtually all of the large cells are neoplastic counterparts of large, transformed lymphocytes. Mixed proliferations usually reflect the presence in the biopsy section of neoplastic lymphocytes at different stages of transformation, but they can also represent a mixture of neoplastic cells and normal, reactive lymphoctyes (for example, areas of proliferating transformed large B cells which are interspersed with areas of normal small T cells).

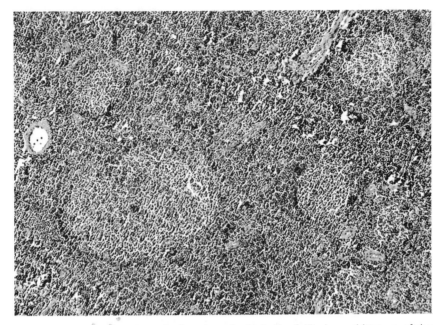

Fig. 18-2. Low-power view of a lymph node. Note the follicular architecture of the proliferative process. On higher power (see Fig. 18-4), the cells within the follicles are seen to be small cleaved follicular center cells. Diagnosis: follicular small cleaved cell lymphoma.

Small cell lymphomas may be lymphomas of small lymphocytes with a low rate of cell turnover, or lymphomas of rapidly dividing cells with a high rate of turnover, for example, the transformed "small" non-cleaved follicular center cell (see below). Therefore, small cell lymphomas may be of either low-grade or high-grade aggressiveness. *Large cell lymphomas* are lymphomas of one of four types of proliferating lymphocytes—large cleaved follicular center cells, large non-cleaved follicular center cells, immunoblasts of B lineage, immunoblasts of T lineage—or, rarely, a lymphoma of true histiocytes. *Large cell lymphomas are always of intermediate or high-grade aggressiveness.*

TYPES OF B CELL LYMPHOMAS

B cell lymphomas, which make up about 75% of all lymphomas, may proliferate in a diffuse or follicular fashion. Most, but not all, diffuse lymphomas of dormant-appearing lymphocytes are of B cell origin. In some, the cells are identical in morphologic and surface marker features to the cell of chronic lymphocytic leukemia and represent a proliferative disorder of a cell whose normal counterpart' is an early "virgin" B cell not yet exposed to antigen (see Chapter 17). Others represent proliferative disorders of cells whose normal cell counterparts are effector B-lymphocytes, "educated" by exposure to antigen and capable of secretion of immunoglobulin (Fig. 18-3). Some of the lymphocytes may have plasmacytoid features, and when such cells are prominent, the lymphoma is called a plasmacytoid lymphoma. (If the plasmacytoid cells secrete large amounts of monoclonal IgM into the serum, the disorder is referred to as Waldenström's macroglobulinemia (see Chapter 20).)

Only B cells home to follicles in normal lymph nodes, and all lymphomas with a follicular architecture will be B cell lymphomas. B cells within normal secondary follicles (see Fig. 14-2) can be divided into four cytologic types representing different stages of transformation after exposure to antigen (Fig. 18-3). These are:

1. Small cleaved follicular center cells. The cells have a variable configuration with irregular, indented, or cleaved nuclei and occasional small nucleoli (Fig. 18-4).
2. Large cleaved follicular center cells. These differ from small cleaved cells in having a nucleus larger than the nucleus of a

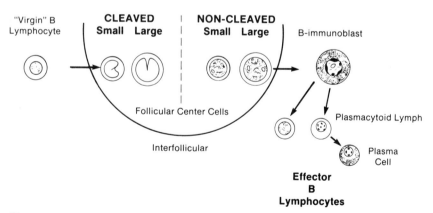

Fig. 18-3. A schematic representation of the sequence of transformation of normal B cells in follicular centers and their subsequent entrance into the interfollicular area to form effector cells capable of secreting immunoglobin. (Modified from Lukes RJ, Collins RD: Immunologic characterization of human malignant lymphomas. Cancer 34:1488, 1974; by permission)

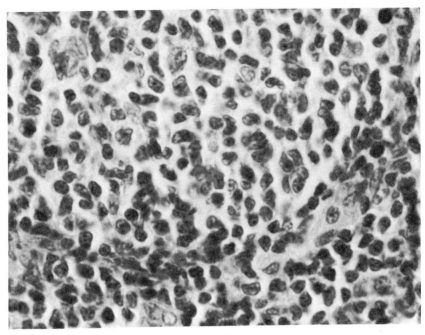

Fig. 18-4. High-power view of the edge of a follicle from the biopsy specimen shown in Figure 18-2. Note that almost all of the cells are small lymphocytes with a variable configuration and irregular, indented, or cleaved nuclei.

reactive histiocyte. Occasional cells will have exaggerated cleavage planes.

3. "Small" non-cleaved follicular center cells. These cells have a round nucleus (called small because it is smaller than the nucleus of a histiocyte) with finely dispersed chromatin and small nucleoli; a moderate amount of pyroninophilic cytoplasm (cytoplasm staining with methyl green pyronine, which means that it contains a large amount of RNA); and cohesive borders that cause the cells to proliferate in a lymphoma in a cohesive pattern (Fig. 18-5).

4. Large non-cleaved follicular center cells. These cells have large, round to oval nuclei; prominent nucleoli, which frequently are noted at the nuclear membrane; and more cytoplasm that the small non-cleaved cell.

Lymphomas representing the neoplastic counterpart of each of these cell types have been recognized. The small *cleaved follicular*

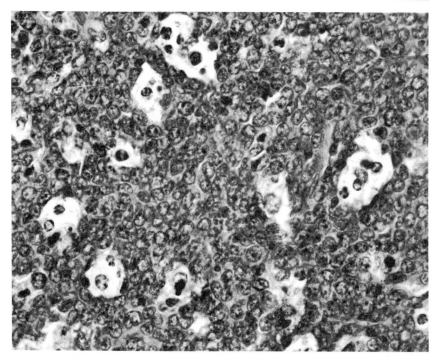

Fig. 18-5. High-power view of a lymph node biopsy in Burkitt's lymphoma. The uniform, primitive-appearing cells have a round, non-cleaved nucleus that is smaller than the nucleus of a histiocyte. The cells are growing in a cohesive pattern. Interspersed large, pale histiocytes produce a "starry sky" appearance.

center cells are cells at early stages of transformation, and they have a low mitotic rate. Lymphomas consisting primarily of small cleaved follicular center cells tend to grow slowly and to retain a follicular (nodular) architecture. The *non-cleaved cells* are the proliferative cells of the follicle. Lymphomas of these cells have numerous mitoses and are fast growing. The great majority grow in a diffuse pattern; in less than 10%, remnants of a follicular architecture may be detected on scanning multiple fields of a biopsy under low power, and these then are classified as follicular (nodular).

After antigen-induced transformation and proliferation within follicles, transformed B cells move out of the follicles and give rise to the plasma cells of the medullary cords of a lymph node (see Fig. 14-2). A large transformed B cell with beginning plasma cell differentiation has been recognized in the interfollicular area of a lymph node. This cell, the *B-immunoblast*, has a large, vesicular (empty-appearing) nucleus with chromatin that has become marginated along the nuclear membrane and prominent nucleoli often centrally placed; its cytoplasm is deeply pyroninophilic and may contain immunoglobulin on immunocytochemical staining. Since the B-immunoblast is not a follicular center cell, a lymphoma of its neoplastic counterpart, B-immunoblastic sarcoma never has a follicular architecture and should not have an accompanying minor population of cleaved cells. (If follicles are seen in a node biopsy, they represent remnants of normal lymphoid tissue in the node.)

TYPES OF T CELL LYMPHOMAS

Twenty percent of lymphomas are T cell lymphomas. T cells are normally found in the paracortical area of lymph nodes; T cell lymphoma arises in this area of a node and never has a follicular architecture. Certain T cells home to subcutaneous tissues, and almost all lymphomas that present with prominent skin manifestations are T cell lymphomas. These T cells tend to have fine folds in the nucleus, which are difficult to see in tissue sections but are readily seen on imprints or blood smears and which give the cell a cerebriform appearance (see Fig. 17-12). About 5% of the diffuse lymphomas of small, dormant-appearing lymphocytes will be T cell lymphomas. At least some of these are related to the Tγ cell leukemia/lymphocytosis syndrome described in Chapter 17.

In another type of uncommon T cell lymphoma, called *lympho-epithelioid lymphocytic lymphoma or Lennert's lymphoma,* clusters of epithelioid cells are seen throughout the lymph node. Lymphocytes may predominate in the intervening tissue or the intervening cell population may be heterogeneous, with varying proportions of lymphocytes, plasma cells, and large, transformed forms. The histopathology may resemble mixed cellularity Hodgkin's disease, but characteristic Reed-Sternberg cells (see Chapter 19) are not found.

Large, transformed T cells are sometimes referred to as T-immunoblasts, and lymphomas containing appreciable numbers of such cells have been called *T-immunoblastic sarcomas.* These lymphomas are frequently pleomorphic, containing a mixture of smaller lymphocytes with irregular, contorted nuclei and larger cells with either round or polylobulated nuclei and abundant, water-clear cytoplasm. Patients with HTLV-I positive adult T cell lymphoma/leukemia (see Chapter 17) may have this histologic pattern on lymph node biopsy, but it is also seen in virus-negative T cell lymphomas. Occasionally, a lymphoepithelioid lymphocytic lymphoma may transform into a T-immunoblastic sarcoma.

CLASSIFICATION OF LYMPHOMAS

Classification systems are still evolving as molecular genetic, surface marker, and viral studies enhance our knowledge of the pathogenesis of lymphoma. Three classification systems are used in the United States, but one—in which lymphomas are classified by cell size into lymphocytic, histiocytic, or mixed—is falling into disuse. As mentioned, the large cell lymphomas referred to in this classification as "diffuse histiocytic lymphoma" almost always represent lymphomas of transformed lymphocytes.

A second classification system, called the Working Formulation of Non-Hodgkin's Lymphomas for Clinical Usage, resulted from a National Cancer Institute international cooperative study. It divides lymphomas by their clinical prognosis into low grade, intermediate grade, and high grade and is based upon the following relations between histopathology and rate of disease progress:

1. Lymphomas with a follicular architecture usually have a more indolent course than lymphomas of the same cell type with a diffuse architectural pattern.
2. Lymphomas of small, dormant-appearing lymphocytes and lymphomas of small cleaved follicular center cells have a low proliferative rate and slow course, whereas lymphomas of large cells are lymphomas of proliferating cells with a more aggressive course.
3. Lymphomas of small lymphocytes with blast-like features and lymphomas of small non-cleaved transformed follicular center cells have a high rate of proliferation and a rapidly progressive course.

A partial, simplified version of the Working Formulation is summarized in Table 18-2; a complete description is found in the reference listed in *Selected Reading.*

A third classification system, that of Lukes and Collins, integrates morphologic and immunologic observations. It divides lymphomas into those of B and T cell origin, and relates lymphomas to stages of transformation of their normal cell counterparts. It stemmed from an early appreciation that lymphomas of follicular center cells, whether

Table 18-2. An Abbreviated Version of the Working Formulation of Non-Hodgkin's Lymphoma

LOW GRADE

ML*, Small lymphocytic
    Consistent with CLL⁺
    Plasmacytoid
ML, Follicular
    Small cleaved cell
    Mixed small cleaved and large cell

INTERMEDIATE GRADE

ML, Follicular
    Large cell
ML, Diffuse
    Small cleaved cell
    Mixed small and large cell
    Large cell

HIGH GRADE

ML, Large cell, immunoblastic
ML, Small non-cleaved cell (Burkitt's or Burkitt-like)
ML, Lymphoblastic

*Malignant lymphoma
⁺Chronic lymphocytic leukemia

of follicular or diffuse architecture, are B cell lymphomas. The Lukes-Collins classification is summarized in Table 18-3.

CLINICAL EVALUATION OF THE PATIENT WITH LYMPHOMA

When a pathologic diagnosis of non-Hodgkin's lymphoma has been made, one must establish the extent of the patient's disease. This provides the added information needed:

1. To predict prognosis. For any given pathologic type, patients with limited disease will usually have a better prognosis than patients with extensive disseminated disease.
2. To plan therapy and to assess its effect.

The tests performed commonly include the following:

1. A blood count, including a platelet count.
2. Bone marrow biopsy at two sites to look for evidence of bone marrow involvement.
3. A blood chemistry panel to include screening tests of liver and renal function and measurement of serum lactic acid dehydrogenase (LDH). Liver and renal function tests are needed, not only to look for evidence of involvement of these organs, but for planning therapy. (For example, one reduces the dose of doxorubicin in patients with hepatocellular disease and should not give high-dose methotrexate to patients with impaired creatinine clearance.) The serum level of LDH is an indicator of extent of disease in patients with intermediate- and high-grade lymphomas.
4. Chest radiographs.

Table 18-3. Lukes-Collins Functional Classification of Lymphomas

I. B CELL

Small lymphocytic (chronic lymphocytic leukemia related)
Plasmacytoid lymphocytic
Follicular center cell (FCC) types

Follicular architecture	Diffuse architecture
Small cleaved cell	Small cleaved cell*
Large cleaved cell	Large cleaved cell
Large non-cleaved cell*	Large non-cleaved cell
—	Small non-cleaved cell (Burkitt's and non-Burkitt types)

Immunoblastic sarcoma (B)

II. T CELL

Small lymphocytic[+]
Convoluted cell (related to T cell acute lymphoblastic leukemia)
Cerebriform cell (mycosis fungoides, Sézary syndrome)
Lymphoepithelioid lymphocytic lymphoma (Lennert's)
Immunoblastic sarcoma (T)

III. HISTIOCYTIC*

---

*Rare
[+]Probably a heterogenous group, including a Tγ cell leukemia related type

5. Abdominal CT scan for evaluation of the retroperitoneum, particularly retroperitoneal lymphadenopathy that could obstruct the ureters.

Additional tests that are sometimes indicated include:

1. Lumbar puncture to look for evidence of CNS involvement in all patients with lymphoblastic lymphoma or small non-cleaved follicular center cell lymphoma and in patients with diffuse large cell lymphoma who have evidence of bone marrow involvement (and, therefore, a high risk for CNS involvement).
2. Gastrointestinal radiographs in patients with gastrointestinal symptoms or in whom occult blood is found on examination of the stool.
3. Isotopic bone scan in patients with bone pain.
4. Serum protein electrophoresis in patients with a pathologic diagnosis of plasmacytoid lymphoma who are at risk for complications of hyperviscosity secondary to an elevated plasma level of IgM.

Laparotomy to look for pathologic evidence of abdominal disease, a staging procedure sometimes still used in Hodgkin's disease, is not indicated in non-Hodgkin's lymphoma. A possible exception is a young patient with a diffuse large cell lymphoma localized to a single nodal area (for example, a cervical node) in whom all other studies reveal no evidence of disease spread and in whom intensive, involved field irradiation therapy is being considered as a curative procedure.

MANIFESTATIONS OF SPECIFIC LYMPHOMAS

Low-Grade Lymphomas

These lymphomas consist of:

1. Diffuse lymphomas of small lymphocytes (chronic lymphocytic leukemia-related) or of plasmacytoid lymphocytes. These make up 10 to 15% of non-Hodgkin's lymphomas.
2. Follicular small cleaved cell and mixed small cleaved and large cell lymphomas. These make up about 40% of non-Hodgkin's lymphomas.

Although indolent, low-grade lymphomas are not presently curable. Occasional patients may live for many years, but most patients die of some complication of their disease within 6 to 10 years of its diagnosis. An individual patient's prognosis is determined by:

1. How advanced the disease is at the time of diagnosis.
2. Whether and when the disease evolves into a lymphoma of a higher grade. This happens in at least 50% of patients with a follicular lymphoma.

DIFFUSE SMALL CELL LYMPHOCYTIC LYMPHOMA (CHRONIC LYMPHOCYTIC LEUKEMIA-RELATED)

This is a disorder of older individuals. Its usual presenting manifestation is unexplained peripheral lymphadenopathy in an otherwise asymptomatic patient. A lymph node biopsy reveals a diffuse proliferation of non-cohesive, small, round lymphocytes with inconspicuous nucleoli, clumped chromatin, and scanty cytoplasm (see Fig. 18-1 and Fig. 18-6). The histologic appearance is indistinguishable from what one would find on biopsy of an involved node in a patient with chronic lymphocytic leukemia. The surface marker features of the cells (see Table 17-3) are also indistinguishable. Thus, the disease, which is less common than chronic lymphocytic leukemia, differs from it primarily in the absence of a marked peripheral blood lymphocytosis and extensive involvement of the bone marrow.

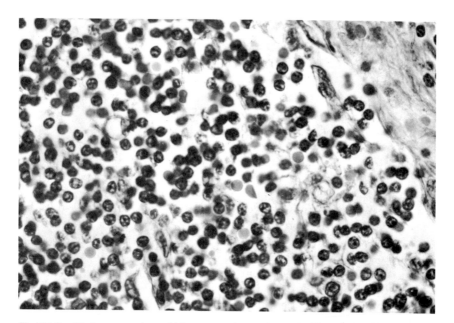

Fig. 18-6. High-power view of biopsy specimen shown in Figure 18-1. Note that the proliferation is made up of small, dormant-appearing lymphocytes with a round nucleus of uniform appearance.

FOLLICULAR SMALL CLEAVED CELL AND MIXED SMALL CLEAVED AND LARGE CELL LYMPHOMAS

These are also lymphomas of older adults (45 to 65 year age range) in which a patient usually presents with evidence of peripheral lymphadenopathy and without systemic symptoms. Occasionally a patient seeks attention because of an abdominal mass due to enlarged mesenteric lymph nodes. Lymph node biopsy (see Fig. 18-2 and Fig. 18-4) reveals a follicular proliferation of either:

1. Small cleaved cells with only a few large non-cleaved cells (follicular small cleaved cell lymphoma), or
2. A mixture of small cleaved cells and from 5 to 15 large non-cleaved cells per high-power field (follicular mixed small cleaved and large cell lymphoma).

The cytologic features of these cells have already been described. *Surface marker analysis* reveals bright staining of the cells (see Fig. 17-8) for surface immunoglobulin of a single light chain type and also staining for CD10 (CALLA). *Cytogenetic study* (not needed for clinical diagnosis) usually discloses a specific karyotypic abnormality, t(14;18), in which a gene, called the *bcl-2* gene, is translocated from chromosome 18 to a site on chromosome 14 where two germ-line gene segments of the heavy chain of immunoglobulin molecules normally combine to generate a productively rearranged heavy chain gene.

Although some patients may initially have lymphadenopathy confined to a single area, the disease is always disseminated. In about three quarters of patients, small areas of paratrabecular (adjacent to a spicule of bone) lymphomatous infiltrates will be found on bone marrow biopsy. In all patients, surface marker studies of peripheral blood lymphocytes will reveal an excess of B-lymphocytes with the same light chain type as that found on the cells of the tissue biopsy. They persist in the circulation after a patient has obtained an apparent complete remission, which fits with the knowledge that essentially all patients eventually relapse. In a few patients, large numbers of lymphocytes with a cleaved nucleus circulate in the blood (see Fig. 17-7), a manifestation referred to as lymphosarcoma cell leukemia.

Initially, one may not treat asymptomatic patients without evidence of bulky peripheral lymphadenopathy, a large abdominal mass, or retroperitoneal lymphadenopathy threatening ureteral obstruction. About one quarter of patients who are just observed spontaneously enter a period of remission. Eventually, however, patients will need treatment, usually because of slowly progressive lymphadenopathy. In one reported study, the median time from diagnosis to beginning treatment was 4 years for patients with small cleaved cell lymphoma but less than 1.5 years for patients with mixed small cleaved and large cell lymphoma.

Patients given a single oral alkylating agent (for example, chlorambucil) have fared as well as patients treated vigorously with total lymphoid irradiation plus combination chemotherapy. Nodes will shrink and most patients will obtain a partial or complete remission that may persist for several years.

A relapse may or may not respond to further treatment with the agents used initially. This depends, at least partly, on whether the disease has evolved into a more aggressive form. A follicular proliferation may convert to a lesion containing residual follicular areas interspersed between areas of diffuse proliferation of large cleaved cells. In about 40% of patients, the disease will transform at some point into a diffuse, large non-cleaved cell lymphoma. The interval between diagnosis and transformation appears independent of whether treatment is initially withheld.

Once follicular lymphoma evolves into a more aggressive disease (in contrast to *de novo* intermediate and high-grade lymphomas, see later), it responds poorly to further chemotherapy. The patient's survival is markedly shortened as compared with the patient in whom transformation has not taken place.

Because of this, a new approach to therapy—treatment with anti-idiotype antibodies—has been explored. The variable region of an immunoglobulin molecule (see Chapter 20) contains an antigen combining site unique for that molecule. This combining site also provides the molecule with an unique antigen profile or *idiotype* to which anti-idiotype antibodies can be raised. Since the cells of follicular lymphomas possess surface immunoglobulin and are of monoclonal origin, it was thought that all of the lymphoma cells of a particular patient should possess an identical, specific surface antigen—the idiotype of their surface immunoglobulin. Anti-idiotype antibodies were therefore prepared from tumor biopsies from individual patients with the hope that they would react with idiotypic antigen on the surface of all of the patient's neoplastic cells and, in so doing, induce a persisting complete remission.

However, in most patients treated to date, only brief, partial remissions have been observed. During the rearrangements of germline gene segments that lead to the formation of functional immunoglobulin chain genes, frame shifts occur in normal B cells that change their idiotypes. This is how normal B cells naturally alter unstable regions (so-called hot spots) in the variable region of the immunoglobulin molecule as they attempt to develop antibodies of increased affinity in response to exposure to antigen. Similar frame shifts apparently occur in the proliferating cells of a B cell lymphoma. Whereas the cells retain a single light chain type and heavy chain class as evidence of their monoclonal ancestry, they are the products of subclones with surface immunoglobulin of different idiotypes. Unfortunately, anti-idiotype antibody therapy will probably require preparation of a panel of antibodies for individual patients, a task curtailing its general use.

Diffuse Large Cell Lymphomas

TYPES

These lymphomas, which are of intermediate- and high-grade aggressiveness, include:

1. Follicular center cell lymphomas of a diffuse architecture without evidence of residual nodularity:
   a. Mixed cell type (a lymphoma made up of large and small cleaved cells and of large non-cleaved cells).
   b. Large cleaved cell.
   c. Large non-cleaved cell (Fig. 18-7).
2. Large cell lymphomas of non-follicular center cell origin
   a. B-immunoblastic sarcoma (Fig. 18-7).
   b. T-immunoblastic sarcoma.
3. Rare true histiocytic lymphoma.

Determining into which category a large cell lymphoma fits is often difficult, and pathologists frequently disagree. Special histochemical stains (for example, methyl green pyronine, nonspecific esterase for the rare histiocytic lymphoma), immunocytochemical stains for cytoplasmic immunoglobulin, and surface marker studies of frozen sections with B and T lineage-specific monoclonal antibodies may all be needed to establish the correct pathologic diagnosis.

MANIFESTATIONS

Most patients are middle aged, but individual patients vary in age from the late teens to the eighth decade. Patients seek help because of:

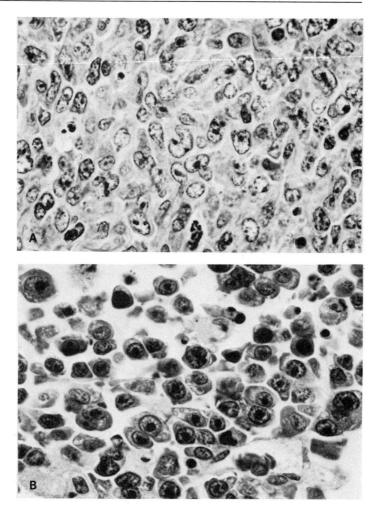

Fig. 18-7. Lymph node biopsy specimens, magnification 800×, stained with hematoxylin and eosin to illustrate the different cytologic features of the cells in two types of large B cell lymphoma: *(A)* a large noncleaved follicular center cell lymphoma and *(B)* a B cell immunoblastic sarcoma. As seen in *A,* the nuclei of the large noncleaved follicular center cells vary in size and shape and have finely dispersed nuclear chromatin with thin nuclear membranes and small nucleoli on or near the nuclear membrane. The cytoplasm is lightly stained, is limited in amount, and lacks plasmacytoid features. As seen in *B,* the nuclei of the B immunoblasts have an accumulation of nuclear chromatin at the nuclear membrane that results in a thickened, prominent nuclear membrane. Nucleoli are large. The cytoplasm is plentiful, is stained densely, and has plasmacytoid features (*e.g.,* in a few cells one can see a clear area [hof], which represents a prominent Golgi complex). (Provided through the generosity of Dr. Robert J. Lukes, Professor of Pathology, University of California at Irvine)

1. Peripheral lymphadenopathy.
2. Constitutional symptoms—weight loss, night sweats, or fever — in about one half of patients.
3. Pain, which is usually abdominal or bone pain.

Occasional patients will give a history of earlier autoimmune or other immunologic disease (for example, chronic thyroiditis, Sjögren's syndrome, chronic urticaria, systemic lupus erythematosus). They will usually be found to have an immunoblastic sarcoma.

Most patients have widespread disease when first seen. Some will have evidence of extranodal disease, for example, a gastrointestinal lesion or bone marrow involvement. An occasional patient may present with a evidence of a pulmonary lesion. Although uncommon on initial examination, CNS disease develops later in about 10% of patients, particularly in patients presenting with bone marrow infiltration.

COURSE AND TREATMENT

Untreated or treated suboptimally, patients with large cell lymphomas succumb much more rapidly to their disease than do patients with the low-grade lymphomas described in the preceding section. However, a substantial percentage of patients with diffuse large cell lymphomas given intensive combined chemotherapy enter a complete remission, which, if maintained for over 2 years, carries only a minimal risk of later relapse. Thus, whereas the goal of treatment of low-grade lymphomas is palliation, the goal of treatment of diffuse large cell lymphomas is cure.

Intensive treatment with multiple drugs is started without delay. The objective is to give the most medication within the shortest time, that is, to kill all of the neoplastic cells before the otherwise inevitable, rapid emergence of drug-resistant subclones. In patients with evidence of widespread tumor (high serum LDH, bone marrow infiltrates), CNS therapy should be added as soon as it is clear that the patient is entering a remission. The intensive chemotherapy inevitably causes toxicity, for example, mucositis, granulocytopenia, dysesthesias, and extremity muscle weakness, but this does not deter one from giving as much chemotherapy as possible without creating an unacceptable risk of death from infection. (Thus, in one current protocol, chemotherapy is deferred only if the granulocyte count falls below 100 per μL.) Patients given such intensive therapy must be watched by physicians thoroughly familiar with its use.

If initial chemotherapy produces a complete remission, one hopes that the patient is cured, but this remains only a hope until a period of at least 2 years has elapsed without evidence of recurrance of disease. If chemotherapy produces only partial or no remission, patients in large reported series have all died within 24 months.

Whether the pathologic type is an important determinant of curability with intensive chemotherapy is not yet known. When less intensive chemotherapy was used, it appears from some studies that patients with lymphoma of large non-cleaved follicular center cells have had a substantially higher percentage of persisting remission than patients with lymphoma of other large cell types. Regardless of cell type, patients in whom a diffuse large cell lymphoma arises *de novo* respond more favorably to chemotherapy than do patients in whom a large cell lymphoma is known to have evolved from a lower grade lymphoma (for example, a B-immunoblastic sarcoma from an earlier plasmacytoid lymphocytic lymphoma or a diffuse large non-cleaved cell lymphoma from a follicular small cleaved cell lymphoma).

Certain clinical findings were related to outcome in patients treated with earlier chemotherapy regimens. A predictive combination of four factors was identified:

1. Sex (males have a worse prognosis than females).
2. The presence or absence of:
   a. Constitutional symptoms.
   b. A large abdominal mass (greater than 10 cm in diameter) that involves the gastrointestinal tract.
   c. Infiltration of the bone marrow.

Other factors were also prognostic indicators, for example, a level of serum LDH above 250 U and the presence of hepatic involvement affected prognosis adversely. However, these findings did not add to the prediction of survival defined from the first four factors.

Small Non-Cleaved Follicular Center Cell Lymphomas

These are high-grade lymphomas of rapidly proliferating cells. They have been divided on the basis of the morphologic appearance of the cells into Burkitt's lymphoma and non-Burkitt's lymphoma type. Their clinical presentation may vary somewhat.

BURKITT'S LYMPHOMA

Burkitt's lymphoma is endemic in tropical Africa; nonendemic, sporadic cases are seen elsewhere throughout the world. Its tumor doubling time of 24 to 48 hours makes it the fastest growing human cancer. Histopathologic examination reveals a diffuse, monotonous-appearing proliferation of cells growing in a cohesive pattern with interspersed histiocytes that produce a "starry sky" appearance (see Fig. 18-5). The cells have small, uniform nuclei containing finely dispersed chromatin and one to three small nucleoli. On Wright's stained lymph node imprints or marrow aspirate smears, the cells have a nucleus with reticular chromatin and well-defined nucleoli and cytoplasm that is deeply basophilic and contains multiple vacuoles. (This is the morphology of the rare L3 cell type of acute lymphoblastic leukemia, which is the leukemic form of Burkitt's lymphoma.)

Marker studies confirm that the cells are transformed B cells. Thus, despite their primitive morphologic appearance, they possess monoclonal surface immunoglobulin and do not contain TdT, which is present in lymphoblasts before their processing into B or T cells. As discussed in Chapter 15, the cells possess a characteristic karyotypic finding—a translocation involving the c-*myc* locus on chromosome 8 and a structural gene locus for an immunoglobulin chain, which, depending upon the chain, may involve chromosomes 2, 14, or 22.

An unexplained link exists between the African form of Burkitt's lymphoma and Epstein-Barr (EB) viral infection (see Chapter 21). African patients have high titers of EB viral antibodies and their tumor cells contain multiple copies of the EB viral genome. The polyclonal expansion of B cells that follows EB viral infection somehow appears to set the stage for emergence of a malignant clone of transformed B-lymphocytes. In contrast, an association with EB viral infection has not been found in nonendemic Burkitt's lymphoma. (Patients with AIDS or AIDS-related disease who develop small non-cleaved cell lymphoma of either Burkitt's or non-Burkitt's type are an exception in that copies of the EB viral genome have been detected in the lymphoma cells of some of these patients.)

Burkitt's lymphoma produces large, extranodal tumors. In about 50% of African patients, the disease presents as a massive tumor of the jaw in a small child. In the United States, the disease most often presents in children or young adults as an intra-abdominal tumor arising in the wall of the terminal ileum or in mesenteric lymph nodes. Sometimes the kidneys or ovaries are involved. The tumor spreads to the bone marrow in up to one quarter of patients, but the cells rarely circulate since their growth in a cohesive pattern impedes their release into the circulation. Patients usually do not present with CNS involvment; however, the CNS is frequently involved in patients who relapse after chemotherapy.

When a large abdominal mass is found at surgery, as much of the tumor as possible is removed; the less left, the greater the chance that chemotherapy can kill all remaining tumor cells. Because of the tumor's rapid doubling time, multiagent chemotherapy should be started quickly. However, one must be certain first that renal function is adequate to excrete the large amounts of uric acid, potassium, and phosphorous that will be liberated from the tumor cells, which are initially exquisitely sensitive to chemotherapy. The patient is given large amounts of intravenous fluids, sodium bicarbonate to make the urine alkaline, a diuretic at times, and allopurinol.

Two-year disease-free survival (tantamount to cure in such a fast-growing tumor) varies from close to 90% for patients with disease in a single extra-abdominal site to less than 20% for patients with a large intra-abdominal tumor and also involvement of multiple extra-abdominal sites.

NON-BURKITT'S TYPE

This form of small non-cleaved follicular center cell lymphoma differs in histologic appearance from Burkitt's lymphoma in that the proliferating cells have more nuclear variation and prominent nucleoli. Moreover, in the past, the patients usually have been middle-aged adults who have presented with nodal rather than extranodal disease. However, most of the increasing number of new patients with small non-cleaved follicular center cell lymphoma being seen today have developed lymphoma in the setting of infection with HTLV-III (see Chapter 21). In these patients, regardless of whether the tumor has the histologic appearance of Burkitt's lymphoma or of non-Burkitt's lymphoma, the disease presents at extranodal sites.

Principles of therapy are the same as for patients with Burkitt's lymphoma. The prognosis for patients with underlying HTLV-III infection has been dismal.

Lymphoblastic Lymphoma

Lymphoblastic lymphoma (convoluted T cell lymphoma) is a high-grade lymphoma of older children or young adults. It differs from the other non-Hodgkin's lymphomas in that the malignant cell is not the neoplastic counterpart of a differentiated lymphocyte that has then undergone transformation but is the neoplastic counterpart of a lymphoblast that is evolving into a T cell. Thus, it is closely related to acute T cell lymphoblastic leukemia (see Chapter 17). When lymphoblastic lymphoma spreads to the marrow, as it often quickly does, the disease may be indistinguishable from a form of acute T cell lymphoblastic leukemia in which a patient is first seen with a high circulating lymphoblast count, diffusely infiltrated marrow, a mediastinal mass, and often, bulky lymphadenopathy and splenomegaly.

Pathologic examination reveals a diffuse proliferative process that often invades surrounding tissue. Interspersed, phagocytic reactive histiocytes may create a "starry sky" appearance as in Burkitt's lymphoma. However, unlike Burkitt's lymphoma, the cells proliferate in a noncohesive pattern and vary in size and nuclear configuration. The nucleus may be round or lobulated with finely dispersed chromatin, inconspicuous nucleoli, and fine linear subdivisions. In many patients, deep linear indentations give the nucleus a convoluted appearance (Hence, one name for the disease—convoluted T cell lymphoma). The cells have a surface marker pattern of early thymic pre-T cells.

In 50% to 75% of patients, the disease presents with symptoms or signs caused by a mediastinal mass. These may be emergent due to compression of intrathoracic structures (for example, superior vena caval syndrome) or to pericardial effusion secondary to spread of the lymphoma to the pericardium. A high proportion of patients will have evidence of marrow involvement at presentation in either a focal or diffuse pattern. If the latter, the WBC count will be high due to circulating lymphoblasts of either L1 or L2 morphology (see Chapter 17) and, as already mentioned, the disease may be called, not lymphoblastic lymphoma, but acute T cell lymphoblastic leukemia. CNS involvement is usually not present initially but will develop in about one third of patients not given CNS prophylactic therapy.

The neoplastic cells are usually sensitive to chemotherapy and, as with Burkitt's lymphoma, one must make sure that the patient has a urinary output sufficient to excrete the products of tumor cell lysis. Treatment must be aggressive with multiple drugs and early prophylactic CNS therapy. In one regimen, patients have been treated initially with cyclophosphamide, doxorubicin, vincristine, and prednisone; then they receive L-asparaginase and also high-dose intravenous methotrexate, which with additional intrathecal methotrexate, provides CNS prophylaxis; and then they are given a long course of further treatment with 6-mercaptopurine and methotrexate.

Even with intensive chemotherapy, many patients relapse and die of their disease.

MANIFESTATIONS OF EXTRANODAL LYMPHOMAS

Lymphoma presenting at extranodal sites is becoming more common because the lymphoma that develops in patients with acquired disorders impairing immune function usually presents in this way. Thus, the high-grade B cell lymphomas seen with increasing frequency in homosexual patients with evidence of HTLV-III infection (see Chapter 21) commonly involve the brain, gastrointestinal tract, mucocutaneous sites, and the bone marrow. Lymphoma developing in patients receiving immunosuppressive drugs after renal or cardiac transplant have usually been B-immunoblastic sarcomas of the CNS. In addition, lymphoma may arise in extranodal tissues subjected to chronic immune stimulation, for example, in the thyroid gland of a patient with chronic thyroiditis or in the wall of the jejunem of a patient with long-standing celiac disease (gluten-induced enteropathy). Specific extranodal lymphomas are described further below.

Cutaneous T Cell Lymphomas

The cutaneous T cell lymphomas—mycosis fungoides and Sézary's syndrome—have been initially discussed in Chapter 17 in relation to T cell leukemias. Although mycosis fungoides and Sézary's syndrome differ in their clinical manifestations, they are thought to be variants of the same proliferative disorder of a CD4 (T4) positive T-lymphocyte with a tropism for skin. Mycosis fungoides, in particular, may appear initially confined to the skin, but in both, visceral disease eventually becomes overt, and most patients eventually succumb to some complication of visceral disease. Unlike the rapidly fatal disorder, adult T cell leukemia, which also involves the skin, infection with HTLV-I cannot be demonstrated in patients with mycosis fungoides or Sézary's syndrome.

MYCOSIS FUNGOIDES

Mycosis fungoides is a slowly progressive, proliferative disorder whose first manifestation may be a nonspecific, scaling, itching erythematous eruption, indistinguishable in clinical appearance or on biopsy from an inflammatory dermatosis. This stage is followed after months to several years by the development of characteristic, indurated plaques. Biopsy of an indurated plaque reveals an infiltrate with these diagnostic features:

1. *Distribution*: in the upper dermis in a band hugging the basement membrane of the epidermis and, in areas, infiltrating the epidermis to form small aggregates called Pautrier's abscesses.
2. *Composition*: polymorphous, consisting of a mixture of lymphocytes, plasma cells, histiocytes, and eosinophils.
3. *Characteristic abnormal cells*: a scattering of large cells with dark, hyperchromatic nuclei (so-called mycosis cells) plus small clusters of atypical lymphocytes with highly convoluted nuclei containing overlapping folds and deep clefts (cerebriform cells).

As mycosis fungoides progresses, nodules and fungating tumors develop in the skin. These ulcerate, become infected, and may give rise to episodes of life-threatening staphylococcal septicemia. By this time, visceral involvement is evident in lymph nodes and often in other organs such as the spleen, lung, bone marrow, liver, and myocardium.

Electron beam radiotherapy is often used as an initial treatment for mycosis fungoides because high doses of radiation can be directed to the skin alone. Long remissions may follow electron beam therapy. The alkylating agent, nitrogen mustard, has also been applied topically to control disease in the skin. Patients with evidence of visceral disease are treated with systemic chemotherapy.

SÉZARY'S SYNDROME

Sézary's syndrome is a more aggressive disorder characterized by:

1. A diffuse, intensely itching, erythematous, exfoliative erythroderma.
2. Peripheral lymphadenopathy, in which one can often demonstrate paracortical infiltrates of atypical, cerebriform neoplastic lymphocytes. With early nodal involvement, biopsy of an enlarged node may be reported as showing only dermatopathic changes, but DNA hybridization techniques (see Chapter 15) will demonstrate an expanded monoclonal population of T cells in the node.
3. Sézary cells with a typical cerebriform nucleus in the peripheral blood (see Fig. 17-12).

Skin biopsy is similar to that of mycosis fungoides, but clusters of atypical cerebriform lymphocytes may be more prominent.

Management usually requires systemic chemotherapy. New approaches to therapy currently being evaluated include the use of interferon, deoxycoformycin, and monoclonal anti-T cell antibodies.

Primary Splenic Lymphoma

A few patients are seen in whom lymphoma appears to arise in the spleen or in whom neoplastic cells arising elsewhere home to and preferentially proliferate in the spleen. Such patients, who are said to have primary splenic lymphoma, exhibit the following disease manifestations:

1. A very large spleen without accompanying peripheral lymphadenopathy.
2. A peripheral blood count that is often normal. When abnormal, the WBC count, platelet count, or both may be moderately depressed or a modest lymphocytosis may be present.
3. A bone marrow biopsy that may be either normal or show lymphocytic infiltrates.
4. Evidence, often from biopsy material obtained at the time of splenectomy of:
   a. Accumulations of lymphocytes in portal areas of the liver indicative of some degree of liver involvement.
   b. At least microscopic involvement by lymphoma of splenic hilar or retroperitoneal lymph nodes.

Splenectomy may be followed by a long period of remission or smoldering disease. In about one half of the patients, the splenic pathology will be that of a diffuse, small lymphocytic lymphoma, with a monotonous proliferation of dormant-appearing small lymphocytes involving all of the malpighian bodies of the white pulp. Patients with this diagnosis appear to have the best prognosis for long-term survival. A substantial proportion of the remaining patients will have a diffuse large cell lymphoma of one pathologic type or another, and many of these patients will die of their disease within several years of the time of diagnosis.

The presenting manifestations of hairy cell leukemia (see Chapter 17) may closely resemble those of a primary splenic lymphoma. However, one can distinguish hairy cell leukemia by the characteristic morphologic appearance of proliferating hairy cells in a bone marrow biopsy (see Fig. 17-9) or in the spleen. Rare patients may also be seen with an unusual form of plasmacytoid lymphocytic leukemia in which massive splenomegaly out of proportion to increased numbers of circulating plasmacytoid lymphocytes causes the disease to resemble primary splenic lymphoma.

Gastric Lymphoma

Lymphoma arising in the stomach is seen primarily in patients over the age of 50 years. Pathologic examination of resected stomach tissue reveals that the lymphoma often arises on a background of chronic gastritis with lymphoid hyperplasia. The lymphomatous proliferation is almost always diffuse lymphoma of a large cell type. Occasionally, large cells of different pathologic types have been seen in histologic sections prepared from different portions of the same tumor. With rare exceptions, gastric lymphomas are B cell lymphomas.

Patients usually complain of pain, vomiting, or gastrointestinal bleeding. Upper gastrointestinal radiographic examination will reveal a mass lesion that often resembles gastric carcinoma. The diagnosis of lymphoma can usually be established by endoscopic biopsy. Treatment is by surgery, followed by irradiation therapy or, in some older patients, by irradiation therapy alone.

Over 50% of patients will be alive 5 years after diagnosis. Prognosis appears to be more related to the extent of the lymphoma at the time of diagnosis than to its pathologic type. Invasion of the muscular layer of the stomach wall, a large tumor mass, or spread to regional lymph nodes are adverse prognostic findings.

Intestinal Lymphoma

Most patients with intestinal lymphoma in western countries present with findings of abdominal pain, intestinal obstruction, or gastrointestinal bleeding. The lymphoma usually arises in follicles in the wall of the distal ileum (Peyer's patches) and is a B cell lymphoma of the diffuse large cell or small non-cleaved cell (Burkitt-like) type. In unusual patients, who will have a history of chronic diarrhea and malabsorption, lymphoma develops on the background of adult celiac disease (gluten-sensitive enteropathy). Then, it will arise in the wall of the upper small intestine.

Often the diagnosis of small bowel lymphoma is made at the time of surgery for findings of an acute abdomen. As already mentioned, as much tumor as possible should be removed at surgery. Intensive multiple drug chemotherapy is indicated and with a minimum of postoperative delay.

In countries of the Mediterranean basin, a form of intestinal lymphoma has been seen in young Arabs or Sephardic Jews in a setting of steatorrhea, abdominal pain, and weight loss secondary to a chronic immunoproliferative small-intestinal disease of unknown cause. Some of the patients have an elevated level of a fragment of the heavy chain of IgA in the serum (and their disease is then sometimes referred to as α heavy chain disease). A jejunal biopsy reveals a dense infiltrate of normal-appearing plasma cells in the lamina propria. When intestinal lymphoma is superimposed upon this background, tumor masses of B-immunoblasts are found in the deeper layers of the jejunal wall and sometimes in the mesentery.

Lymphoma-Related Pulmonary Lesions

Pulmonary lesions are commonly found at autopsy in patients with advanced, widespread lymphoma. Unusual patients are also seen who have a primary pulmonary lesion that is either a prelymphomatous disorder or atypical lymphoma. Two entitites have been delineated— lymphoid interstitial pneumonitis and lymphomatoid granulomatosis.

LYMPHOID INTERSTITIAL PNEUMONITIS

This disorder affects patients over a wide age range and affects women more commonly than men. Patients complain of cough, dyspnea, and weight loss and sometimes of low-grade fever and pleuritic chest pain. An occasional patient also has Sjögren's syndrome (parotid and lacrimal gland enlargement due to intense infiltration with lymphocytes, associated with a dry mouth and dry eyes) or rheumatoid arthritis.

Basilar rales are heard at the lung bases, but the physical examination may be otherwise unremarkable. Chest radiographs usually show basilar infiltrates, which may be coarsely linear or nodular. Some patients have had hypergammaglobulinemia on serum protein electrophoresis; others have had hypogammaglobulinemia.

A diffuse interstitial infiltrate of mature lymphocytes and plasma cells is seen on lung biopsy. The infiltrate distends the interalveolar septa, at times forming small nodules within the septa. A rare patient has also had a pulmonary mass or enlarged hilar lymph nodes at presentation, which on biopsy contain unequivocable lymphoma. What proportion of the remaining patients would eventually develop lymphoma is not clear, since many patients, particularly older patients, have died within a few months of respiratory failure secondary to a progressive diffuse interstitial fibrosis. Patients have been treated with adrenal steroids and some have also been given cyclophospham-ide with variable benefit.

LYMPHOMATOID GRANULOMATOSIS

This disorder, which also occurs over a wide age range, differs both clinically and pathologically from lymphoid interstitial pneu-monitis. Patients are often quite ill when first seen with pulmonary complaints and fever. Up to one half may have skin lesions consisting of an erythematous rash or subcutaneous, painful erythematous nod-ules that resemble erythema nodosum but are located mainly on the trunk rather than the legs. Occasional patients have CNS findings suggestive of a mass lesion, for example, seizures, ataxia, mental confusion, or cranial nerve signs. A few patients may have peripheral lymphadenopathy or splenomegaly when first seen.

Chest radiography reveals multiple nodular lesions, usually bi-lateral, that can look like metastatic tumor to the lungs. Patients with CNS complaints may have evidence of a mass lesion on CT scanning.

Lung biopsy reveals a polymorphous proliferation of lympho-cytes, plasma cells, histiocytes, and atypical mononuclear cells. How-ever, in contrast to lymphocytic interstitial pneumonitis, the infiltrates are centered around small pulmonary vessels whose walls are invaded and destroyed. The infiltrates also spread out from the vessels to involve the pulmonary parenchyma and may be associated with areas of necrosis and fibroblastic reaction. Lesions of similar histologic appearance may be found in extrapulmonary sites, for example, in a skin biopsy or a biopsy of a mass lesion in the brain.

If not treated, the disease transforms in most patients into a clearly recognizable lymphoma within months to several years. In-deed, some pathologists believe that the disease is a lymphoma from the outset, masked by an associated inflammatory reaction. A sub-stantial number of patients treated with long-term corticosteroids and cyclophosphamide have been reported to obtain a long-lasting remis-sion.

HISTIOCYTIC MEDULLARY RETICULOSIS

Histiocytic medullary reticulosis is a true histiocytic neoplasm. Its onset may mimic an acute infection with sudden high fever and variable systemic complaints referable to proliferation of histiocytes in several organs. Lymphadenopathy, hepatomegaly, and splenomegaly are common findings but need not be prominent when the patient is first seen. Some patients develop a rash caused by the proliferation of histiocytes in the skin. Most patients become anemic rapidly. The anemia stems in large part from hemolysis caused by erythrophagocytosis by histiocytes proliferating in the sinusoids of the liver and spleen. Jaundice may develop because of the inability of an infiltrated liver to clear the increased bilirubin load resulting from hemolysis. Leukopenia and thrombocytopenia are common. Occasionally, atypical histiocytes are seen on peripheral blood smears; the same cells are seen more frequently on bone marrow smears. However, a frankly leukemic bone marrow—with an overwhelming infiltration of histiocytes replacing the normal marrow elements—is not found.

A lymph node biopsy reveals a proliferation of histiocytes that permeates the stroma but does not give rise to cohesive sheets of histiocytes. The histiocytes have a tendency to proliferate within sinusoids, forming small aggregates that resemble nests of tumor cells. These intrasinusoidal histiocytes often exhibit erythrophagocytosis. Occasional histiocytes may be seen that resemble Reed-Sternberg cells.

Temporary remissions may be obtained with multiagent chemotherapy, but many patients die within 6 months of the onset of symptoms. Accumulations of histiocytes are found in many organs at autopsy.

IMMUNOBLASTIC LYMPHADENOPATHY

Immunoblastic (angioimmunoblastic) lymphadenopathy is a systemic disease of unknown cause characterized by both hyperimmune responsiveness of the B cell system and an impaired resistance to infection. Although the pathologic features are not those of a neoplasm, the disease has a malignant clinical course. Many patient die within 2 years of disease onset, often of infection. In some patients, the disease evolves into B-immunoblastic sarcoma.

Pathologic Diagnosis

On lymph node biopsy (Fig. 18-8), one finds that the normal architecture of the node is obliterated by a diffuse process with the following features:

1. A prominent immunoblastic proliferation with immunoblasts, plasma cells, and cells intermediate between the two.

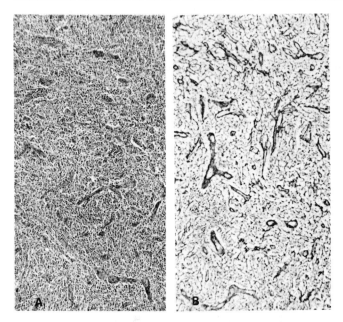

Fig. 18-8. Low-power view of a lymph node biopsy in immunoblastic lymphadenopathy (angioimmunoblastic lymphadenopathy) to show the proliferation of small arborizing vessels characteristic of the lesion. *(A)* Hematoxylin and eosin stain; *(B)* reticulum stain. (Lukes RJ, Tindle BH: Immunoblastic lymphadenopathy. A hyperimmune entity resembling Hodgkin's disease. N Engl J Med 292:1, 1975; reproduced by permission of the New England Journal of Medicine)

2. A proliferation of small arborizing vessels.
3. The presence of an eosinophilic, amorphous interstitial material diffusely distributed throughout the node.

This triad of findings is diagnostic of immunoblastic lymphadenopathy.

In some instances, histiocytes may also be a prominent component of the lesion. This, plus increased numbers of eosinophils may give the lesion a mixed histologic appearance resembling mixed cellularity Hodgkin's disease, with which immunoblastic lymphadenopathy has at times been confused in the past.

Clinical Manifestations

The disease may begin suddenly with large peripheral lymph nodes developing over several days. In some patients, a hypersensitivity response to an allergen, usually a drug, seems to precipitate the disease. Lymphadenopathy may be regional, for example, confined to cervical nodes, but in most patients is generalized. Systemic symptoms accompany the lymphadenopathy—fever, sweats, and weight loss. Many patients also develop a generalized, itching maculopapular rash. A few develop a migratory polyarthritis. Hepatomegaly and splenomegaly are found on physical examination in some but not all patients.

The following laboratory findings are usually present:

1. Polyclonal hypergammaglobulinemia on serum protein electrophoresis (virtually all patients).
2. A positive Coombs' test (over 50% of patients).
3. Smooth muscle antibodies (about 75% of patients). The antibodies appear to be specific for a polypeptide of intermediate filaments of mesenchymal cell cytoskeleton called vimentin.

The WBC count may be elevated, with a decreased percentage of lymphocytes on the differential count but with occasional activated and plasmatoid lymphocytes seen on the blood smear. The absolute number of circulating T cells is reduced.

Course and Treatment

Although a rare patient has obtained a spontaneous remission, the disease usually worsens in an untreated patient. Administering prednisone alone may cause the lymph nodes to diminish but rarely induces a complete remission. A number of patients have now been treated with drug combinations containing prednisone, cyclophosphamide, vincristine, and sometimes other agents. If such therapy fails to induce a remission, the patient will usually die within 1 year. If such therapy induces a remission, it may persist for months to several years, but eventually, most patients will relapse. At that time, the disease may have changed from immunoblastic lymphadenopathy to B-immunoblastic sarcoma.

SELECTED READING

1. Coleman M: Editorial. Chemotherapy for large-cell lymphoma: optimism and caution. Ann Intern Med 103:140, 1985.
2. Cullen MH, Stansfeld AG, Oliver RTD, Lister TA, and Malpas JS: Angioimmunoblastic lymphadenopathy: report of ten cases and review of the literature. Q J Med 48:151, 1979.
3. Fisher RI, Hubbard SM, DeVita VT, Berard CW, Wesley R, Cossman J,

Young RC: Factors predicting long-term survival in diffuse mixed, histiocytic, or undifferentiated lymphoma. Blood 58:45, 1981.

4. Horning SJ, and Rosenberg SA: The natural history of initially untreated low-grade non-Hodgkin's lymphomas. N Engl J Med 311:1471, 1984.

5. Levine AM, Taylor CR, Schneider DR, Koehler SC, Forman SJ, Lichtenstein A, Lukes RJ, Feinstein DI: Immunoblastic sarcoma of T-cell versus B-cell origin: I. Clinical features. Blood 58:52, 1981.

6. Lukes RJ: The immunologic approach to the pathology of malignant lymphomas. Am J Clin Pathol 72:657, 1979.

7. Lukes RJ, and Tindle BH: Immunoblastic lymphadenopathy. A hyperimmune entity resembling Hodgkin's disease. N Engl J Med 292:1, 1975.

8. Raffeld M, Necker L, Longo DL, and Cossman J: Spontaneous alteration of idiotype in a monoclonal B-cell lymphoma. Escape from detection by anti-idiotype. N Engl J Med 312:1653, 1985.

9. Rosen PJ, Feinstein DI, Pattengale PK, Tindle BH, Williams AH, Cain MJ, Bonorris JB, Parker JW, Lukes RJ: Convoluted lymphocytic lymphoma in adults. A clinicopathologic entity. Ann Intern Med 89:319, 1978.

10. The Non-Hodgkins Lymphoma Pathologic Classification Project. National Cancer Institute sponsored study of classification of non-Hodgkin's lymphoma: summary and description of a working formulation for clinical usage. Cancer 49:2112, 1982.

11. Ziegler JL: Burkitt's lymphoma. N Engl J Med 305:735, 1981.

19

Hodgkin's Disease

HISTOPATHOLOGY

The histopathology of Hodgkin's disease differs fundamentally from that of the non-Hodgkin's lymphomas. In the latter, the cell type characterizing the lymphoma predominates and often totally obliterates the normal architecture of a lymph node (see Fig. 18-1). In contrast, in Hodgkin's disease, the Reed-Sternberg cell and its neoplastic mononuclear precursors rarely predominate on the biopsy section and, indeed, are sometimes hard to find. The histologic features of the biopsy vary widely and reflect the ability of the patient to combat the neoplastic proliferation. Only when host resistance fails may a biopsy reveal large clusters of Reed-Sternberg cells and neoplastic mononuclear cells.

The Reed-Sternberg Cell

The diagnostic cell of Hodgkin's disease—the Reed-Sternberg cell—fulfills two morphologic criteria (Fig. 19-1):

1. It is multinucleated, sometimes with mirror-image nuclei.
2. Each of its nuclei contains a giant nucleolus resembling an inclusion body.

As already mentioned, mononuclear cells with neoplastic features are also present in Hodgkin's disease and are considered precursors of the Reed-Sternberg cell. They are sometimes referred to as pre-Sternberg or Hodgkin cells. These mononuclear cells—which will incorporate large amounts of tritiated thymidine into the nucleus and,

345

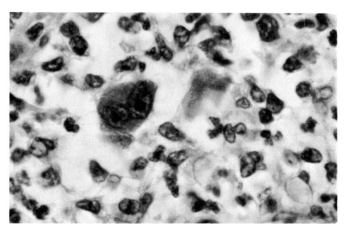

Fig. 19-1. High-power view of a typical Reed–Sternberg cell with mirror-image nuclei, each of which contains a giant nucleolus.

therefore, are actively making DNA—may be the major replicating neoplastic cell of Hodgkin's disease. However, their morphologic features are not distinctive enough to permit a diagnosis of Hodgkin's disease to be made reliably in the absence of typical Reed-Sternberg cells.

Much evidence suggests that the neoplastic cells of Hodgkin's disease are of monocyte-macrophage lineage. They may represent neoplastic transformation of a monocyte-derived cell found in the T cell region of lymph nodes, the interdigitating or dendritic reticulum cell whose normal function is to "present" antigens to T-lymphocytes (see Chapter 14).

Histologic Classification

Since histopathology reflects host resistance and, consequently, prognosis (Fig. 19-2), a pathologic diagnosis of Hodgkin's disease must include an evaluation of the histology of the lesion. A histologic classification, known as the Rye classification (adopted after a conference on Hodgkin's disease at Rye, New York, in 1966), divides Hodgkin's disease into four categories:

1. *Lymphocyte predominance.* Biopsy reveals lymphocytic proliferation plus a variable degree of reactive histiocytic proliferation. Little or no necrosis or fibrosis is seen. Reed-Sternberg cells are infrequent and may sometimes be found only after a

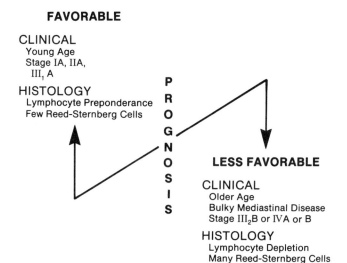

Fig. 19-2.   Relationship of histologic and clinical characteristics to prognosis.

careful search. This pattern (which is most commonly found in a young male patient with localized, high cervical disease) is indicative of strong host resistance and is associated with a good prognosis.

2. *Mixed cellularity.* Biopsy discloses a polymorphous lesion characterized by variable numbers of lymphocytes and reactive histiocytes; by neutrophils, eosinophils, and plasma cells; and by small foci of necrosis and slight to moderate fibrosis which is disorderly and without collagen formation. Reed-Sternberg cells are present in variable numbers but are usually readily apparent. The mixed cellularity pattern, with its combination of a beginning loss of the lymphocyte population of a node plus features of an inflammatory response, is indicative of an intermediate degree of host resistance.

3. *Lymphocyte depletion.* Biopsy reveals that the normal cellular elements of the lymph node have been replaced by loosely cellular, fibrillar connective tissue, disorderly in distribution and without collagen formation. Areas of focal necrosis are seen. Only scattered residual islands of lymphocytes can be found. Reed-Sternberg cells are usually numerous and sometimes are present in clusters. The lymphocyte depletion pattern means that host resistance has broken down and is associated with the least favorable prognosis.

4. *Nodular sclerosis.* This variant of Hodgkin's disease—which is most often seen in younger patients and is twice as frequent in women as in men—usually arises in lymph nodes of the upper mediastinum or cervical region. It is characterized by nodules of lymphoid tissue separated by orderly bands of collagenous connective tissue. On low power (Fig. 19-3), many cells are seen to be within what look like clear spaces. On high power (Fig. 19-4), these cells are found to be large, atypical cells with a prominent nucleolus and cytoplasm artifactually shrunken by formalin fixation to give the appearance of a cell sitting within a clear space. These so-called lacunar cells are considered the diagnostic equivalent of Reed-Sternberg cells. Typical Reed-Sternberg cells (contrast Fig. 19-1 with Fig. 19-4) may be difficult or impossible to find, and, in this exception, a diagnosis of Hodgkin's disease can be made in their absence.

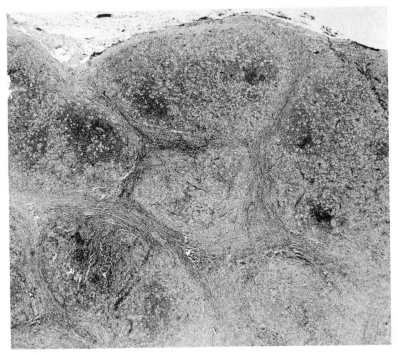

Fig. 19-3. Low-power view of a lymph node biopsy showing nodular sclerosis. Wide bands of collagenous connective tissue separate the nodules of lymphoid tissue. Even at this magnification, cells within clear spaces, or lacunas, can be recognized.

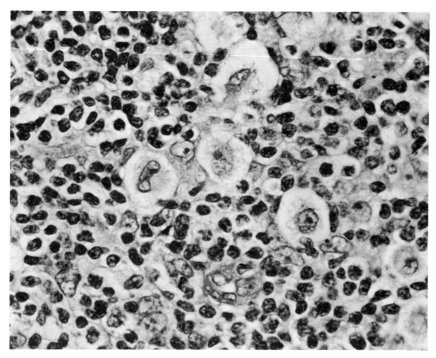

Fig. 19-4. High-power view of the biopsy shown in Figure 19-3. Note characteristics of the variant cells found in lacunas (lacunar cells) in nodular sclerosis.

Nodular sclerosis can be divided according to cellular composition into lymphocyte predominance, mixed cellularity, and lymphocyte depletion subtypes. These cellular patterns appear to have the same relevance for prognosis in nodular sclerosis Hodgkin's disease as they have in non-nodular sclerosis Hodgkin's disease, that is, a good prognosis for lymphocyte preponderance, an intermediate prognosis for mixed cellularity, and a least favorable prognosis for the lymphocyte depletion subtype.

ORIGIN AND SPREAD

In the 1960s and 1970s, large numbers of patients were subjected to careful clinical evaluation followed by a laparotomy to delineate further the extent and distribution of abdominal disease. This provided important information on the origin and spread of Hodgkin's disease. It appears that:

1. Hodgkin's disease arises in a *single* anatomic focus.
2. The disease begins in lymph nodes in over 90% of patients.
3. When the disease begins above the diaphragm, it remains confined to lymph nodes for a variable period, spreading from the original site to lymph nodes in other areas in predictable patterns:
   a. Nodular sclerosis spreads by direct contiguity to adjacent lymph nodes. For example, a lesion arising in the mediastinum will spread first to nodes in the lower neck and to nodes in the upper retroperitoneal area.
   b. The other histologic types may also spread by contiguity, but many lesions first noted in the neck skip the mediastinum and spread, possibly by retrograde flow in the thoracic duct, to upper retroperitoneal nodes. (It is also possible that the disease begins in the upper retroperitoneum but does not become apparent until it spreads to the neck.)
3. Disease spreads to extranodal sites by two processes:
   a. Direct extension, for example, from enlarged hilar lymph nodes to the lungs.
   b. Vascular invasion, which can then result in hematogenous dissemination.
4. Hodgkin's disease in the spleen represents evidence of hematogenous dissemination, and its discovery raises the possibility of hematogenous dissemination to other organs, such as the liver and bone marrow. Conversely, the absence of disease in the spleen makes disseminated disease in other organs unlikely.
5. When the disease begins below the diaphragm, it frequently has spread by hematogenous dissemination to extralymphoid sites by the time the diagnosis is made.

IMMUNOLOGIC ABNORMALITIES

Patients with Hodgkin's disease have evidence of defective cell-mediated immunity. Even in early, localized disease one can demonstrate that the lymphoblastoid transformation of T cells exposed in vitro to lectins is diminished. Patients with more extensive disease but still in good clinical condition frequently exhibit impaired delayed hypersensitivity, for example, negative skin tests with multiple antigens, such as tuberculin, coccidiodin, histoplasmin, and mumps antigen. Patients with advanced disease may be lymphopenic as a reflection of a generalized depletion of tissue lymphocytes. Since the degree of impaired cellular immunity rises with increasing extent of disease, it would appear that disturbed cellular immunity follows rather than precedes the development of Hodgkin's disease.

The untreated patient usually makes normal amounts of humoral antibodies; an occasional patient has polyclonal hypergammaglobu- linemia ("broad-based" pattern on serum protein electrophoresis, see Fig. 20-3). However, treatment with either extensive radiotherapy or combination chemotherapy depresses antibody synthesis; evidence of impaired synthesis, for example, failure to develop an adequate titer of antibodies after administration of pneumococcal vaccine, may persist for several years afterwards.

Because of these immunologic abnormalities, patients with Hodgkin's disease have an increased susceptibility, not only to bac- terial infections, but also to disseminated fungal and herpes virus infections. At particular risk are:

1. Patients with advanced disease and lymphocyte depletion.
2. Patients who have received both radiotherapy and combination chemotherapy within the past year.

Autoimmune hemolytic anemia and autoimmune thrombocyto- penia also occur in Hodgkin's disease but do so less commonly than in non-Hodgkin's lymphoma or chronic lymphocytic leukemia. Rare patients may develop a nephrotic syndrome or jaundice with liver function tests mimicking obstructive jaundice as probable manifes- tations of disturbed immune function.

CLINICAL MANIFESTATIONS

Hodgkin's disease may develop at any age from early childhood to advanced old age. A bimodal curve of age incidence is found with a peak in the United States in the mid to late 20s, a fall in incidence between age 30 and 50 years, and a second rise after age 50 years. In young children, Hodgkin's disease occurs primarily in boys. The young adult peak is composed equally of men and women; in the peak after age 50 years, men exceed women. Disease developing in women under the age of 30 is usually of the nodular sclerosis type.

The most frequent initial complaint is progressive, painless swelling of a peripheral lymph node or nodes, usually in the neck.

An occasional patient presents because of the discovery of a mediastinal mass on a routine chest film or on a film taken because of symptoms such as persistent cough. The patient may have no other complaints or he or she may have systemic symptoms referable to the disease—fever, night sweats, or weight loss.

When the disease arises in the retroperitoneal area, the patient may present with a history of a prolonged, high fever. Sometimes, lymphadenopathy, hepatomegaly, splenomegaly, or a combination of these findings is discovered on physical examination, but the examination results are often negative except for the fever. Nevertheless, these patients usually have extensive retroperitoneal disease.

Only rarely will a patient have initial complaints attributable to an extranodal lesion, for example, hemorrhage secondary to a gastrointestinal lesion or pain secondary to involvement of bone.

Diagnosis

As already discussed, the diagnosis is made by finding either typical Reed-Sternberg cells or "lacunar cells" in an appropriate histologic setting. This almost always requires lymph node biopsy. Only rarely has the diagnosis been made from other biopsy material, for example, from a bone marrow biopsy. Diagnostic difficulty may arise when the histologic features of a biopsy are compatible with Hodgkin's disease but convincing Reed-Sternberg cells cannot be found (as may occur, for example, in immunoblastic lymphadenopathy, see Chapter 18).

MANAGEMENT

The goal of management is cure. Several factors influence prognosis:

1. Host resistance, which, as discussed, is reflected in the histologic appearance of the biopsy.
2. The extent of disease at presentation and the presence or absence of systemic symptoms.
3. Age, probably because older age is associated with both decreased host resistance and a poorer tolerance for aggressive therapy.
4. Sex, with women having a better prognosis then men. This may reflect the influence of two factors—the proclivity for young women to have nodular sclerosis (which has a lower likelihood of early noncontiguous dissemination to extranodal sites) and the higher male-to-female ratio of older patients.

As discussed later, cure is attainable in most young adult patients, but most patients over 50 years of age will die of their disease within 5 years of diagnosis.

Determining Extent of Disease

Extent of disease strongly influences choice of therapy and, therefore, must be carefully assessed in each new patient.

INITIAL CLINICAL EVALUATION

A systematic initial workup should include:

1. A detailed clinical history, from which one establishes the presence or absence of fever, night sweats, or weight loss, and a complete physical examination.
2. A blood count that includes a platelet count and an erythrocyte sedimentation rate.
3. Liver function tests, particularly the serum alkaline phosphatase level.
4. Urinalysis and renal function tests.
5. Radiographic studies.
   a. To look for thoracic disease
      (1) Posteroanterior and lateral chest films.
      (2) If chest films are abnormal, whole lung tomograms to look for pulmonary infiltrates.
   b. To look for abdominal disease
      (1) CT scan of the abdomen, which can visualize lymph node enlargement in upper para-aortic, splenic hilar, celiac, and portal hepatis areas that cannot be seen on lymphangiogram and may also visualize tumor nodules in the spleen and liver.
      (2) Lymphangiography, a procedure in which dye is injected into lymphatic channels in both feet. This is performed because Hodgkin's disease may disrupt the internal structure of a lymph node, and so produce an abnormal appearance of the node on lymphangiography, without enlarging the node to a degree that it is recognized as abnormal on CT scan. (Lymphangiography is contraindicated, however, if a patient is known to have extensive retroperitoneal disease or if the patient has pulmonary parenchymal disease, which may be aggravated by multiple small emboli of dye that reach the lung as a consequence of the procedure).

6. Bilateral bone marrow biopsy to obtain histologic sections of a core of marrow. This is sometimes omitted in young patients with a favorable histologic pattern on lymph node biopsy and who appear to have clinical stage IA or IIA (see below) disease.

CLINICAL STAGING

When the initial evaluation is completed, the extent of the patient's disease is staged as follows (modified Ann Arbor staging system):

Clinical Stage (CS) I—Involvement of a single lymph node region.

CS II—Involvement of two or more lymph node regions on the same side of the diaphragm.

CS III—Involvement of lymph node regions on both sides of the diaphragm but disease still confined to lymphoid tissue. This stage may be divided further into:

CS III$_1$—Disease below the diaphragm is limited to the upper abdomen, that is, the spleen, splenic hilar nodes, celiac nodes, porta hepatis nodes.

CS III$_2$—Disease below the diaphragm includes para-aortic, mesenteric, iliac, or inguinal nodal involvement with or without upper abdominal disease.

CS IV—Diffuse or disseminated involvement of one or more extralymphatic organs or tissues, for example, the liver or bone marrow. (Direct extralymphatic extension of disease, as from mediastinal lymph nodes to the lung, has a different prognostic meaning than hematogenous dissemination of disease and so is not classified as stage IV. It is delineated by adding the subscript E to whatever the stage would be from the extent of lymph node involvement. Thus, if only mediastinal nodes were enlarged in the example just cited, the disease would be staged as CS I$_E$.)

All stages are also given the letter A to indicate the *absence* of systemic symptoms or the letter B to indicate the *presence* of fever, night sweats, or weight loss exceeding 10% of body weight in the 6 months prior to evaluation. B symptoms probably result from release of interleukin I and tumor necrosis factor (TNF) from large numbers of activated, reactive monocytes-macrophages and, therefore, represent evidence of more active, progressive disease. For each stage of the disease, the presence of B symptoms diminishes the statistical chance for cure as contrasted to patients with the same stage but no B symptoms.

LAPAROTOMY AND PATHOLOGIC STAGING

Formerly, patients without obvious stage IV disease after clinical study were routinely subjected to a staging laparotomy that included splenectomy, biopsy of lymph nodes from multiple abdominal sites, and biopsies from both lobes of the liver. Extent of disease was then reclassified with these added data to yield a pathologic stage (PS). As data from large numbers of patients accumulated, it became clear that:

1. Substantial numbers of patients in CS IA and IIA (25% in one series) will have involvement of abdominal nodes, the spleen, or both, that is, will be in PS IIIA. Moreover, occasional patients will have disease in the spleen without disease in upper abdominal nodes.
2. As many as 50% of patients with CS IB and IIB will be reclassified as PS IIIB after laparotomy.
3. Absence of splenic disease means, with only a rare exception, that the liver is also free of disease, whereas presence of more than three nodules of disease in the spleen makes liver involvement likely.

Until recently, radiotherapy was the primary treatment for all stages of Hodgkin's disease except stage IV and stage IIIB. However, combination chemotherapy—which will treat Hodgkin's disease throughout the body—has replaced radiotherapy in many centers for all patients with B symptoms and for increasing numbers of patients with stage IIIA disease. This diminishes the need for staging laparotomy.

Moreover, a British National Lymphoma Investigation Group, which now treats all patients with stage III disease with chemotherapy, has recently concluded that laparotomy is rarely justified even in CS IA and IIA patients. The group believes that a subset of CS IA and IIA patients with an increased risk for early relapse after radiotherapy, and who might therefore benefit from initial treatment with combination chemotherapy rather than radiotherapy, can be identified without resorting to laparotomy. They recommend use of a prognostic index that relies heavily on the histopathologic classification of the biopsy but also takes into account age, sex, the erythrocyte sedimentation rate, and the presence or absence of mediastinal involvement.

In contrast, many groups in the United States and other countries still rely on the information provided by laparotomy to plan therapy for patients with clinical stage IA or IIA disease.

Therapeutic Options

As the above indicates, opinion differs as to whether certain patients should be treated initially with irradiation or combination chemotherapy. If it were not for a substantial incidence of late acute leukemia and non-Hodgkin's lymphoma when irradiation and chemotherapy are used together (combined modality therapy), both might well be given as initial therapy to many if not most patients with disease other than upper cervical stage I disease of favorable histology. This would assure the sterilization of small foci of disease that might be present outside radiation fields and would also assure the effective treatment of bulky disease, in which radiotherapy may be needed to kill all the neoplastic cells in a large mass lesion.

However, because using MOPP (see below) chemotherapy, either with or without irradiation, has a higher risk than radiotherapy for late second malignancies (and also because chemotherapy with MOPP causes infertility in males), most patients with stage IA or IIA disease above the diaphragm are treated initially with radiotherapy. When laparotomy is performed, the following guidelines are frequently used:

1. If no abdominal disease is found, radiation therapy is given to a supradiaphragmatic mantle field and to a subdiaphragmatic field that extends to the pelvic brim.
2. If disease is found in upper abdominal nodes but not or only minimally in the spleen, total nodal radiation is given to include the pelvic and inguinal nodes.
3. If disease is found in lower abdominal nodes or if more than minimal disease is found in the spleen, combination chemotherapy is given, either alone or with radiotherapy.

Patients with stage IA or IIA disease who present with a large mediastinal mass greater than one-third the diameter of the chest are also given combined modality therapy. Spread of disease to the lung and difficulty in shielding the lung while providing tumoricidal irradiation to the mediastinal mass prevent effective therapy with irradiation alone.

Patients with stage IB or stage IIB have a substantially higher risk of relapse after radiation therapy than do patients with stage IA or stage IIA disease, and patients with B symptoms are also often treated with combined chemotherapy rather than with radiation therapy. If the latter is chosen, laparatomy to rule out abdominal disease is indicated, since the superiority of combination chemotherapy over radiation therapy for stage IIIB disease has been clearly established.

Virtually everyone agrees that patients with stage III_2A, IIIB, or IV disease should receive combination chemotherapy. MOPP (nitrogen mustard, vincristine, procarbazine, and prednisone) given in 28-day cycles for six courses or longer (two courses beyond evidence of residual disease on restaging) has been the standard regimen. However, a second combination called ABVD (doxorubicin, bleomycin, velban, and dacarbazine) is now also being increasingly used for initial combined chemotherapy. It is equivalent to MOPP in controlling disease, is less likely to cause male infertility, and so far does not appear to increase the risk for late acute leukemia. However, ABVD produces such severe vomiting in some patients that they refuse to continue therapy. MOPP and ABVD are non-cross-resistant regimens. In a recent study, alternating MOPP and ABVD for a total of 12 cycles significantly improved the likelihood of cure in patients with stage IV disease as contrasted with giving 12 cycles of MOPP alone.

Therapeutic Responses

The care of many patients requires the combined efforts of an experienced hematologist–oncologist, pathologist, surgeon, and radiotherapist. Such patients often benefit from referral to a center for therapy.

As mentioned, irradiation should cure most young patients with stage IA or IIA disease. The actuarial statistics for *10-year disease-free survival* reported from one center where such patients receive irradiation to a field that extends to the pelvic brim are:

1. For stage IA patients, 88%.
2. For stage IIA patients, 76%.

Patients with stage III disease treated with irradiation alone fare less well. A retrospective collaborative study yielded the following values for *5-year disease-free survival* after total nodal irradiation:

1. For stage III_1 patients, 63%.
2. For stage III_2 patients, 32%.

Despite these statistics, patients with stage III_1A disease and no or only minimal splenic involvement are often initially treated with radiotherapy. Chemotherapy with MOPP is relied upon to salvage the one third of patients who will relapse after radiotherapy. However, MOPP chemotherapy, with or without irradiation, has now replaced irradiation in most centers as the initial treatment for patients with stage III$_2$A disease.

In stage IIIB or IV disease, chemotherapy with MOPP may be expected to induce 10-year disease-free survival in about 50% of patients. However, older patients do poorly; the median survival of one group of patients over 60 years of age given combination chemotherapy with or without irradiation was 39 months.

Late Complications

LATE RELAPSE

In a large series of young patients with Hodgkin's disease of all histologic types and stages:

1. Ninety-six percent obtained an initial complete remission.
2. At 3 years, 70% were still in remission.
3. At 20 years, about 60% were still in remission.

These data suggest that 10% to 15% of all young patients in complete remission at 3 years (including some patients presenting with only stage I disease) will later relapse. In the reported series, most of the patients with late relapse had nodular sclerosis.

Therefore, patients in remission after therapy—regardless of the stage of disease at presentation and particularly if they have nodular sclerosis—should be examined periodically for up to 20 years for evidence of relapse. Unexplained fever in a patient in long-term remission should raise concern for renewed disease activity.

SECOND MALIGNANCY

As already mentioned, patients treated with irradiation plus MOPP are at increased risk of developing a second malignancy, particularly acute non-lymphocytic leukemia and non-Hodgkin's lymphoma. Estimated risks are: for acute leukemia at 7 years, 4%; for non-Hodgkin's lymphoma at 10 years, 4% to 5%.

NON-MALIGNANT COMPLICATIONS OF THERAPY

Non-malignant late complications of high-dose irradiation include:

1. Chronic pericardial disease, with signs of constrictive pericarditis, which may first become evident several years after irradation without an earlier, recognized episode of effusive pericarditis.
2. Hypothyroidism, which will eventually develop in most patients receiving irradiation to cervical nodes. Therefore, a TSH (thyroid stimulating hormone) level, which is a sensitive screening test for hypothyroidism, should be measured periodically for at least 6 years after such therapy.

SELECTED READING

1. Austin-Seymour MM, Hoppe RT, Cox RS, Rosenberg SA, and Kaplan HS: Hodgkin's disease in patients over sixty years old. Ann Intern Med 100:13, 1984.
2. Bonadonna G, Valagussa P, and Santoro A: Alternating non-cross-resistant combination chemotherapy or MOPP in stage IV Hodgkin's disease. A report of 8-year results. Ann Intern Med 104:739, 1986.
3. DeVita VT Jr, Jaffe ES, and Hellman S: Hodgkin's disease and the non-Hodgkin's lymphomas. IN DeVita VT Jr, Hellman S, and Rosenberg SA (eds): Cancer. Principles and Practice of Oncology. Ed. 2. Philadelphia, Lippincott, 1985.
4. Haybittle JL, Easterling MJ, Bennett MH, Vaughan Hudson B, Hayhoe FGJ, Jelliffe AM, Vaughan Hudson G, and MacLennan KA: Review of British National Lymphoma Investigation studies of Hodgkin's disease and development of prognostic index. Lancet 1:967, 1985.
5. Herman TS, Hoppe RT, Donaldson SS, Cox RS, Rosenberg SA, and Kaplan HS: Late relapse among patients treated for Hodgkin's disease. Ann Intern Med 102:292, 1985.
6. Kaplan HS: Hodgkin's disease: biology, treatment, prognosis. Blood 57: 813, 1981.
7. Keller AR, Kaplan HS, Lukes RJ, and Rappaport H: Correlation of histopathology with other prognostic indicators in Hodgkin's disease. Cancer 22:487, 1968.

20

Immunoglobulins and Malignant Immunoproliferative Disorders

STRUCTURE AND FUNCTION OF IMMUNOGLOBULINS

Immunoglobulins (also called gamma globulins because they are found in the gamma position on serum protein electrophoresis, see Fig. 20-3) are proteins with antibody activity. Each molecule will bind preferentially to one of literally millions of possible antigenic determinants. Binding to antigen alters the molecule, and it then can participate in effector functions, which include:

1. Binding and activation of complement.
2. Binding to a receptor on macrophages with consequent phagocytosis of the antigen-antibody complex.
3. Triggering the release of the granule contents of mast cells and possibly of eosinophils.

All immunoglobulin molecules are made up of a basic structural unit (Fig. 20-1) consisting of two smaller polypeptide chains, called light chains, and two larger polypeptide chains, called heavy chains. The chains are held together by interchain disulfide bonds.

Both light and heavy polypeptide chains have two major structural segments:

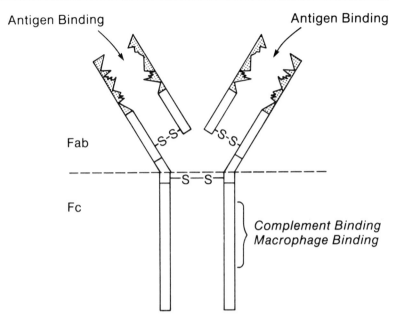

Fig. 20-1. An IgG molecule, consisting of two identical light chains and two identical heavy chains held together by disulfide bonds. The shaded area of the chains represents the variable region. The irregular areas in the variable region denote hypervariable regions. Papain splits the molecule into two Fab fragments and one Fc fragment (see text).

1. An amino-terminal segment, known as the variable region because each molecule arising from a different B cell/plasma cell clone will differ in amino acid sequences in certain of its subsegments (called hypervariable regions or "hot spots"). These differences in amino acid sequences confer on antibody molecules their preferential ability to bind to specific antigens. As shown in Figure 20-1, a basic four polypeptide antibody unit possesses two antigen binding sites—each identical to the other and arising from a specific conformation of a binding pocket produced by the variable region of one light chain and of one heavy chain.

2. A carboxy-terminal segment, known as the constant region. The constant region of a light chain consists of a single domain, whereas that of a heavy chain is made up of several domains. The binding sites for the effector functions of an antibody mol-

ecule are located on domains of the constant region of its heavy chains.

In any given immunoglobulin molecule, the two light polypeptide chains are identical and the two heavy polypeptide chains are identical. Most immunoglobulin molecules are monomers of the basic unit, but some are polymers of either two or five units. Such polymers consist of identical basic units linked by an additional chain, called a J chain, which is also synthesized by B-lymphocyte/plasma cells.

The enzyme papain cleaves the basic antibody unit at a region of the heavy chain called the hinge (see Fig. 20-1). This gives rise to three fragments:

1. Two identical Fab fragments, made up of a whole light chain plus part of a heavy chain. Each Fab fragment contains an antigen binding site.
2. One Fc fragment, which is made up of the remaining carboxy-terminal domains of both heavy chains. The Fc fragment contains the binding sites for the effector functions of the molecule.

Types of Light Chains

Patients with multiple myeloma may excrete in the urine proteins called Bence Jones proteins, which were first recognized because of their unusual thermal properties. These proteins turned out to be immunoglobulin light chains. Studies with antisera to Bence Jones proteins from different patients led to the discovery of two antigenically different types of light chains. These were named kappa (κ) and lambda (λ) light chains.

Kappa and lambda light chains are coded for by different germline genes, which are located on different chromosomes. A functional light chain gene is formed by rearrangement of germ-line DNA segments in which different segments of a number of alternative gene segments for different portions of the variable region are combined. These rearrangements, plus frame shifts at combining sites during rearrangement, make it possible for a relatively limited number of germ-line segments to code for a polypeptide chain segment of virtually infinitely variable amino acid sequences. The rearranged variable region DNA segment then combines with a single germ-line DNA segment for the constant region of the κ chain gene or with one of six duplicated germ-line segments for the λ chain gene. Therefore, the amino acid composition of the constant region—the carboxy-segment of the light chain—differs only minimally (because of allelic genes, see below) for all light chains of the same type. However, the amino acid sequences of the constant region of κ and λ light chains differ substantially from each other. This is responsible for the antigenic differences that originally led to the recognition of the two light chain types.

Each progenitor of a functional B cell possesses two (one from each parent) germ-line κ chain genes and two germ-line λ chain genes. During processing, the cell tries first to rearrange one of its germ-line κ chain genes into a functional light chain gene and, if this fails, the other of its κ chain genes. If both fail, the cell then tries to rearrange one and then the other of its λ chains. If all rearrangements fail, the cell dies during processing (see Chapter 14). Once a light chain gene is successfully rearranged, further attempts cease. This is why:

1. Each individual antibody molecule will contain either two κ or two λ light chains but not one of each.
2. The antibodies normally found in plasma, which arise from multiple B cell/plasma cell clones, are a mixture of molecules containing κ light chains and molecules containing λ light chains. However, because the κ chain gene has the first chance at rearrangement, there are more molecules with κ chains than molecules with λ chains.

Classes of Heavy Chains

There are five major kinds of heavy polypeptide chains. First recognized because of antigenic differences in their constant regions, they were given the Greek letter names: γ (gamma), α (alpha), μ (mu), δ (delta), and ε (epsilon).

Immunoglobulins are divided into classes based upon the kind of heavy chain they possess. Each class of immunoglobulin contains molecules with either κ or λ type light chains but with the same single class of heavy chain (Fig. 20-2). A standard nomenclature is used in which the symbol Ig (for immunoglobulin) is followed by a letter denoting the class, for example, IgG for the class containing γ heavy chains, IgA for the class containing α heavy chains, and so on. The logic of dividing the immunoglobulins into classes based upon differences in the constant region of the heavy chain lies in the observation that the different classes have different biologic activities.

The germ-line gene for a heavy chain differs from the germ-line

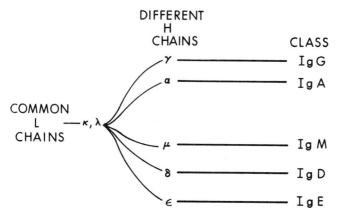

Fig. 20-2. Common light chains and different heavy chains of the classes of immunoglobulins.

genes for the light chains. In addition to multiple alternative DNA segments for the different portions of the variable region, a heavy chain germ-line gene also contains a series of constant chain DNA segments—one for each of the heavy chain classes (and subclasses, see below). During different stages of B cell processing and differentiation (see Chapter 14), heavy chains are made in which the variable region combines with constant regions of different classes. Through complex mechanisms involving RNA splicing for some switches and DNA splicing for others:

1. The B cell first combines its heavy chain variable region with the μ chain constant region to make IgM and then also with the δ chain constant region to make IgD. These initial IgM and IgD molecules become embedded in the cell surface membrane where they serve as recognition sites for the specific antigenic determinants to which the cell, by its germ-line DNA rearrangements, has become committed to respond.

2. The fully processed B cell—as it responds to exposure to the antigenic determinant it recognizes and so begins both secreting circulating antibody and differentiating into a plasma cell—first secretes IgM molecules but then switches to combine its variable region with the constant region for IgG, for IgA, or, rarely, for IgE. Hybrid molecules are not made. As mentioned, any given immunoglobulin molecule will contain only one class of heavy chains.

Further Subdivisions of Immunoglobulins

The immunoglobulin classes can be divided further into subclasses based upon serologic and physicochemical differences in the class-specific constant regions of their heavy chains. Thus, there are two subclasses of IgM (μ_1, μ_2), two subclasses of IgA (α_1, α_2), and four subclasses of IgG (γ_1, γ_2, γ_3, γ_4). A heavy chain gene contains a separate DNA segment for each constant region subclass, which is alternatively available to support synthesis of an immunoglobulin molecule of that subclass. Antibody molecules of different IgG subclasses vary in their biologic activities. For example, antibodies of IgG_1 or IgG_3 subclass, after reacting with antigen, have a greater capacity to bind complement and also a greater binding affinity for macrophage Fc receptors than do antibodies of the IgG_2 or IgG_4 subclass.

ISOTYPES

The two types of light chains and the classes and subclasses of heavy chains are present in every member of the human species. Therefore, the plasma of every individual will contain a spectrum of immunoglobulin *isotypes*, made up of each possible combination of a type of a light chain and a subclass of a heavy chain.

ALLOTYPES

Immunologic differences have also been delineated between immunoglobulin isotypes of different individuals. In different populations, several *allotypes* may exist for a particular isotype. They result from the existence of alternative genes (alleles) in different individuals at the chromosomal loci for the constant regions of the γ chain subclasses (Gm system), of the α chain (Am system), and of the κ chain (Inv system). Sensitization to an IgA allotype through prior transfusions has been shown to cause one type of plasma transfusion reaction with itching, urticaria, and wheezing.

IDIOTYPES

Each immunoglobulin synthesized by a different B-lymphocyte/plasma cell clone differs antigenically because of differences in the amino acid sequences of its hypervariable regions. The same structural differences that allow the antibody to bind preferentially to an antigenic determinant also confer on the antibody a unique antigen profile. This antigen profile, called its *idiotype*, is made up of a mixture of antigenic determinants from the hypervariable regions, each of which is referred to as an idiotypic determinant. Monoclonal antibodies can be made to an immunoglobulin that will react only with a specific idiotypic determinant of that immunoglobulin. Such antibodies, which are known as anti-idiotype antibodies, are being used experimentally in the treatment of some types of lymphoma (see Chapter 18).

Properties of the Immunoglobulin Classes

All classes of immunoglobulins except IgM are found in serum as the basic four-chain unit. Although traces of IgM may be detected as a four-chain monomer, IgM exists primarily as a macroglobulin made of five identical four-chain units held together by a J chain. When the IgA level in serum is markedly elevated, as in IgA myeloma, substantial amounts of IgA may circulate as a dimer of two four-chain units. Some properties of the immunoglobulin classes are summarized in Table 20-1.

IgM are antibodies that B-lymphocytes can secrete before they differentiate fully into plasma cells and are the first antibodies secreted on initial exposure to an antigen. Although IgM is present in only a low concentration in normal plasma, several IgM antibodies are of clinical importance, including:

1. The anti-A and anti-B isohemagglutinins.
2. Cold agglutinins.
3. Rheumatoid factor.

Table 20-1. Properties of the Immunoglobulin Classes

	IgG	IgA	IgM	IgD	IgE
Molecular weight (daltons)	150,000	170,000	900,000	180,000	200,000
Plasma concentration (mg/dL)	700–1500	250	100	3	0.03
Biologic half-life (days)	21	6	5	3	2
Intravascular distribution (% of total body pool that is intravascular)	45	40	75	75	50
Placental transfer	Yes	No	No	No	No

4. The heterophil antibody of infectious mononucleosis (see Chapter 21).

IgM cannot cross the placental barrier. Therefore, elevated levels of IgM in cord blood have been taken to indicate intrauterine infection (for example, congenital cytomegalic inclusion disease, congenital rubella).

IgG is the major antibody of plasma and extravascular fluid. It can fix complement, cross the placental barrier, and sensitize the skin for passive cutaneous anaphylaxis.

IgA, a lesser plasma component, is the major antibody of the external secretions (tears, respiratory tract secretions, gastrointestinal tract secretions). IgA exists in secretions as a dimer of two four-chain units plus another protein, structurally and genetically unrelated to immunoglobulins, which is called the secretory piece. IgA antibodies play an important role in combating respiratory and intestinal tract infections.

As already mentioned, IgD embedded in the surface membrane of the B cell functions as an antigen recognition site. Functions for the small amounts of IgD that circulate have yet to be identified.

IgE is present in plasma in such a low concentration that it is expressed in nanograms (ng) per mL. Its levels may be increased in patients with helminthic infections and in some patients with allergic disorders. IgE antibodies bind to the surface of tissue mast cells by their Fc region. Subsequent binding of antigen to their antigen binding sites causes the mast cells to discharge their granules. This may provoke an immediate hypersensitivity reaction (anaphylaxis, acute asthmatic attack, urticaria).

TESTS REFLECTING SERUM PROTEIN ALTERATION

In each dL of normal plasma are 6.5 to 8.5 g of a complex mixture of proteins made primarily by liver cells (albumin, fibrinogen, many globulins) and by plasma cells and lymphocytes (the immunoglobulins). Disease frequently alters the serum proteins. Common clinical tests that reflect these alterations include:

1. The erythrocyte sedimentation rate.
2. Chemical determination of albumin and globulin levels.
3. Electrophoresis of serum proteins.
4. Tests combining electrophoresis and immunoprecipitation, for

example, immunoelectrophoresis and immunofixation electrophoresis.
5. Examination of serum for cryoglobulins.

These tests are particularly useful in the workup of hematologic patients for the information they provide about the immunoglobulins.

Erythrocyte Sedimentation Rate

The rate that RBCs settle as blood stands in vitro depends on the concentration of plasma substances that aggregate RBCs and the concentration of the RBCs. The major plasma proteins facilitating aggregation are:

1. *Fibrinogen.* Its increased synthesis as part of the acute phase response is responsible for the fast sedimentation rate found in a wide variety of disorders—tissue injury, inflammation, acute infections, neoplasia.
2. *Immunoglobulins.* Their elevation contributes to the fast sedimentation rate found in chronic disorders with increased polyclonal gamma globulin synthesis, for example, chronic infections, autoimmune disorders—and in immunoproliferative disorders with increased levels of a plasma monoclonal immunoglobulin, for example, multiple myeloma.

Anemia of any cause (except sickle cell disorders) also increases the erythrocyte sedimentation rate because a fall in RBC concentration increases the ratio of plasma aggregating substances to RBCs in blood.

Finding a fast sedimentation rate in a patient with complaints of illness of a significance difficult to evaluate—for example, the recent onset of excessive fatigue and arthralgia, or the recent onset of backaches—and no objective evidence of disease on physical examination leads one to search further for evidence of significant underlying disease. Finding a normal sedimentation rate in such a patient, although making certain disorders such as temporal arteritis or early multiple myeloma very unlikely, unfortunately may not rule out other serious disorders, such as a cancer before it has grown large or spread by metastases.

Albumin and Globulin Levels

Albumin can be separated from all of the other plasma proteins, the globulins, by its differential solubility in a salt solution. Normal values for serum proteins determined in this way are albumin, 3.5 to 4.5 g per dL, and globulins, 2.5 to 4.0 g per dL. A low serum albumin means that a patient is chronically ill. A high serum globulin indicates increased production of immunoglobulins.

Serum Protein Electrophoresis

Because their isoelectric points differ, the serum proteins separate in an electrical field. At the pH commonly used for serum protein electrophoresis, albumin moves farthest towards the positive pole and gamma globulin moves least. The other globulins fall between. When cellulose acetate is used as a supporting medium, the electrophoretic pattern for normal serum looks like that shown on strip A of Figure 20-3. When the intensity of protein staining of the different bands is measured with an instrument called a densitometer, tracings such as those shown in Figure 20-3 are obtained.

Serum protein electrophoresis has been particularly useful in distinguishing so-called broad-based, or polyclonal, hypergammaglobulinemia (strip B of Fig. 20-3) from narrow band, or monoclonal, hypergammaglobulinemia (strip C of Fig. 20-3).

CAUSES OF POLYCLONAL HYPERGAMMAGLOBULINEMIA

The pattern shown in strip B of Figure 20-3 results from an increased synthesis of heterogenous immunoglobulins by many clones of plasma cells. Such a pattern is found in:

1. Chronic infections—infective endocarditis, chronic osteomyelitis, disseminated granulomatous disease. Very high levels may be found in occasional patients with chronic infections causing persistent antigenic stimulation (for example, in a patient with a chronic draining sinus due to actinomycosis).
2. Chronic parenchymal liver disease of any etiology.
3. Some patients with autoimmune disorders, such as systemic lupus erythematosus, rheumatoid arthritis, and chronic thyroiditis.

CAUSES OF MONOCLONAL HYPERGAMMAGLOBULINEMIA

The pattern shown in strip C of Figure 20-3 results from the synthesis of increased amounts of a single homogeneous immunoglobulin by plasma cells or lymphocytes originating from a single clone. This pattern may be found in:

1. Multiple myeloma.
2. Plasmacytoid lymphocytic lymphoma. The monoclonal protein is usually (although not invariably) IgM, and if its concentration

A   ALB α_1 α_2 β γ

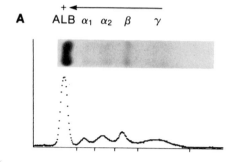

B

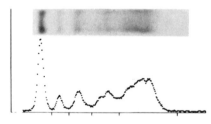

Fig. 20-3. Serum protein electrophoresis on cellulose acetate. The arrow indicates direction of migration, which is toward the positive pole. A densitometer tracing of staining intensity of bands is shown beneath each strip. (Strip A) Normal pattern. (Strip B) The diffuse, "broad-base" pattern of polyclonal hypergammaglobulinemia. (Strip C) The "narrow-band" or sharp peak pattern (on the densitometer tracing) of monoclonal hypergammaglobulinemia.

C

is high, the plasmacytoid lymphoma is often referred to as *macroglobulinemia of Waldenström.*

3. Primary amyloidosis.
4. A surprisingly large number of elderly patients who may initially have no evidence of a causal underlying disease. These patients are said to have *monoclonal gammopathy of undetermined significance (MGUS).* In most, the disorder is benign. The concentration of the homogeneous immunoglobulin, which

is usually IgG, remains below 2 g per dL and no findings suggestive of multiple myeloma, plasmacytoid lymphocytic lymphoma or primary amyloidosis appear over years of observation. However, in some patients, who are indistinguishable initially from the others, the concentration of homogeneous immunoglobulin slowly increases over months to several years and findings of multiple myeloma become evident.

Immunoelectrophoresis and Immunofixation Electrophoresis

These techniques are primarily used in hematologic diagnosis to characterize the composition of serum monoclonal immunoglobulins, or of free light chains or heavy chains excreted in the urine. In *immunoelectrophoresis*, the proteins in a test sample are separated by electrophoresis in agar gel and an antiserum specific for a light chain type or heavy chain class is placed in a trough in the agar gel and allowed to diffuse into the gel. A precipitin line forms at the site of interaction between an immunoglobulin and an antiserum directed against its light chain type or heavy chain class (Fig. 20-4). In *immunofixation electrophoresis*, proteins in a test sample are first resolved by electrophoresis in several lanes of agarose gel and then each lane is overlaid with a different specific antiserum. The resultant antigen-antibody complexes precipitate. The unreacted soluble proteins are washed away, and precipitated antigen–antibody complex is visualized by staining.

Cryoglobulins

Cryoglobulins are serum proteins that are insoluble at 4°C. To test for cryoglobulins, one clots blood at 37°C and separates the serum by centrifuging in a warmed centrifuge cup. The serum is then allowed to stand in a refrigerator for 24 hours and examined for either a gel or a white precipitate. Two kinds of cryoglobulins have been identified:

1. *Pure cryoglobulins.* These are found in occasional patients with malignant immunoproliferative disease, as pure IgG cryoglobulin in multiple myeloma, and as pure IgM cryoglobulin in macroglobulinemia of Waldenström.
2. *Mixed cryoglobulins.* These are antigen–antibody complexes that contain IgG immunoglobulin and either an IgG or an IgM

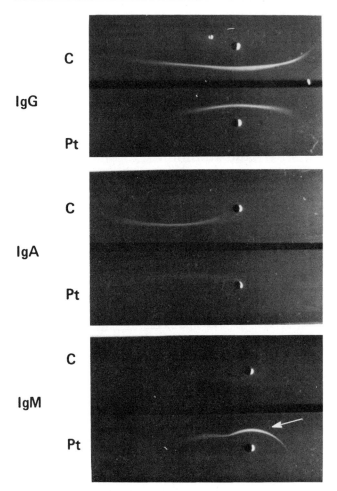

Fig. 20-4. The immunoelectrophoretic pattern found in macroglobulinemia of Waldenström. Three agarose gels are shown. In each, normal plasma, placed in the upper well, and patient's plasma, placed in the lower well, have been subjected to electrophoresis. The trough in the agar contains antiserum to a heavy chain: in the upper gel, anti-γ chain antiserum; in the middle gel, anti-α chain antiserum; in the lower well, anti-μ chain antiserum. In the upper and middle gels one notes a less heavy precipitin line for the patient's plasma than for normal plasma, denoting a reduced concentration of IgG and IgA in the plasma. In the lowermost well, one notes a markedly increased precipitin line for the patient's plasma, which contains a "blip" characteristic of a monoclonal immunoglobulin.

immunoglobulin with anti-IgG activity. They may also contain complement. Mixed cryoglobulins have been identified in disorders associated with prolonged, increased IgG synthesis (for example, systemic lupus erythematosus, rheumatoid arthritis, and certain infections, such as leprosy or chronic hepatitis due to hepatitis B virus) which serves to stimulate the synthesis of autoantibodies against the IgG in sufficient quantity to form circulating immune complexes. Besides precipitating in the cold in vitro, these immune complexes may also precipitate in vessels in vivo, producing a syndrome of purpura, arthralgia, and progressive glomerular damage with hematuria.

MULTIPLE MYELOMA

Multiple myeloma is a uniformly fatal malignancy in which neoplastic plasma cells proliferate in nodules or diffusely throughout the bone marrow. Plasma cells also proliferate in the spleen, liver, and lymph nodes, although these organs are usually not clinically enlarged. Frequently, a few plasma cells spill over into the peripheral blood; rarely, large numbers of plasma cells escape into the peripheral blood. The patient is then said to have *plasma cell leukemia*.

Over 80% of patients with multiple myeloma have increased amounts of a monoclonal immunoglobulin in the serum. Since multiple myeloma results from the neoplastic proliferation of a single clone of plasma cells, each patient's monoclonal protein presumably represents a different antibody of the millions of specific antibodies that the B cell/plasma cell population of normal peripheral lymphoid tissue is programed to make. For the typical patient, the time from the malignant transformation of a single cell to the accumulation of a tumor burden sufficient to produce clinically evident disease throughout the bone marrow is thought to be 1 to 2 years.

Pathogenesis of Clinical Disease

Important clinical manifestations of myeloma result from the following pathologic processes:

1. Release of products from the myeloma cells, which may include:
   a. A monoclonal immunoglobulin, whose plasma level reflects the extent of the tumor cell mass.

b. Free light chains, which

(1) May be partially catabolized and deposited in the tissues as amyloid with resultant tissue damage.

(2) May be excreted in the urine as Bence Jones protein with the potential for inducing renal failure.

c. A material called osteoclast activating factor (OAF) that activates osteoclasts in areas adjacent to myeloma cells and leads to bone destruction. (An antibody to interleukin 1 was recently reported to neutralize the activity of OAF in in vitro systems.) Bone destruction causes many of the serious clinical manifestations of myeloma discussed below.

2. Impaired hematopoiesis, which, as the disease progresses, can lead to increasingly severe anemia, neutropenia, and thrombocytopenia. Worsening pancytopenia often reflects both increasing occupancy of the marrow by myeloma cells and cumulative toxicity from chemotherapy.

3. Impaired production of humoral antibodies, which along with neutropenia and immobilization from pain or fractures, enhances the patient's risk of serious infection.

4. Organ or tissue damage from expanding local areas of myeloma tissue, for example, spinal cord compression from myeloma in vertebral marrow that breaks through into the extradural space.

Manifestations

CLINICAL FINDINGS

Most patients are between 50 and 70 years of age; the disease is rare in patients under 40 years of age. A common initial complaint is *skeletal pain*, for example, severe back pain of sudden onset following a compression fracture of a vertebral body. (Because roentgenograms may show only diffuse osteoporosis without punched-out lytic lesions, an occasional patient with back pain has been first thought to have senile osteoporosis.) The patient may also seek medical attention because of a pathologic fracture of other bones, for example, a fracture of the hip following minimal trauma.

For unknown reasons, occasional patients are free of pain. They may present a problem in the differential diagnosis of anemia, uremia, or hypercalcemia. An uncommon patient is first seen because of the sudden onset of findings of impending paraplegia secondary to spinal cord compression by extradural myelomatous tissue.

The patient often looks pale. Unless infected, he or she is afebrile. He or she may resist movement because of pain. The spine, ribs, and bony pelvis are often tender. Splenomegaly and peripheral lymphadenopathy are uncommon but are occasionally found. Rarely, a large soft tissue mass is discovered—a tumor usually formed by plasma cells that have broken through the cortex of an underlying bone. Deposits of amyloid are sometimes noted in the mouth, tongue, or soft tissues of the extremities. Amyloid deposited in joint capsules may produce pain and swelling of the hands, mimicking rheumatoid arthritis. An infrequent patient may have findings of a peripheral neuropathy.

LABORATORY FINDINGS

1. *Peripheral blood count.* A normochromic, normocytic anemia is present almost without exception. The WBC count is frequently low—4000 to 5000 per µL. The platelet count is usually initially normal. The erythrocyte sedimentation rate is typically rapid, but occasionally may be abnormally slow because of hypogammaglobulinemia (see below).

   Rouleaux (Fig. 20-5), plus an infrequent plasma cell, are often observed on the peripheral blood smear. (This combination on a blood smear always makes one highly suspicious of multiple my-

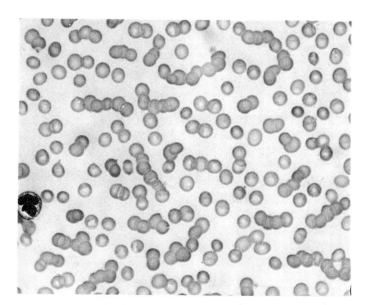

Fig. 20-5. Rouleaux on a peripheral blood smear from a patient with multiple myeloma.

eloma.) Rarely, when the marrow is heavily infiltrated, the blood smear may show evidence of a leukoerythroblastic reaction—scattered normoblasts and immature myeloid forms and large, abnormal platelets.

2. *Bone marrow.* The bones are soft in multiple myeloma. To avoid fracturing the sternum or pushing a needle through the sternum into the mediastinum, one should aspirate marrow only from the posterior iliac spine if multiple myeloma is suspected.

Marrow smears contain increased numbers of plasma cells. In most patients, a number of cells will look malignant with large, bizarre nuceoli (Fig. 20-6), marked variation in size, and multi-nucleated forms. In a few patients, the cells may be morphologi-cally indistinguishable from the reactive plasma cells found in increased numbers in the marrow in nonmalignant disorders as-sociated with hypergammaglobulinemia. Clusters or sheets of plasma cells are usually seen on a bone marrow biopsy section.

3. *Bone radiographs.* Lesions appear primarily in those bones that contain red marrow: the skull, ribs, sternum, spine, pelvis, clavi-

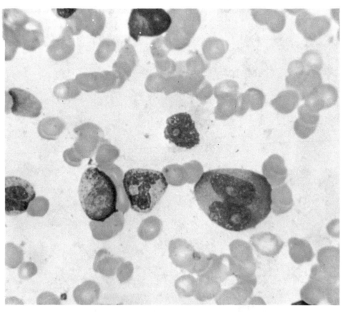

Fig. 20-6. High-power view of a bone marrow smear from patient with multiple myeloma. Note binucleated plasma cell containing large, malignant-appearing nucleoli.

cles, and upper ends of the long bones of the extremities. Punched-out lytic lesions, diffuse osteoporosis, or both may be seen. Occasionally, bone films are negative early in the disease. Osteoblastic lesions or lytic lesions with sclerotic borders are not seen (except for an extremely rare, indolent variant of the disease whose features include osteosclerosis and a high frequency of peripheral neuropathy). Because of the lack of an osteoblastic reaction, radionuclide bone scans are less sensitive than radiographs and are not indicated in looking for bone lesions in multiple myeloma.

4. *Serum proteins.* To understand the serum and urine protein abnormalities that may be found, one must remember the following:
   a. Malignant plasma cells may synthesize:
      (1) A whole immunoglobulin molecule—usually IgG, sometimes IgA, and only rarely IgM, IgD, or IgE.
      (2) A whole immunoglobulin molecule plus an excess of light chains, which, because of their low molecular weight, are not retained in the serum but excreted in the urine as Bence Jones protein.
      (3) Only light chains, that is, only Bence Jones protein.
   b. Immunoglobulin synthesis by plasma cells other than the malignant clone is markedly reduced. The reason is poorly understood, but the consequence is a functional deficiency of humoral antibodies.

Therefore, either of the following serum protein abnormalities may occur in multiple myeloma:
   a. Marked hypergammaglobulinemia with a narrow immunoglobulin band on serum protein electrophoresis (strip C of Fig. 20-3). This is the common finding.
   b. Hypogammaglobulinemia, which occurs when the malignant plasma cell synthesizes only light chains or a small amount of whole immunoglobulin (as in the rare IgD myeloma). Since homogeneous immunoglobulin does not accumulate in the plasma, serum protein electrophoresis reflects only the suppression of normal immunoglobulin synthesis.

What multiple myeloma never causes is hypergammaglobulinemia with a broad-based, diffuse pattern on electrophoresis indicative of increased immunoglobulin synthesis by many clones of plasma cells. Discovery of this pattern of polyclonal hypergammaglobulinemia eliminates multiple myeloma from further diagnostic consideration.

5. *Urine proteins.* Proteinuria is common in multiple myeloma and may result from:

a. The excretion of Bence Jones protein alone, without associated renal damage and resultant excretion of large serum proteins. Bence Jones protein was originally identified by its thermal properties, which cause it to precipitate from acidified urine at 50°C and redissolve when the urine is boiled. It is now more reliably recognized by electophoresis of a concentrate of urine, which reveals a single narrow band in the gamma globulin area. Bence Jones protein in the urine may be missed if one uses only a dipstick test to screen for proteinuria.

b. The excretion of large serum proteins, primarily albumin and whole immunoglobulin, secondary to renal damage. Bence Jones protein is often present also. The electrophoretic pattern of the urine may resemble that of plasma with an albumin band and a single narrow band in the gamma area corresponding to a whole monoclonal immunoglobulin. Sometimes one finds two narrow bands in the gamma area, one representing the whole immunoglobulin molecule and the other extra band representing Bence Jones protein.

6. *Blood chemistries.* Several alterations in blood chemistries should be looked for in the patient with multiple myeloma:

a. *Hypercalcemia,* which results from bony decalcification.

b. Hyperuricemia.

c. Elevated levels of blood urea nitrogen and creatinine secondary to renal failure.

Diagnosis

If the bone marrow aspirate contains large numbers of bizarre, malignant-looking plasma cells, the diagnosis of myeloma is established. If, however, a bone marrow aspirate contains increased numbers of normal-appearing or atypical, but not obviously malignant, plasma cells, the diagnosis requires at least one of the following added findings:

1. Hypergammaglobulinemia with a high concentration (over 2 g per dL) of a homogeneous "narrow band" immunoglobulin on serum protein electrophoresis.

2. Bence Jones proteinuria.

3. Lytic bone lesions.

An occasional patient may be discovered with a monoclonal immunoglobulin in the plasma in the 2 g per dL range, no or minimal anemia, minimally increased numbers of plasma cells in the bone marrow, and no bone lesions or only moderate osteoporotic changes on bone radiographs. Observation over months to years will settle whether such a patient has:

1. Early active myeloma.
2. A slowly progressive, smouldering variant of myeloma that may require no treatment for several years.
3. A non-progressive, truly benign monoclonal gammopathy.

An infrequent patient may present with evidence of a mass more suggestive of a carcinoma than of multiple myeloma (for example, a solitary nodule in the lung), a moderately increased monoclonal immunoglobulin band on serum protein electrophoresis, and increased numbers of plasma cells in the bone marrow of questionable significance. The monoclonal gammopathy should not distract one from the need to proceed without delay to establish by biopsy whether the mass lesion is carcinoma.

Complications

The wide variety of complications that may develop in multiple myeloma include the following:

1. *Infection.* Patients are prone to bacterial infections, particularly pneumonia, because of the combination of impaired synthesis of normal immunoglobulins, neutropenia, and immobilization. The two-month period immediately after the start of chemotherapy and the late stage of the disease, when the patient is severely neutropenic and refractory to further treatment, are periods of particularly high risk for infection.
2. *Renal damage.* Excretion of light chains (Bence Jones protein) is the major cause of renal insufficiency in multiple myeloma. This may result from two mechanisms:
   a. A direct toxic effect upon the tubule cells, resulting from reabsorption and catabolism of light chains.
   b. Precipitation of light chains in the renal tubules with resultant tubular obstruction. Dehydration may precipitate acute renal failure by this mechanism in the patient with Bence Jones proteinuria.

   Not all light chains are equally nephrotoxic; in general, patients excreting λ light chains are at greater risk for renal damage than patients excreting κ chains. Microscopic examination of the kidney of patients with renal insufficiency secondary to Bence Jones proteinuria reveals dense protein casts with accompanying peculiar giant cells in the tubules. These findings on a histologic section of the kidney are pathognomonic of multiple myeloma. *Hypercalcemia* may also lead to renal insufficiency secondary to tubule damage and nephrocalcinosis. Prompt treatment of hypercalcemia may reverse beginning renal failure from this cause. Deposition of *amyloid* within the glomeruli is another important, although less frequent, cause for renal insufficiency in multiple myeloma. It may give rise to a nephrotic syndrome.

3. *Pathologic fractures.* Bone radiographs should always include the upper femur and upper humerus to identify large lytic lesions in these areas that may cause a disabling pathologic fracture. Radiation therapy to such lesions can prevent fracture.

4. *Neurologic complications.* These may be grouped into three categories:

    a. Mental changes—confusion, somnolence, or even coma— which should alert one to the possibility of

        (1) Hypercalcemia.

        (2) Hyperviscosity of the blood.

    b. Spinal cord or cauda equina compression symptoms. Increasing radicular pain, sensory changes, or weakness in the legs requires careful neurologic evaluation for impending cord or cauda equina compression. This is reversible if relieved early but may result in irreversible paraplegia if allowed to progress untreated.

    c. Peripheral neuropathy, an uncommon complication, which, in some but not all patients, is associated with amyloidosis.

5. *Hypercalcemia.* This may produce a syndrome of severe nausea and vomiting, obstipation, dehydration with polyuria, and a fluctuating semi-comatose state.

6. *Hyperviscosity syndrome.* Although usually a complication of macroglobulinemia of Waldenström (see later), clinical manifestations of hyperviscosity also occur in multiple myeloma when the monoclonal protein concentration is high. This is particularly true for IgA myeloma in which individual immunoglobulin molecules have an increased tendency to polymerize. Hyperviscosity gives rise to the following clinical findings:

    a. Abnormal bleeding, particularly purpura and bleeding from mucous membranes.

b. Visual disturbances with dilitation and segmentation of retinal veins, hemorrhages, and sometimes papilledema (Fig. 20-7).

c. Central nervous system symptoms, for example, vertigo, syncope, somnolence, sometimes convulsions.

d. Marked distention of dependent veins and capillary beds secondary to an increased plasma volume, often with peripheral edema.

e. Dyspnea from distention of the pulmonary capillary bed and from congestive heart failure.

7. *Amyloidosis.* This develops in about 10% of patients and may result in nodular deposits of amyloid in the skin and subcutaneous tissues, enlargement of organs (tongue, liver), and failure of organ function (renal failure, congestive heart failure) due to infiltration by amyloid.

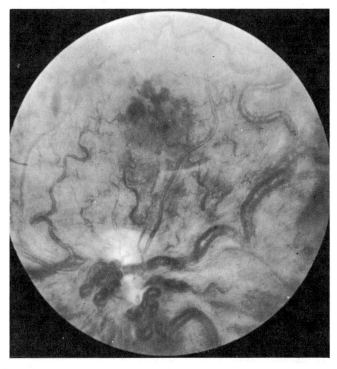

Fig. 20-7. Papilledema, hemorrhages, and dilated, tortuous, veins in the optic fundus of a patient with macroglobulinemia of Waldenström.

Prognosis

Most patients with multiple myeloma used to die within 1 year after the diagnosis was made. Chemotherapy has definitely improved survival, and median survival is now between 2 and 3 years, with a small but not insignificant percent of patients living beyond 5 years. A number of related factors affect an individual patient's progress:

1. *The inherent growth rate of the tumor* at the time of diagnosis. As mentioned, an infrequent patient may have smouldering disease that progresses only very slowly over several years. (Such patients should be observed without treatment.)
2. *The type of light chain and immunoglobulin class of the monoclonal protein.* Patients with λ light chain myeloma do less well as a group than patients with κ light chain myeloma, possibly because the excretion of λ light chains in the urine increases the risk for renal failure and for complicating amyloidosis. The rare IgD myeloma, which is almost always of λ light chain type and is frequently associated with uremia, amyloidosis, and severe anemia, has a short median survival. IgA myeloma tends to be more aggressive than IgG myeloma and has a greater tendency for development of extraosseous tumors. Although grim for all, survival statistics are least grim for patients with κ light chain IgG myeloma.
3. *Extent of disease.* As would be expected, patients with less extensive myeloma at presentation usually live longer than patients with more extensive myeloma. Clinical findings can be used to classify disease extent as follows:

   Stage I (early disease). Evidence of all of the following:
   a. Low production of monoclonal protein.
      (1) Monoclonal protein less than 5 g per dL if IgG or less than 3 g per dL if IgA.
      (2) Urine light chains, less than 4 g excretion in 24 hours.
   b. No significant bone destruction.
      (1) Normal bone structure on radiographs (or only a solitary lytic bone lesion).
      (2) Serum calcium no higher than 12 mg per dL.
   c. Minimal anemia with hemoglobin greater than 10 g per dL

   Stage II (intermediate disease). Findings fitting neither Stage I nor Stage III.

Stage III (extensive disease). Any one of the following:
a. Evidence of high production of monoclonal immunoglobulin.
   (1) Monoclonal protein greater than 7 g per dL if IgG, or greater than 5 g per dL if IgA.
   (2) Urine light chains, greater than 12 g excretion in 24 hours.
b. Evidence of extensive bone destruction.
   (1) Radiographic evidence of advanced lytic lesions.
   (2) Serum calcium greater than 12 g per dL.
c. More severe anemia, with Hgb less than 8.5 g per dL.

This system of classifying disease extent has proved particularly useful in assuring that treatment groups are comparable in protocol studies of different therapeutic regimens.

Serum levels of β_2 microglobulin—which is the shed light chain of the class I histocompatibility determinants found on most cells (see Chapter 14) and which has areas of homology with the constant region domains of immunoglobulins—are elevated in multiple myeloma. The degree of elevation correlates well with disease extent, and measurement of serum β_2 microglobulin appears to be an additional useful predictor of survival in multiple myeloma.

4. *Presence or absence of renal disease.* Patients with abnormal renal function on presentation (serum creatinine over 2.0 mg per dL) have a shorter median survival than do patients presenting with normal renal function.
5. *Responsiveness to chemotherapy with an alkylating agent.*

Treatment

The majority of patients given intermittent high-dose chemotherapy with an alkylating agent, either melphalan or cyclophosphamide, and prednisone will improve initially.

Manifestations of improvement include:

1. Relief of bone pain, which presumably results from a decrease of pressure from expanding marrow lesions.
2. Fall in the serum level of the monoclonal protein.
3. Fall in the excretion of light chains in the urine.
4. Rise in the hemoglobin level.
5. Failure of bone lesions to progress on radiographic examination. (Healing of existing bone lesions is rare.)
6. Fall in the serum β_2 microglobulin level.

Patients whose monoclonal immunoglobulin level falls rapidly after treatment may relapse sooner and therefore not survive as long as patients whose abnormal protein production decreases slowly. This probably means that "fast responders" have a more aggressive tumor with fewer resting cells.

Oral melphalan and prednisone (for example, melphalan, 9 mg per m^2 of body surface area and prednisone, 80 mg for 4 successive days each 28 days) is a standard initial therapy used for many patients. Recent studies suggest that more complicated regimens using additional drugs such as BCNU, vincristine, and doxorubicin may yield better response rates but possibly at the cost of greater risk of toxicity and of greater inconvenience for the patient.

Therapy is continued as long as the plasma concentration of the monoclonal protein is decreasing. How long to continue therapy thereafter is not clear. Some physicians continue for a full 2 years, despite an increasing risk of acute leukemia with continuing long-term alkylating agent chemotherapy.

Various types of secondary therapy have been tried, usually in vain, for patients who fail to respond to initial therapy or who relapse while continuing to receive an alkylating agent. However, a regimen of cycles of continuous intravenous doxorubicin and vincristine over 4 days, along with high-dose adrenal steroid therapy, was recently reported to induce remission in a substantial percentage of patients with advanced disease resistant to alkylating agents.

Other important points in management include the following:

1. If manifestations of the hyperviscosity syndrome are present when the patient is first seen, the serum protein level may need to be reduced immediately by plasmaphoresis to gain time for chemotherapy to take effect. Similarly, plasmaphoresis may be needed as an immediate measure to reduce the excretion of light chains in the urine in patients with heavy Bence Jones proteinuria and evidence of increasing renal failure.

2. Patients with marked hypercalcemia should be treated with large amounts of intravenous fluids, furosemide, and adrenal steroids. They may also need treatment with calcitonin and, rarely, with mithramycin.

3. Patients should be kept out of bed as much as possible to minimize decalcification of bones. They should drink 2 to 3 L of fluid daily to prevent dehydration.

4. Patients with painful local lesions or with large lytic lesions

that could lead to a pathologic fracture should receive supplemental radiation therapy to these lesions.

5. Patients who develop fever should be seen without delay. Appropriate cultures should be taken and treatment with antibiotics started while awaiting results.

Late Course

Patients with advanced disease may enter an aggressive terminal phase characterized by increasingly severe pancytopenia, an accelerated rate of rise of the plasma monoclonal immunoglobulin, and a marrow packed with myelomatous infiltrate. Such patients succumb to some complication of their disease, usually infection, within a short period.

Chemotherapy of myeloma carries a major risk for subsequent acute, non-lymphocytic leukemia which approaches 20% at 4 years. A preleukemic syndrome, characterized by leukopenia and a refractory sideroblastic anemia, often precedes the appearance of frank leukemia.

PLASMA CELL NEOPLASIA RELATED TO MULTIPLE MYELOMA

Solitary Myeloma of Bone

Solitary myeloma of bone usually presents as a single osteolytic lesion of the spine, pelvis, or femur (sometimes of a multicystic "soap-bubble radiologic appearance instead of a sharply demarcated lytic lesion), which on biopsy is shown to be a plasma cell tumor. A random sample of bone marrow is normal. Serum protein electrophoresis may be normal or show a small amount of a monoclonal immunoglobulin. Although local surgical therapy, radiotherapy, or both will usually control the local lesion, the disease eventually progresses to multiple myeloma. This occurs within 5 years of diagnosis in many patients, but in a few patients only after a period of up to 20 years.

Extramedullary Plasmacytoma

This is a solitary plasma cell tumor arising in tissue other than bone marrow, most often in the subepithelium of the upper airway, for example, of the paranasal sinuses. Upper airway disease spreads by local extension with damage to surrounding tissues and sometimes local erosion of bone, and by lymphatic drainage to cervical lymph nodes. The disease may also metastasize to bone, including unusual sites, such as the distal tibia, which do not contain red marrow and are therefore not involved in typical multiple myeloma. Aggressive therapy of local disease may induce prolonged survival. Unlike solitary myeloma of bone, which appears to be a variant of what later turns into typical multiple myeloma, extramedullary plasmacytoma is a disease of different biologic behavior than multiple myeloma.

MACROGLOBULINEMIA OF WALDENSTRÖM

Macroglobulinemia of Waldenström is a variant of plasmacytoid lymphocytic lymphoma in which the neoplastic cells synthesize large amounts of a monoclonal IgM molecule. As a result, a high concentration of this macroglobulin protein is found in the plasma. In a small but not insignificant number of patients, the IgM may be shown to possess antibody activity, either as a cold agglutinin or as an anti-IgG antibody with rheumatoid factor activity.

Some patients with chronic cold agglutinin disease (see Chapter 9)—a disorder in which small amounts of a monoclonal macroglobulin with potent cold agglutinin activity triggers episodes of hemolysis—later develop high plasma macroglobulin levels and other findings of full-blown macroglobulinemia of Waldenström. One infers from this that other patients may have an early or precursor stage of macroglobulinemia of Waldenström that smoulders for years but goes unrecognized because the particular macroglobulin synthesized does not produce symptoms at a low concentration.

Manifestations

CLINICAL FINDINGS

The patient with fully developed disease is usually an older man. The most common initial complaints are weakness and fatigue, manifestations of abnormal bleeding (for example, recurrent epistaxis or rectal bleeding), and blurring of vision. Funduscopic examination frequently reveals a characteristic lesion produced by hyperviscosity of the blood: dilated, tortuous retinal veins with sausage-like segmentation, microaneurysms, retinal hemorrhages, and, often, papilledema (see Fig. 20-7). Moderate lymphadenopathy and hepatosplenomegaly are commonly discovered. Bone pain and tenderness are not found.

LABORATORY FINDINGS

1. *Peripheral blood count.* A normochromic, normocytic anemia with a normal or low reticulocyte count is usually observed. In some patients, the anemia may be severe. The low hemoglobin level results partly from a reduced RBC mass and partly from a marked increase in plasma volume secondary to the increased protein in the serum. The WBC count is usually normal. Mild thrombocytopenia is found in a small number of patients.
2. *Bone marrow.* Bone marrow is often difficult to aspirate. Aspirate smears may be hypocellular but contain increased numbers of small lymphocytes, of lymphocytes with plasmacytoid features, and frequently, of plasma cells. Increased numbers of tissue mast cells are also noted. Marrow biopsy sections show nodular areas of hypercellularity or are diffusely hypercellular. The hypercellularity results from the same admixture of small lymphocytes, plasmacytoid lymphocytes, and plasma cells noted on the smears. Occasional cells with accumulations of periodic acid-Schiff (PAS)-positive material that overlie the nucleus (Dutcher bodies) can be found in some patients.
3. *Serum protein electrophoresis* reveals a narrow band of homogenous protein usually located between the β and γ areas. This is identified as IgM by its reaction with anti-μ chain serum on immunoelectrophoresis (see Fig. 20-4) or immunofixation electrophoresis. Electrophoresis of the urine will reveal excretion of free light chains in some patients.
4. *Coagulation studies.* The *bleeding tendency* in macroglobulinemia (and probably also in the hyperviscosity syndrome arising in multiple myeloma) mainly stems from the coating of platelets by the monoclonal protein. This prevents the platelets from forming hemostatic plugs normally in vivo and causes a long bleeding time. The coated platelets will not aggregate normally when ADP or other aggregating agents are added to platelet-rich plasma in vitro. A rare patient may bleed abnormally from another cause—an acquired deficiency of von Willebrand factor (see Chapter 26).
5. *Bone radiographs.* Films do not show lytic lesions in macroglobulinemia of Waldenström. As in many older persons, generalized osteoporosis may be noted.

Complications and Treatment

Patients with macroglobulinemia occasionally present as an emergency because of severe manifestations of hyperviscosity: persistent mucosal bleeding, congestive heart failure with pronounced dyspnea, severe visual disturbances, confusion, or even coma. Reducing the macroglobulin concentration by plasmaphoresis usually corrects these abnormalities promptly. Patients with evidence of significant hyperviscosity and anemia should not be given RBC transfusions until the hyperviscosity is reduced by plasmaphoresis, since increasing RBC concentration increases whole blood viscosity and will worsen manifestations of the untreated hyperviscosity syndrome.

The administration of an oral alkylating agent, usually chlorambucil, may control disease activity for periods as long as several years. The macroglobulin level in the serum will fall, and the hemoglobin level often rises. Patients whose disease is resistant to oral alkylating therapy should be managed by chronic plasmaphoresis therapy. In some patients, the disease transforms into an aggressive lymphoma, namely, a B cell immunoblastic sarcoma.

HEAVY CHAIN DISEASES

Whereas urinary excretion of free light chains is common in multiple myeloma and macroglobulinemia, urinary excretion of free heavy chains is virtually never found. However, a few patients with other disorders have been identified who do excrete free heavy chains in the urine. A free heavy chain is detected by its migration as a narrow band in the gamma region on electrophoresis of urine and by its reaction with an anti-heavy chain antiserum but not with an anti-light chain antiserum. When the structure of such free heavy chains has been studied, they have been found to be abnormal, usually because of internal deletions near the combining site of the variable region and the first constant region domain of the chain.

Patients who excrete heavy chains are said to have a heavy chain disease. Three types of heavy chain disease have been described, each due to the excretion of a different class of heavy chain.

1. γ *Heavy chain disease,* in which the patient excretes an abnormal heavy chain of IgG. Most patients have been over the age of 40 years. Many have presented with a syndrome of weakness, weight loss, fever, waxing and waning lymphadenopathy, and hepatosplenomegaly. Swelling of the uvula and palatal

edema may be noted because of involvement of tonsillar lymphoid tissue (Waldeyer's ring). Patients are anemic and sometimes leukopenic. Increased numbers of eosinophils and scattered plasmacytoid lymphocytes may be noted on the peripheral smear. A Coomb's positive autoimmune hemolytic anemia is present in many patients. Plasma cells, plasmacytoid lymphocytes, and eosinophils may be prominent in the bone marrow. The serum protein electrophoretic pattern has varied. In some patients it is normal; in others it reveals hypogammaglobulinemia; and in still others, narrow or broader based bands with a mobility ranging from α_1 to slow γ are found. A lymph node biopsy is sometimes diagnostic of lymphoma but more often a nondiagnostic, hyperplastic histologic pattern is seen with increased numbers of plasma cells and plasmacytoid lymphocytes. Features of the clinical course in many patients, including a variable but usually poor prognosis, resemble those of immunoblastic lymphadenopathy (see Chapter 18).

2. α *Heavy chain disease*, in which the patient excretes an abnormal heavy chain of the IgA molecule. These patients are a subset of patients with the Mediterranean form of intestinal lymphoma (see Chapter 18) and differ from other patients with this disease only in the excretion of free heavy chain in the urine.

3. μ *Heavy chain disease*, These patients have an atypical form of chronic lymphocytic leukemia in which they excrete, not only heavy chain in the urine, but also large amounts of free light chain (Bence Jones protein). The latter finding, plus the presence of unusual vacuolated plasma cells on an aspirate smear of bone marrow, should alert one to the possibility of μ heavy chain disease.

AMYLOIDOSIS

Amyloid is a homogenous, amorphous extracellular material as seen on light microscopy. It is eosinophilic when stained with hematoxylin-eosin and has an apple-green birefringence when stained with Congo red and examined with a polarizing microscope. On electron microscopic examination, amyloid has a fibrillar structure.

Amyloid may be found as local deposits in a single organ, for example, the thyroid gland or pancreas, or as infiltrates in many organs and tissues throughout the body. If the latter, the infiltrates often eventually induce fatal organ damage.

All amyloid is made up of low molecular weight proteins that have been precipitated in a tissue or tissues because of chronic exposure of the tissue to an excess of the protein (or of a precursor that undergoes partial catabolization to an insoluble lower molecular weight form). For example, amyloid deposits in the pancreas of a patient with an insulinoma have properties of insulin, and amyloid deposits in the thyroid in medullary carcinoma have properties of calcitonin.

If one excludes rare hereditofamilial forms (in which the precipitated protein is related to pre-albumin), one may divide generalized amyloidosis into two categories:

1. *Reactive systemic amyloidosis (AA type).* The precipitated low molecular weight protein of the amyloid deposit, called amyloid protein A, is derived from the catabolism of a much larger precursor protein of serum, called serum amyloid A-related (SAA) protein. SAA protein is an acute phase protein. Reactive systemic amyloidosis occurs in disorders associated with excess production of acute phase proteins over a long period, for example, chronic infections (chronic osteomyelitis or leprosy), rheumatoid arthritis, inflammatory bowel disease, and Hodgkin's disease.

2. *Amyloid secondary to an immunologic-related disorder (AL).* The precipitated low molecular weight material consists of a catabolic product of the variable region of a light chain (hence the abbreviation, AL). The insoluble material frequently contains amino acid sequences that are the product of a particular alternative DNA gene segment that codes for a certain portion of the variable region of λ light chains. AL may occur as a complication of multiple myeloma or macroglobulinemia of Waldenström, but may also develop in patients without evidence of underlying lymphocytic or plasma cell neoplasia. Then, it is called *primary amyloidosis.*

The overlapping relation between primary amyloidosis, monoclonal gammopathy of undetermined significance (MGUS), and multiple myeloma is illustrated in Figure 20-8. MGUS, which is relatively common in the elderly (3% of individuals over 70 years in one survey), represents the limited expansion of a plasma cell clone that makes a small to moderate amout of a monoclonal protein. In most patients, this monoclonal protein has no adverse effects and the disorder is benign. If, however, the protein of the expanded clone contains light chains whose catabolic products form precipitates in the tissue, then

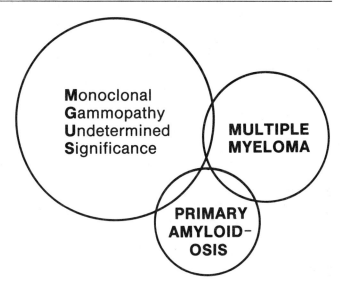

Fig. 20-8. A schematic representation of the overlap of monoclonal gammopathy of unknown significance, multiple myeloma, and primary amyloidosis.

an otherwise benign disorder becomes a fatal disease, *primary amyloidosis.* If the plasma cell clone continues to expand, then MGUS becomes multiple myeloma, and if catabolic products of its light chains are deposited in the tissues, then the multiple myeloma is complicated by amyloidosis.

In primary amyloidosis, as in multiple myeloma, amyloid tends to be deposited in joint capsules and ligaments, the tongue and other skeletal muscles, the heart, the gastrointestinal tract, around peripheral nerve fibers, and sometimes in the liver and kidney. Serum protein electrophoresis in most, but not all patients, will reveal a small peak of a monoclonal immunoglobulin. Clinical manifestations may include peripheral neuropathy, orthostatic hypotension from autonomic nervous system dysfunction, chronic diarrhea, pain and swelling of the wrists and hands (carpal tunnel syndrome), and cardiac failure. Purpura and other abnormal bleeding frequently occur. This stems from increased fragility of small vessels containing amyloid in the walls, from increased fibrinolytic activity, and, in occasional patients, from an acquired deficiency of factor X due to its binding to amyloid in the extracellular tissues. Death often results from refractory congestive heart failure or from a cardiac arrhythmia. It is not clear whether treatment with an alkylating agent and prednisone, as for multiple myeloma, can alter the course in any way except to increase the risk for acute leukemia. Yet, because prognosis for long-term survival of the untreated patient is dismal, such treatment is often tried.

SELECTED READING

1. Barlogie B, Smith L, and Alexanian R: Effective treatment of advanced multiple myeloma refractory to alkylating agents. N Engl J Med 310:1353, 1984.
2. Franklin EC: Amyloidosis. In Williams WJ, Beutler E, Erslev AJ, and Lichtman MA (eds): Hematology. Ed. 3. New York, McGraw-Hill, 1983.
3. Kyle RA: Monoclonal gammopathy of undetermined significance. Natural history in 241 cases. Am J Med 64:814, 1978.
4. Kyle RA, Greipp PR, and Banks PM: The diverse picture of gamma heavy-chain disease. Report of seven cases and review of literature. Mayo Clin Proc 56:439, 1981.
5. Oken MM: Multiple myeloma. Med Clin North Am 68:757, 1984.
6. Wiltshaw E: The natural history of extramedullary plasmacytoma and its relation to solitary myeloma of bone and myelomatosis. Medicine 55:217, 1976.

21

Viral Infections of Lymphocytes and Other Disorders with Prominent Hematologic Findings

GENERAL COMMENTS ON INFECTION OF LYMPHOCYTES BY VIRUSES

The relation between viral infection of lymphocytes and abnormal immune responses and lymphoproliferative malignancies is a matter of current intense study. Two types of viruses infect lymphocytes: a family of human T cell lymphotrophic retroviruses (HTLV-I through V) and two members of the herpesvirus group, Epstein-Barr (EB) virus and cytomegalovirus.

HTLV are RNA viruses, that is, they encode their genetic information in RNA. HTLV infect mature helper/inducer T cells possessing the T4 surface antigen, an antigen present on a surface recognition unit required for T cells to recognize Class II histocompatibility antigens (see Chapter 14). This surface recognition unit apparently can also function as a receptor for HTLV viruses, permitting them to infect the helper/inducer subpopulation of T-lymphocytes. Within infected lymphocytes, HTLV use a viral enzyme, reverse transcriptase, to copy their genetic information into DNA, which is then integrated randomly into the DNA of the cell.

An unknown but substantial proportion of persons infected with HTLV will eventually succumb to its effects. Infection with HTLV-I can, after a long latent period, lead to the emergence of a clone of malignant T4-positive T cells and resultant adult T cell leukemia. HTLV-I has been reported from many geographic areas: Africa, Japan, the Caribbean, and the Southeast United States. HTLV-II has been isolated so far only from rare patients, usually with a T cell form of hairy cell leukemia. HTLV-III (HIV-I) is widespread in East Africa and in high-risk groups in the United States and many other countries. It causes the acquired immunodeficiency syndrome (AIDS). HTLV-IV (HIV-II) has been found as yet only in West Africa; its potential for causing AIDS is not clear. HTLV-V has recently been isolated from some patients with cutaneous T cell lymphomas.

The second type of viruses to infect lymphocytes, the EB virus and cytomegalovirus, are DNA viruses of the same group that includes the herpes simplex virus and the varicella zoster virus. They are ubiquitous; virtually all humans will have antibodies to EB virus in their serum as evidence of past infection by the time they reach mid-adult life. A high proportion will also have antibodies to cytomegalovirus. Except for the circumstances discussed later, infection with these viruses does not result in fatal disease.

A surface receptor for a fragment of the complement protein C3, called C3d, also functions as a receptor for the EB virus. This receptor is present on B but not T-lymphocytes and, therefore, the EB virus can infect only B-lymphocytes. In low socioeconomic groups, infection occurs primarily in early childhood and usually does not produce recognized disease. In higher socioeconomic groups, infection occurs primarily in adolescence or young adult life. About one half of the infections are unrecognized; the other half present as an acute illness with characteristic findings, namely, infectious mononucleosis.

Infection with EB virus rarely produces long-lasting or serious hematologic consequences because the continued proliferation of EB virus in lymphocytes is suppressed by activated T cells. However, EB virus persists in a latent form in B-lymphocytes and oropharyngeal epithelium for the rest of the person's life. Maintenance of latency requires continuous T cell surveillance. If T cell immune responses are severely impaired (for example, by intensive immunosuppressive therapy in a patient with a renal transplant), EB virus within B-lymphocytes can reactivate and initiate a polyclonal proliferation of B cells. If unchecked, this can lead to a fatal polyclonal proliferative disorder with a polymorphous histologic appearance or to the emergence of a dominant B cell clone and the development of a monoclonal high-grade B cell lymphoma.

INFECTION WITH HTLV-III (HIV)

Epidemiology

Infection by HTLV-III virus (also very recently given the name human immunodeficiency virus or HIV) has reached epidemic proportions in high-risk groups in the United States. These include homosexual or bisexual men, men or women who abuse drugs intravenously, and hemophiliacs given pooled clotting factor concentrates before 1985, when procedures diminishing the risk of transmitting HTLV-III by blood products were introduced. Surveys for HTLV-III antibody have yielded seropositivity rates of between about 25% and 75% in homosexual men in the United States and of over 75% in persons with hemophilia A.

The virus can be recovered in the body fluids of an infected individual: semen, blood, saliva, and even tears. The presence of antibody to the virus in body fluids apparently does not diminish their infectivity. The disease has been transmitted primarily as a venereal disease of homosexual men or by a blood-borne route (shared contaminated needles, transfusion of blood or blood products). However, the disease has also been found in the female sexual partners of affected men. An infected mother may transmit the disease to the fetus in utero or to the newborn infant.

The high prevalence of intravenous drug abuse in prostitutes assures the spread of the virus into this epidemiologic group. Since the proportion of asymptomatic infected persons to ill patients is high, promiscuous heterosexual individuals will be increasingly exposed to the virus. They will constitute a new high-risk group, since it is now clear that the disease can also be transmitted by sexual intercourse with an infected woman. The disease is not transmitted by casual contact, but rare instances of infection of hospital personnel caring for patients with AIDS have recently been reported.

The Spectrum of Manifestations of HTLV-III Infection

Many individuals infected with HTLV-III have so far remained asymptomatic; others have developed a syndrome characterized by persistently enlarged lymph nodes; still others have developed AIDS with lymphopenia, atrophy of lymph nodes, and paralysis of virtually all immune responses. Why a selective infection of T4 helper/inducer lymphocytes may remain asymptomatic in one person and trigger destruction of the immune system of another is unknown. It probably does not stem from differences in the virus itself, since transfusion of blood from individuals who have remained asymptomatic carriers has produced fatal AIDS in recipients.

THE ASYMPTOMATIC CARRIER

The interval between infection, for example, a needle stick injury, and the development of a positive blood test for antibody (HIV-seroconversion) is thought to be between 3 and 12 weeks. Most patients discovered to have a positive antibody test will be asymptomatic, although many will have an abnormally low ratio of peripheral blood T4 (helper/inducer) lymphocytes to T8 (suppressor/cytotoxic) lymphocytes due to a selective reduction of T4-lymphocytes.

The risk of an asymptomatic carrier developing AIDS persists for years. The incubation period for AIDS in patients developing AIDS following blood transfusion has varied from 15 months to nearly 9 years, with a mean interval of over 2 years. In different studies, from 5% to 20% of homosexual men with retrospectively determined seropositivity of an earlier serum sample developed AIDS within 2 to 5 years. Another 25% developed other AIDS-related conditions.

Virus has been grown from the blood of asymptomatic seropositive individuals and all asymptomatic seropositive individuals must be considered capable of transmitting the infection.

AIDS-RELATED COMPLEX (ARC)

Chronic Lymphadenopathy. A number of patients with HTLV-III seropositivity develop chronically enlarged lymph nodes at two or more sites (cervical, occipital, axillary, epitrochlear, inguinal). The nodes are moderately enlarged (1 to 3 cm) and usually painless. Some patients may have no other findings; others experience fatigue, low-grade fevers, and weight loss. The WBC count is usually normal but may be moderately decreased; the T4:T8 ratio is usually reduced. About one fourth of patients will be anergic on skin testing.

Lymph node biopsy has usually shown an intense follicular hyperplasia. Unless continued growth of nodes arouses suspicion of lymphoma, lymph node biopsy rarely helps in the patient's clinical management. Increasingly prominent fever and night sweats, continuing weight loss, and the development of oral candidiasis (thrush) heighten concern for early progression to AIDS. In some series, about

10% of homosexual males with chronic lymphadenopathy observed for 1 to 2 years developed AIDS. What will happen to most patients with HTLV-III seropositivity and persistent lymphadenopathy is as yet unknown, but their prognosis is worrisome.

Thrombocytopenic Purpura. An increased prevalence of thrombocytopenic purpura has been noted in promiscuous homosexual men and it reflects infection with HTLV-III. Clinical findings resemble those of idiopathic thrombocytopenic purpura (see Chapter 25). Thus, the patient is afebrile, the spleen is not enlarged, RBC morphology on the peripheral blood smear does not show fragmented RBCs, and the marrow contains normal to increased numbers of megakaryocytes and no evidence of an underlying hematologic disease (for example, lymphoma). However, levels of immunoglobulin bound to the circulating platelet (platelet-associated IgG) are reportedly higher than those usually found in adult ITP in other settings. This suggests that the thrombocytopenia stems from coating of platelets with immune complexes rather than binding to platelets of a platelet-antigen specific autoantibody (see Chapter 25).

Patients with this syndrome may respond to treatment with adrenal glucocorticosteroids, danazol, or both, but one worries about more than the temporary use of these drugs, which depress macrophage and lymphocyte function, in patients already at risk for progressive deterioration of immune responses. Platelet counts may rise after splenectomy, but the effect of splenectomy on the long-term course of such patients is not yet known.

AIDS

Diagnosis. The diagnosis of AIDS is made when a patient with a positive serologic or virologic test for HTLV-III develops one of the following:

1. A serious infection with a microorganism that would not cause disease or would cause only limited disease in a person with normal cellular immune function (opportunistic infection).
2. Certain types of malignancies:
   a. Kaposi's sarcoma, which are multicentric tumors of endothelial cells that usually present as multiple purplish lesions of the skin and sometimes also as nodular lesions involving the mouth, gastrointestinal, or tracheobronchial mucosa.
   b. A lymphoma of B cell phenotype and, usually high-grade, ag-

gressive histology (immunoblastic sarcoma, Burkitt-like lymphoma).
3. CNS findings indicative of an encephalitis.

Clinical Manifestations. The findings in AIDS frequently involve the lungs, gastrointestinal tract, and CNS. Pulmonary findings commonly result from infection with Pneumocystis, Cryptococcus, or cytomegalovirus. Pneumocystis infection can produce disabling dyspnea and hypoxia, despite only minimal findings on physical or radiographic examination of the chest. *Gastrointestinal syndromes,* with malabsorption and unremitting diarrhea, usually result from parasitic infection (Cryptosporidium, Isospora), mycobacterial infection *(Mycobacterium avium-intracellulare),* or viral infection (cytomegalovirus infection), but occasionally may result from involvement of the gastrointestinal tract by Kaposi's sarcoma or lymphoma.

CNS findings include persisting headache, confusion, stupor that may progress to dementia, and, in some patients, focal neurologic defects. These findings may stem from primary infection by HTLV-III of neural or glial cells, which apparently possess a surface membrane receptor for the virus; from secondary infection, for example, by toxoplasma or cryptococcus; or from development of a cerebral lymphoma. Discovery of an intracerebral mass on CT scan usually means either an abscess due to toxoplasmosis or a cerebral lymphoma.

Chronic fever and wasting out of proportion to findings of disease in a particular organ system may be encountered in some patients. These findings may stem from disseminated disease secondary to atypical mycobacterial infection *(Mycobacterium avium-intracellulare),* histoplasmosis, or cytomegalovirus.

Laboratory Manifestations. Peripheral blood findings include the following:

1. Anemia, which is usually moderate and with findings characteristic of the anemia of chronic disease (see Chapter 12).
2. Leukopenia, reflecting a marked lymphopenia, but, sometimes, also reflecting an associated granulocytopenia.
3. A normal to moderately reduced platelet count. Occasional patients may have severe thrombocytopenia.
   (Many patients with AIDS who are treated with trimethoprim-sulfamethoxazole for Pneumocystis infection develop a hypersensitivity reaction with a fall in granulocytes, platelets, or both in addition to fever and rash.)

Bone marrow is often aspirated in patients with AIDS, usually for culture but sometimes because of granulocytopenia or thrombocytopenia. The marrow typically contains adequate numbers of megakaryocytes and granulocytic precursors. In an infrequent patient, an infiltrate of lymphocytes suggestive of lymphoma may be found.

Tests to evaluate immune function reveal:

1. A ratio below 1 of T4 to T8 lymphocytes and, as the disease progresses, reduced total numbers of circulating lymphocytes (lymphopenia).
2. Polyclonal hypergammaglobulinemia associated, paradoxically, with an impaired antibody response to specific antigenic stimulation. The hypergammaglobulinemia may result from stimulation of B cells secondary to reactivation within the cells of EB virus.
3. Loss of delayed hypersensitivity responses to all skin test antigens (for example, tuberculin, histoplasmin, coccidioidin, mumps antigen, Candida antigen).

Association with Lymphoma. A number of patients have been seen with aggressive B cell lymphomas either arising during the course of established AIDS or presenting as the initial manifestation in a person with a positive serology for HTLV-III. These lymphomas frequently involve extranodal sites—the CNS, lungs, retroperitoneum, gastrointestinal tract, bone marrow, or subcutaneous tissues. In some patients, a biopsy discloses a polymorphous (many different types of cells) infiltrate made up of immunoblasts, activated lymphocytes, plasmacytoid lymphocytes, and plasma cells. This reflects a failure of T cells to check the proliferation of transformed B cells. The proliferative process at this stage is polyclonal. In some instances, EB viral DNA has been demonstrated in the proliferating cells, which implicates EB virus as the B cell transforming agent.

In other patients, the initial biopsy—or a further biopsy in a patient with an initially polymorphous lesion—reveals a monomorphous proliferation of either immunoblasts (immunoblastic sarcoma) or of small noncleaved cells of either the Burkitt's or non-Burkitt's type (see Chapter 18). Such lesions, which apparently can evolve from a polymorphous proliferative process, reflect emergence of a predominant population of rapidly proliferating cells of monoclonal origin. Multiple copies of EB viral genome can also be demonstrated in DNA isolated from most of these high-grade lymphomas.

Chemotherapy induces only partial, transient remission in most patients with lymphoma associated with AIDS, regardless of whether the biopsy reveals a polymorphous or monomorphous lesion.

EB VIRAL INFECTION

Infectious Mononucleosis

Infectious mononucleosis is an acute febrile illness fulfilling the following diagnostic criteria in the typical patient:

1. Fever, sore throat, and cervical lymphadenopathy.
2. An absolute lymphocytosis with many atypical activated lymphocytes in the peripheral blood (Fig. 21-1).
3. A positive heterophil antibody test (Monospot test).

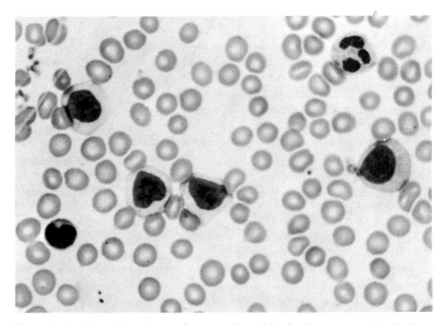

Fig. 21-1. Peripheral blood smear from a patient with infectious mononucleosis. Note appearance of activated lymphocytes found in this disease. Some lymphocytes have irregular, indented nuclei and most cells have an increased amount of cytoplasm. The nucleus is frequently eccentric. The increased basophilia of the cytoplasm is difficult to illustrate in a black-and-white photomicrograph.

EPIDEMIOLOGY

EB virus infects two types of cells: B-lymphocytes and epithelial cells of the oropharynx. Virus can be found in the saliva of patients with infectious mononucleosis and sometimes is shed into the saliva intermittently for months to years afterwards. Exposure to EB virus in saliva, often as a result of kissing, is the usual mode of transmission of the disease. The incubation period is 30 to 50 days. Infectious mononucleosis is rare after the age of 40 years, because by then virtually everyone has been exposed to the virus.

PATHOGENESIS

Virus infecting oral epithelium causes the sore throat of infectious mononucleosis. The virus reproduces itself (replicates) within the oral epithelium, with resultant death of cells and shedding of virus into the saliva.

Virus infecting B-lymphocytes does not replicate but produces viral proteins that transform the quiescent B cell into an activated, proliferating cell. B cell activation is associated with an outpouring of IgM antibodies—not only antibodies specific for EB viral antigens but also a variety of unrelated antibodies, for example, the heterophil antibody, antibody to the i antigen of cord blood RBCs, and sometimes antibody to cardiolipin (the antigen used in the VDRL test for syphilis).

When B cells are infected with EB virus in vitro, the B cells become "immortal," that is, they develop into permanent cell lines that continue to proliferate indefinitely. This would also happen in the body except that T cells mount an intense immune response to suppress the continued proliferation of virally transformed B-lymphocytes. Activated cytotoxic T cells recognize and kill B-lymphocytes that possess a viral protein (called lymphocyte-derived membrane antigen or LYDMA) that becomes inserted into the cell membrane of infected B cells.

Thus, the lymphadenopathy and splenomegaly of infectious mononucleosis result from a dual proliferation of virally infected B cells and of T cells activated to suppress the B cells. A lymph node biopsy reveals an intense hyperplasia that can be confused with a lymphomatous proliferation. Moreover, cells indistinguishable from the Reed-Sternberg cell of Hodgkin's disease have occasionally been noted. The atypical lymphocytes that appear in the peripheral blood are primarily activated, cytotoxic T cells.

As the T cell response succeeds in controlling the proliferation of transformed B cells, the acute illness subsides. However, dormant EB virus persists in some B-lymphocytes. It remains dormant in most patients, who never develop recognizable infectious mononucleosis again. In a few patients, virus may apparently reactivate to give rise to a syndrome of chronic or recurrent infectious mononucleosis (see below).

In patients with disorders that seriously impair cellular immune function, T-lymphocytes may be unable to check the proliferation of EB virus-infected B-lymhocytes. Then, either after initial infection in a patient with a hereditary disorder or later, as cells containing dormant virus escape from control in a patient with an acquired disorder, a fatal lymphoma may arise.

MANIFESTATIONS

Clinical Findings. Infectious mononucleosis usually begins gradually with increasing fever, malaise, and sore throat. Headache, photophobia, and pain on movement of the eyes are sometimes prominent symptoms.

Common findings include:

1. Lymphadenopathy, which is present in almost 100% of cases. The cervical glands are almost always enlarged; the axillary and inguinal glands are also frequently enlarged.
2. Pharyngitis, which is present in over three fourths of patients and which may be severe, occasionally even with ulceration and a membrane. A transitory fine petechial rash on the palate is frequently seen. A peculiar gelatinous appearance of the soft palate and uvula has been described.
3. Edema of the eyelids which has been noted in about one third of patients.
4. Splenomegaly, which is found in more than one half of patients.
5. A palpable liver edge, which is present in about one quarter of patients.

Rarely, the patient may develop jaundice, a skin rash, or evidence of CNS involvement (meningoencephalitis, cranial nerve palsies, optic neuritis).

Laboratory Findings.

1. *Peripheral blood count.* The total WBC count may be low, normal, or high. Low counts are encountered early in the illness

and rise as the disease progresses. At sometime during the illness, the percentage of mononuclear cells usually exceeds 60% of the differential count. Characteristic, activated lymphocytes with eccentric or irregular nuclei, increased cytoplasm, and, often, radiating folds of increased blueness (basophilia) of the cytoplasm are found in large numbers. (These are activated T-lymphocytes). A few lymphocytes may also be seen that have fine nuclear chromatin, prominent nucleoli, and homogeneous dense blue cytoplasm. (These are probably transformed B-lymphocytes.)

Anemia and thrombocytopenia are rare. When a patient with an established diagnosis of infectious mononucleosis becomes anemic, one of two serious complications is likely:

a. An autoimmune hemolytic anemia, associated with a positive direct Coombs' test.

b. A ruptured spleen with bleeding into the capsule or the peritoneal cavity.

2. *Heterophil antibody test.* As mentioned, a primary infection with EB virus stimulates B cells to make a variety of IgM antibodies, including one that reacts with sheep, beef, and horse RBCs. Because it reacts with cells of other species, this antibody is called a heterophil antibody. Its detection became the primary serologic test for the diagnosis of infectious mononucleosis long before EB virus was identified as the causative agent. A heterophil antibody test (the Monospot test) has remained the mainstay of the serologic diagnosis because of its simplicity and the lack of general availability of tests for antibodies to EB viral antigens. Although it may need to be repeated if initially negative, a heterophil antibody test will be positive at some time during the illness in over 95% of patients with infectious mononucleosis.

3. *Liver function tests.* Infectious mononucleosis regularly produces an anicteric hepatitis, with mild elevations of values for SGOT (aspartate aminotransferase, or AST), SGPT (alanine aminotransferase or ALT), and alkaline phosphatase. An occasional patient develops hyperbilirubinemia sufficiently severe to produce clinical jaundice.

4. *Urinalysis.* The urine is usually clear, but a rare patient may develop proteinuria or hematuria.

DIFFERENTIAL DIAGNOSIS

Diagnosis presents little difficulty in most patients. However, diagnostic problems may arise in the following situations:

1. When the smear reveals a prominent lymphocytosis with atypical lymphocytes, but the heterophil antibody test is repeatedly negative. One must then consider the following possibilities:
   a. Heterophil antibody negative infectious mononucleosis. One suspects this diagnosis if all other clinical findings are typical for infectious mononucleosis, that is, the patient has fever, sore throat, cervical lymphadenopathy, abnormal liver function tests. Making an unequivocal diagnosis requires demonstrating a pattern of EB viral antibodies in serum indicative of current EB viral infection (see below). Because these serologic tests are not readily available, this is not commonly done.
   b. The cytomegalovirus mononucleosis syndrome. In this syndrome, patients may have fever, malaise, and abnormal liver function tests but usually do not have sore throat or cervical lymphadenopathy. Diagnosis is made by demonstrating a rising titer of IgM antibodies for cytomegalovirus along with negative serologic tests for current EB viral infection.
   c. Other infectious disease—rubella, toxoplasmosis, adenovirus infection, viral hepatitis.
   d. A drug hypersensitivity reaction that produces lymph-adenopathy and circulating, activated lymphocytes (see Chapter 22).
   e. Poorly differentiated lymphocytic lymphoma with the escape of atypical, poorly differentiated lymphocytes into the blood (see Chapter 18).
   Cytomegalovirus mononucleosis and heterophil-negative infectious mononucleosis will account for most of the above type of patients.
2. When a patient presents with fever, severe pharyngitis, and cervical lymphadenopathy, but a lymphocytosis with atypical lymphocytes is not found on the first blood count. Then, the possibility of a bacterial pharyngitis, for example, a beta-hemolytic streptococcal pharyngitis requiring antibiotic treatment, must be considered and a throat culture should be taken. A second blood count in patients whose illness persists may reveal the atypical lymphocytes.
3. When the patient is jaundiced. Then the findings may closely resemble viral hepatitis caused by one of the hepatitis viruses.
4. When the disease presents with a prominent CNS manifestation, for example, meningitis, optic neuritis.

COURSE, COMPLICATIONS, AND TREATMENT

The acute illness usually subsides within 2 to 4 weeks. However, lymphadenopathy occasionally persists for many weeks and decreasing numbers of atypical lymphocytes may still be found on blood smears weeks to months later. Slight malaise and an increased fatiguability may persist for a number of weeks. Serious complications of acute mononucleosis are rare. They include:

1. Rupture of the spleen. The onset of abdominal pain with left shoulder tip radiation, an unexplained tachycardia, or a sudden fall in hemoglobin level alert one to the possibility of this dangerous complication that requires immediate surgery.
2. Severe neurologic involvement, for example, encephalitis with coma or polyneuronitis with extensive flaccid paralysis.
3. Autoimmune hemolytic anemia (Coombs' test positive) or thrombocytopenia.

No specific therapy exists. An antibiotic is indicated if the throat becomes secondarily infected, but ampicillin should be avoided because it often causes a rash in patients with infectious mononucleosis. Corticosteroids are usually given to patients with severe neurologic manifestations, hemolytic anemia, or thrombocytopenia.

Unusual Manifestations of Epstein-Barr Virus Infection

CHRONIC EB VIRUS INFECTION

Occasional young adults are seen with a syndrome of recurrent episodes of profound fatigue, myalgia, tender cervical lymphadenopathy, and mild pharyngitis. The syndrome may develop after an episode of acute infectious mononucleosis from which the patient appears not to recover fully or may develop in patients without a recognized earlier episode of acute infectious mononucleosis. Since fatigue, listlessness, and feelings of depression may be profound and out of proportion to objective physical findings, the syndrome may be difficult to distinguish from a primary neuropsychiatric illness.

Serologic studies may help to identify patients in whom such findings result from chronic, active EB virus infection. In these patients, one may demonstrate a pattern of EB viral antibodies similar to that seen in acute infectious mononucleosis, namely:

1. Persisting IgM antibodies to viral capsid antigens, a high titer of IgG antibodies to viral capsid antigens, or both.
2. Persisting antibodies to the so-called early antigen complex (antigens that are probably viral enzymes).

In addition and possibly of greater diagnostic significance, some patients will *lack antibodies* that arise later in infectious mononucleosis and are thought to be associated with bringing the disease under control. These are:

1. Antibodies to viral antigens that become inserted in the membrane of B-lymphocytes (for example, the LYDMA antigen).
2. Antibodies to at least two EB viral proteins that are found in the nuclei of infected B-lymphocytes (EB viral nuclear antigens, or EBNA).

As yet, however, a diagnosis of chronic EB virus infection is extremely difficult to establish. Only a handful of laboratories can reliably measure the different EB viral antibodies and criteria for the interpretation of test results need substantiation.

FATAL EPSTEIN-BARR VIRUS-RELATED LYMPHOPROLIFERATIVE DISEASE

Very rare patients with hereditary disorders affecting immune function (usually male children with an X-chromosome-linked hereditary immunologic deficiency) do not recover from infectious mononucleosis but develop a fulminant, fatal lymphoproliferative disease with features of a malignant lymphoma. A similar fatal proliferation of donor cells that contained latent EB virus has been reported in bone marrow transplant recipients in whom a monoclonal antibody against T-lymphocytes was used to treat graft-versus-host disease.

A number of instances of lymphoma, often involving the CNS, have been reported in patients receiving continuous immunosuppressive drugs after kidney or heart transplant and, as discussed earlier, in patients with AIDS. In some patients, EB virus has been implicated in the pathogenesis of the lymphoma by demonstration of elevated titers of EB viral antibodies, immunofluorescent staining of tumor tissue for EB nuclear antigen, and the finding by DNA hybridization techniques of EB viral genomes in the tumor tissue.

It is clear, therefore, that recovery from a primary EB virus infection (infectious mononucleosis) requires not only that T cells suppress the proliferation of EB virus-infected B cells during the acute illness but that T cells maintain continuous surveillance to prevent reactivation of latently infected B cells throughout life thereafter.

CYTOMEGALOVIRUS INFECTION

Unlike EB virus, which infects only B cells and oropharyngeal epithelium, another herpesvirus, cytomegalovirus, infects multiple types of cells. Because these include granulocytes and lymphocytes, in which the virus may persist in a latent form, transmission of cytomegalovirus by blood transfusion has become a cause for concern in certain types of patients (see below).

Manifestations in Normal Adults

A high proportion of adults possess plasma antibodies to cytomegalovirus as evidence of past infection and about 5% excrete virus in the urine. Most seropositive adults will not have had a recognized past infection. A few will have experienced a recognized mononucleosis syndrome characterized by:

1. Fluctuating fever of 2 to 6 weeks duration.
2. An anicteric hepatitis with mildly abnormal liver function tests.
3. A normal to slightly elevated WBC count with a lymphocytosis and prominent numbers of atypical lymphocytes.
4. A rising titer of antibodies to cytomegalovirus.
5. Excretion of virus in the urine.

The syndrome differs from infectious mononucleosis in that pharyngitis, lymphadenopathy, hepatomegaly, and splenomegaly are usually absent. However, as in infectious mononucleosis, a variety of IgM antibodies may be produced transiently during the acute infection. These may include cold agglutinins which, in a rare patient, may cause acute hemolysis.

One setting in which a cytomegalovirus mononucleosis syndrome has been recognized is several weeks after a surgical procedure in which a patient received large amounts of blood, for example, cardiopulmonary bypass surgery. In this setting, splenomegaly is often part of the syndrome.

Congenital Cytomegalovirus Infection

Although many seropositive women excrete cytomegalovirus in the urine during pregnancy, activation of cytomegalovirus replication during pregnancy in a patient with a past primary infection does not cause serious disease of the newborn infant. In contrast, if a previously seronegative woman develops a primary cytomegalovirus infection during pregnancy, then the infant may be born with serious congenital cytomegalovirus infection. Such infants may have severe neurologic damage, hepatosplenomegaly, hemolytic anemia, and thrombocytopenia.

Cytomegalovirus Infection in Transplant Patients

Four to 12 weeks after bone marrow transplantation, a substantial number of recipients develop life-threatening interstitial pneumonitis due to cytomegalovirus. Such infections reflect continuing immunosuppression in the recipient. Recovery is dependent upon the emergence of donor T-lymphocytes cytotoxic for cells infected with the virus.

Patients receiving immunosuppressive therapy after renal transplantation may also develop serious interstitial pneumonitis due to cytomegalovirus.

Implications for Transfusion Therapy

Evidence of cytomegalovirus infection can be found in a high percentage of patients following blood transfusion, for example, in a reported 30% of patients receiving transfusions during surgery. The virus is apparently transmitted by infected leukocytes in blood from an asymptomatic donor. It can cause:

1. A primary infection.
2. A superinfection with a new strain of cytomegalovirus.
3. A reactivation, by an unknown mechanism, of latent endogenous cytomegalovirus infection in the recipient.

In most patients, infection after transfusion is asymptomatic and is recognized only by a rise in viral antibody titer. As mentioned, an occasional postoperative patient may develop a transient post-transfusion mononucleosis syndrome. However, in a patient with impaired T cell immune function, transfusion-induced cytomegalovirus infection may have serious or even fatal consequences. Indications for the use of seronegative donors to prevent serious cytomegalovirus infection after transfusion are not yet fully defined. However, it appears prudent to obtain seronegative donor blood (or carefully washed RBCs that are depleted of leukocytes) for the following types of patients:

1. A seronegative pregnant woman, in order to prevent primary infection and consequent congenital infection of the fetus.
2. A seronegative low-birth-weight infant. Premature infants have a limited storage pool of granulocytes and are sometimes given granulocyte transfusions to combat serious infection. If the premature infant is seronegative, the granulocyte donor should also be seronegative to prevent superimposed serious neonatal cytomegalovirus infection.
3. A seronegative transplant recipient receiving an organ from a seronegative donor. Such a patient will not be at risk for serious post-transplant cytomegalovirus infection if only seronegative donors are used for blood, granulocyte, or platelet transfusions.

NEUTROPENIAS

Causes

A transient neutropenia accompanies some acute infectious diseases (for example, some gram-negative infections, viral infections). Manifestations of infection are usually obvious and, unless the neutropenia is extreme, the patient does not present as a primary hematologic problem. However, in an alcoholic patient with infection and neutropenia, the possibility of impaired effective granulopoiesis secondary to folate deficiency arises, and such patients may benefit from folate given therapeutically.

When evaluating a patient because of a *persisting neutropenia,* one attempts to answer the following questions:

1. Is the patient taking a drug that causes neutropenia (see Chapter 22)?
2. Has the patient had fever and lost weight? If so, one must consider the following possibilities:
   a. A chronic infection, for example, a mycobacterial infection.
   b. A lymphoma, for example, abdominal Hodgkin's disease.
   c. An autoimmune disorder, such as systemic lupus erythematosus.

3. Does the patient have evidence of chronic liver disease? (Neutropenia in chronic liver disease may stem from congestive splenomegaly with increased sequestration of neutrophils in an enlarged spleen or, in some patients with chronic hepatitis, from suppression of granulopoiesis by T-lymphocytes in the bone marrow.)

4. Does the patient have an enlarged spleen and, if so, why? Finding an enlarged spleen raises the possibility of:
   a. Congestive splenomegaly with neutropenia secondary to splenic sequestration (for example, in cirrhosis or Gaucher's disease)
   b. A lymphoma or aleukemic lymphocytic leukemia with neutropenia reflecting suppression of granulopoiesis secondary to abnormal immune function or marrow infiltration by lymphomatous cells (for example, in hairy cell leukemia, see Chapter 17)

5. Does the patient have physical findings or laboratory abnormalities suggestive of rheumatic disease—systemic lupus erythematosus, rheumatoid arthritis, polymyositis?

6. Does the patient's peripheral blood smear reveal evidence of a myelodysplastic syndrome (see Chapter 11)? Such evidence might include:
   a. Dysplastic changes in neutrophils, for example, diminished granulation of the cytoplasm, presence of bilobed granulocytes (pseudo Pelger-Huët cells).
   b. RBC abnormalities—an elevated MCV, scattered, large round or oval macrocytes on the blood smear, basophilic stippling.
   c. Large platelets that appear pale blue in color because of a deficient content of granules.

Chronic Idiopathic Neutropenia

Occasional patients, usually women, may be seen in whom an underlying disorder cannot be found to account for a persisting neutropenia with absolute neutrophil counts below 2000 per µL and frequently below 1000 per µL. Such patients are said to have chronic idiopathic neutropenia. Physical examination is unremarkable. The RBC and platelet counts are normal. The neutrophil count is depressed, but the WBCs are otherwise normal, except for a slight monocytosis in some patients. In the bone marrow one finds plentiful numbers of early myeloid precursors but reduced numbers of late metamyelocytes and mature granulocytes. When looked for, antineutrophilic antibodies in the serum have been the exception, not the rule. In one study, T cells suppressing granulopoiesis were demonstrated in the marrow of 9 of 25 patients.

The disorder usually persists for many years with a benign course not requiring treatment in most patients. Occasional patients with severely reduced counts (for example, neutrophil counts persistently below 500 per μL) have experienced troublesome infections. A few patients with neutrophil counts approaching zero and with repeated infections have been cautiously treated with alternate day prednisone, despite its risk of further impairing resistance to infection and of masking manifestations of inflammation.

Felty's Syndrome

Felty's syndrome is a complication of rheumatoid arthritis with the following manifestations:

1. Arthritis, often severe and long-standing and sometimes in a burned-out stage.
2. Splenomegaly, which may be minimal to massive.
3. Severe neutropenia.
4. Serologic abnormalities which may include:
   a. An elevated gamma globulin level associated with a high titer of *rheumatoid factor*.
   b. The presence of antinuclear antibodies.
   c. Evidence of mixed cryoglobulins (which are cold precipitable immune complexes).
5. A bone marrow that usually appears normocellular or hypercellular with increased numbers of early myeloid forms.

Although the appearance of the bone marrow suggests increased granulocyte production, in some patients, granulopoiesis may be depressed. Thus, the bone marrow of some patients contains T-lymphocytes that suppress normal marrow granulocyte colony growth in vitro. These patients are now thought to have a variant of the Tγ cell leukemia/lymphocytosis syndrome (see Chapter 17).

In other patients, increased amounts of immunoglobulin bound to the granulocytes have been demonstrated, as well as increased amounts of immunoglobulin in the serum that can bind to the granulocytes of other individuals. In these patients, an accelerated clearance of immunoglobulin-coated neutrophils and supression of granulopoiesis by serum immunoglobulins reacting with granulocytic precursors in the marrow could be causes for the neutropenia.

Patients with severe neutropenia and repeated serious infections have been subjected to splenectomy, which causes granulocyte levels to rise briefly in virtually all patients. Unfortunately, in many patients it falls again within a few weeks.

EOSINOPHILIAS

Eosinophils in blood normally do not exceed 350 per μL. Eosinophilia with counts above 1000 per μL directs attention to the following possible disorders:

1. Helminthic infection by worms that migrate through tissues (Ascaris, hookworm, Strongyloides) or that persist in tissues (Schistosoma, Trichinella).
2. A sensitivity reaction to a drug (for example, phenytoin).
3. Skin disorders (for example, dermatitis herpetiformis, pemphigus).
4. Allergic states (hay fever, asthma).
5. An underlying malignancy (for example, Hodgkin's disease, non-Hodgkin's lymphoma, occasional patients with carcinoma).
6. Pulmonary infiltrative diseases with eosinophilia (see below).
7. The hypereosinophilic syndrome (see below).

The mechansisms responsible for eosinophilia in these disorders are only partially understood. In the eosinophilias of parasitic infections, T-lymphocytes may interact with tissue-fixed antigens (for example, antigens of larvae that migrate into the lungs, liver, or muscles) to liberate a substance stimulating eosinopoiesis. Tissue mast cells contain materials chemotatic for eosinophils. These materials are liberated when mast cells degranulate and may be responsible for the eosinophilia of peripheral blood and tissues found in some hypersensitivity reactions. Antigen-antibody complexes and an activated fragment of complement, $C5_a$, are chemotactic for both neutrophils and eosinophils and may stimulate the eosinophilia that accompanies some types of skin disease and vasculitis. A substance chemotactic for eosinophils has also been isolated from tumor tissue of a patient with an eosinophilia associated with a pulmonary carcinoma.

Pulmonary Infiltrative Diseases

A hypersensitivity reaction in the lung producing eosinophilia and pulmonary infiltrates on radiographs may occur in:

1. Infectious disease involving the lung.
   a. Helminthic disease in which larva migrate to the lungs—tropical eosinophilia (filaria), invasion of the lungs by larva of Ascaris, Strongyloides, or hookworm.
   b. Fungal disease.
      (1) Bronchopulmonary aspergillosis, a disorder of asthmatic patients in which the fungus colonizes the bronchial tree with resultant wheezing, fever, thick mucoid sputum, pulmonary infiltrates on radiographs that tend to be segmental and central, precipitating plasma antibodies to Aspergillus and eosinophilia of sputum and blood.
      (2) Coccidioides, in which patients may develop a hypersensitivity syndrome with a pulmonary infiltrate, fever, arthralgia, erythema nodosum, and eosinophilia.
2. Hypersensitivity reactions to molds in grain dust (farmer's lung) and other types of dusts. (In some patients, eosinophils may be present in lung biopsies without a peripheral blood eosinophilia.)
3. Chronic eosinophilic pneumonia—a severe, chronic illness of unknown etiology with fever, weight loss, pulmonary infiltrates that are characteristically found in the peripheral lung fields on radiographs, and a mild to moderate eosinophilia in the blood. Asthmatic symptoms and eosinophilis in the sputum may or may not be present. The pulmonary infiltrates disappear promptly after beginning treatment with adrenal corticosteroids.
4. Löffler's syndrome—a mild illness of unknown etiology with transient pulmonary infiltrates and eosinophilia.
5. Disorders in which pulmonary infiltrates are one manifestation of a generalized hypersensitivity disease.
   a. Allergic granulomatosis, a systemic vasculitis with many features in common with periarteritis nodosa but with the additional findings of asthma, pulmonary infiltrates, and eosinophilia.
   b. Sarcoidosis, which is suspected when bilateral hilar adenopathy is found.

Visceral Larva Migrans

This disorder occurs in children who eat dirt and become infected with eggs of nematodes whose natural host is the dog (*Toxocara canis*) or cat (*Toxocara cati*). Larvae migrate to the tissues and produce a serious illness with fever, intense eosinophilia, wheezing, pneumonitis, hepatomegaly, and splenomegaly. The nematode cannot complete its life cycle in the human, and the disorder may gradually subside if the child can be kept from reinfecting himself or herself.

The Hypereosinophilic Syndrome

This disorder of unknown etiology or etiologies has been described under several names: disseminated eosinophilic collagen disease, Löffler's fibroplastic endocarditis, and eosinophilic leukemia. It primarily affects adult males. Its manifestations include combinations of the following:

1. Prominent and persistent eosinophilia with WBC counts between 15,000 and 150,000 per μL and differential counts of from 30% to 70% predominantly mature eosinophils. An anemia of varying severity is also found; platelet counts are usually normal. The bone marrow is hypercellular and, as expected, contains many eosinophils and eosinophilic precursors.
2. Intermittent or persistent fever, which may be low grade.
3. Prominent cardiac findings: cardiomegaly, significant murmurs, abnormal EKGs, echocardiograms showing left ventricular wall thickening and mural thrombi, congestive heart failure.
4. Peripheral embolic phenomena from mural thrombi in the left heart.
5. Hepatomegaly, splenomegaly, or both.
6. Pulmonary infiltrates and, occasionally, pleural effusions.
7. Neurologic dysfunction, most commonly manifest as a sensory polyneuropathy, but sometimes presenting as an encephalopathy or as ischemic CNS episodes due to emboli.

The findings reflect the effect of eosinophilic infiltration of organs and resultant tissue damage by materials liberated from eosinophils (for example, major basic protein). Treatment consists of attempting to check the proliferation of eosinophils, initially with adrenal glucocorticosteroids and, if that fails, with hydroxyurea. Patients with mural thrombi should also be given an oral anticoagulant to prevent emboli.

The progressive course, the extreme eosinophilia that occasionally develops, and the terminal appearance of circulating immature WBC in a few patients suggest that at least some instances of this disorder represent a true eosinophilic leukemia. However, cytogenetic study of bone marrow cells does not reveal the Ph[1] chromosomal abnormality of chronic myelogenous leukemia. A number of patients succumb to cardiac failure, and in such patients, an autopsy often reveals striking endomyocardial fibrosis and large mural thrombi in the left ventricle. Eosinophilic infiltrates are found at autopsy in the heart, liver, spleen, and many other organs.

GAUCHER'S DISEASE

Pathogenesis

Cell membranes contain compounds called globosides and gangliosides. These are made up of a molecule of sphingosine to which are attached a long chain fatty acid (at the amino group) and a series of sugar molecules (at the hydroxy group). The sphingosine-fatty acid complex, called ceramide, is common to all of the compounds, whereas the series of sugar molecules (oligosaccharide chains) differ in their number and arrangement in the different globosides and gangliosides.

During normal catabolism, specific enzymes cleave successive sugar molecules from these compounds, beginning at the distal end of the oligosaccharide chain and working toward the ceramide core. Defective function of different enzymes gives rise to a group of hereditary disorders known as the *lipidoses*. Their clinical manifestations vary widely, a reflection, in part, of differing patterns of accumulation of the incompletely metabolized glycolipids in the tissues. Several disorders, for example, Tay-Sachs disease, present in small infants as catastrophic disorders of the nervous system.

Throughout life, the mononuclear phagocytes of the spleen, liver, and bone marrow remove senescent RBCs from the circulation by phagocytosis and must break down the globosides of the RBC membrane. The major RBC globoside contains a chain of four sugar molecules; the innermost, that is, the sugar attached to the sphingosine, is a glucose molecule. In Gaucher's disease, reduced function of a glucosidase called glucocerebrosidase impedes the splitting of the glucose from the sphingosine. Consequently, glucosyl ceramide (also called glucocerebroside) accumulates in the mononuclear phagocytes, producing lipid-filled macrophages with cytoplasm that has a characteristic wrinkled appearance on light microscopy (Fig. 21-2). Large numbers of these cells, known as Gaucher's cells, accumulate in the organs in which senescent RBCs are destroyed—the spleen, liver, and bone marrow. Lesser numbers may also be found in other organs, for example, the lymph nodes and lung, due to the accumulation of glucosyl ceramide from WBC.

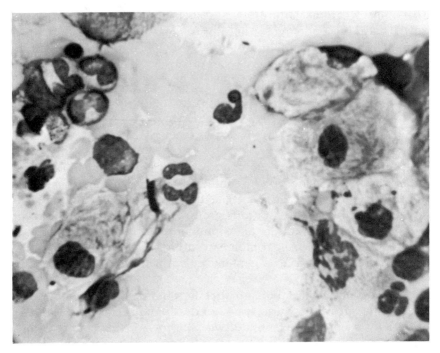

Fig. 21-2. High-power view of a bone marrow smear to show Gaucher's cells. Note large size of cells compared with granulocytic elements and the characteristic wrinkled, tissue paper look of the cytoplasm.

Gaucher's disease is inherited as an autosomal recessive disorder, usually of patients of European (Ashkenazic) Jewish ancestry. Heterozygote carriers are asymptomatic but can be identified by demonstrating reduced activity of one of the glucosidase enzymes in peripheral blood WBC.

Two forms of Gaucher's disease exist: a severe, infantile form in which neurologic dysfunction usually leads to death before the age of 3 years; and a less severe, chronic form compatible with a normal life span. Since the two forms do not occur in the same family, they must stem from different genetic defects.

Manifestations of the Chronic Form

The disease may be first recognized at any age from early childhood until late adult life. Often, the discovery of an enlarged spleen provides the first clue to the diagnosis. The major clinical manifestations are:

1. Splenomegaly, which may be massive.
2. Hepatomegaly.
3. Bone changes due to expansion of the marrow cavity. Thinning of the bony cortex produces a characteristic radiographic finding in the distal end of the femur—the so-called Erlenmeyer flask deformity.

Some patients also develop skin pigmentation and pingueculae (yellowish-brown discolorations of the conjunctiva on either side of the cornea).

The hematologic manifestations largely reflect sequestration of blood cells in an enlarged spleen with hyperactive phagocytic activity (hypersplenism) and consist of:

1. A mild to moderate anemia.
2. Mild leukopenia (some patients).
3. Minimal to moderate thrombocytopenia (many patients) to pronounced thrombocytopenia (rare patients).

Most patients also have a high serum level of acid phosphatase, which escapes from lysosomal granules of the enormously increased number of lipid-filled tissue macrophages.

Course of the Chronic Form

Some patients live a normal life span with little difficulty from their disease. In other patients, a massively enlarged spleen produces disabling symptoms. Children may experience episodes of acute infarction of bone, causing bone pain and fever that mimics acute osteomyelitis. This apparently results from masses of Gaucher's cells compromising blood flow in end arteries leading to the epiphyseal plate. Thinning of the bony cortex may lead to pathologic fractures of long bones.

Splenectomy has been performed in some patients to relieve pressure symptoms or to alleviate thrombocytopenia. However, removing the splenic site of RBC breakdown accelerates the accumulation of Gaucher's cells in other organs and may lead to massive hepatomegaly and increased severity of bone lesions. Therefore, a patient with moderate thrombocytopenia, who has little risk of serious bleeding, should not be subjected to splenectomy.

SELECTED READING

AIDS

1. Broder S, and Gallo RD: A pathogenic retrovirus (HTLV-III) linked to AIDS. N Engl J Med 311:1292, 1984.
2. Curran JW, Morgan WM, Hardy AM, Jaffe HW, Darrow WW, and Dowdle WR: The epidemiology of AIDS: Current status and future prospects. Science 229:1352, 1985.
3. Gottlieb MS: Nonneoplastic AIDS syndromes. Semin Oncol 11:40, 1984.

Infectious Mononucleosis

1. Epstein MA, and Achong BG: Pathogenesis of infectious mononucleosis. Lancet 2:1270, 1977.
2. Horowitz CA, Henle W, Henle G, Polesky H, Balfour HH Jr, Seim RA, Borken S, and Ward PCJ: Heterophil-negative infectious mononucleosis and mononucleosis-like illnesses. Laboratory confirmation of 43 cases. Am J Med 63:947, 1977.
3. Niederman JC: Editorial: Chronicity of Epstein-Barr virus infection. Ann Intern Med 102:119, 1985.
4. Snydman DR, Rudders RA, Daoust P, Sullivan JL, and Evans AS: Infectious mononucleosis in an adult progressing to fatal immunoblastic lymphoma. Ann Intern Med 96:737, 1982.

Cytomegalovirus Infection

1. Adler SP: Transfusion-associated cytomegalovirus infections. Rev Infect Dis 5:977, 1983.
2. Quinnan GV Jr, Kirmani N, Rook AH, Manischewitz JF, Jackson L, Moreschi G, Santos GW, Saral R, and Burns WH: Cytotoxic T cells in cytomegalovirus infection. HLA-restricted T-lymphocyte and non-T lymphocyte cytoxic responses correlate with recovery from cytomegalovirus infection in bone marrow transplant recipients. N Engl J Med 307:7, 1982.

Neutropenias

1. Bagby GC, Lawrence HJ, and Neerhout RC: T-lymphocyte-mediated granulopoietic failure. In vitro identification of prednisone-responsive patients. N Engl J Med 309:1073, 1983.
2. Blumfelder TM, Logue GL, and Shimm DS: Felty's syndrome: effects of splenectomy upon granulocyte count and granulocyte-associated IgG. Ann Intern Med 94:623, 1981.
3. Dale DC, Guerry D IV, Wewerka JR, Bull JM, and Chusid MJ: Chronic neutropenia. Medicine 58:128, 1979.
4. Kyle RA: Natural history of chronic idiopathic neutropenia. N Engl J Med 302:908, 1980.

Eosinophilias

1. Butterworth AE, and David JR: Current concepts: eosinophil function. N Engl J Med 304:154, 1981.
2. Carrington CB, Addington WW, Goff AM, Madoff IM, Marks A, Schwaber JR, and Gaensler EA: Chronic eosinophilic penumonia. N Engl J Med 280:787, 1969.
3. Chusid MJ, Dale DG, West BC, and Wolff SM: The hypereosinophilic syndrome: analysis of fourteen cases with review of the literature. Medicine 54:1, 1975.
4. Parillo JE, Fauci AS, and Wolff SM: Therapy of the hypereosinophilic syndrome. Ann Intern Med 89:167, 1978.

Gaucher's Disease

1. Peters SP, Lee RE, and Glew RH: Gaucher's disease. A review. Medicine 56:425, 1977.

22

Hematologic Reactions to Drugs

Drugs can produce a wide variety of hematologic reactions (Table 22-1). When faced with an unexplained hematologic abnormality, one must never overlook the possibility that it stems from a drug.

MARROW APLASIA

This most serious of all hematologic drug reactions results from suppression or destruction of hematopoietic stem cells in the bone marrow and in the sites of potential extramedullary hematopoiesis (spleen, liver, and lymph nodes). When caused by an antimetabolite, the aplasia is usually transitory. When caused by other drugs, the damage is all too often permanent.

The patient presents with pancytopenia—severe anemia with a depressed reticulocyte count, severe leukopenia, and thrombocytopenia. The spleen, liver, and lymph nodes are not enlarged. Usually, the bone marrow is empty—with an increased amount of fat and residual cells consisting of lymphocytes, plasma cells, tissue mast cells, macrophages, and fibroblasts.

As mentioned in Chapter 11, marrow aplasia from drugs falls into two categories:

1. Aplasia secondary to drugs, such as alkylating agents and anti-metabolites, whose therapeutic effect stems from interference with vital cell processes. Used to destroy malignant cells, the

TABLE 22-1. A List of Hematologic Reactions Induced by Drugs

A. Marrow aplasia with pancytopenia
B. Reactions primarily affecting RBCs
  1. Impaired erythropoiesis
    a. Drug-induced selective erythroid aplasia (very rare)
    b. Drug-induced megaloblastic anemia (see Chapter 4)
  2. Hemolysis
    a. Secondary to oxidation of hemoglobin in patients with intrinsic RBC
      defects
      (1) G6PD deficiency or other rare deficiencies limiting the supply or
         availability of GSH for reducing H_2O_2 (see Chapter 7)
      (2) Unstable hemoglobins (see Chapter 5)
    b. Secondary to an immune reaction
      (1) Reactions in which an antibody damages RBCs only in the presence of
         the drug
         (a) Drug adsorption type
         (b) Immune complex type
      (2) Reactions in which a drug-induced antibody interacts with RBC
         antigens in the absence of the drug (alpha methyldopa, L-dopa)
C. Reactions primarily affecting WBCs
  1. Agranulocytosis
    a. Immunologic
    b. Toxic depression of granulopoiesis
  2. Neutropenia
D. Reactions primarily affecting platelets
  1. Drug-induced immunologic thrombocytopenic purpura
  2. Drug-induced impairment of platelet function (see Chapter 26)
E. Hypersensitivity reactions
  1. With lymphadenopathy and atypical lymphocytes in the blood
  2. With a lupus-like reaction
  3. With eosinophilia

drugs also damage normal bone marrow cells. Their effect on hematopoietic tissue depends upon the dose. *Every patient will develop marrow aplasia if given enough drug.*

2. Aplasia secondary to drugs that do not seriously damage the hematopoietic tissue of the vast majority of patients. *Aplasia results from a unique sensitivity of the patient's hematopoietic tissue to the drug or its metabolites.*

    Chloramphenicol (Chloromycetin), *phenylbutazone* (Butazolidin), and *oxyphenbutazone* (Tandearil) lead the list of drugs causing this type of aplasia. Others include: *indomethacin* (Indocin), *methylphenylethylhydantoin* (Mesantoin), *trimetha-*

dione (Tridione), *carbamazepine* (Tegretol), and gold compounds.

Chloramphenicol may produce two probably unrelated hematologic syndromes:

1. Pharmacologic depression of hematopoiesis, which occurs in most patients receiving large doses (4 to 12 grams daily) of drug over several days. This is characterized by:
   a. A gradually developing anemia with reticulocytopenia, a high serum iron, a disappearance of late normoblasts from the bone marrow, and the appearance of cytoplasmic vacuoles in pronormoblasts.
   b. Moderate leukopenia, which is sometimes associated with vacuolated myeloid precursors in the marrow.
   c. Moderate depression of the platelet count.
   Hematopoiesis promptly recovers when the drug is stopped and residual evidence of marrow damage is not found.
2. Permanent marrow aplasia, which occurs rarely (an estimated 1 in 30,000 risk) but often ends fatally. Aplasia is unrelated to duration of therapy or dosage. Pharmacologic depression is not a known precursor of aplasia, which may be first detected several months after the drug has been stopped. *Because one cannot predict which patient will become aplastic, chloramphenicol should be used only in seriously ill patients with infection not controllable by other antibiotics.*

DRUG-INDUCED HEMOLYSIS

When the possibility arises that a drug has caused hemolysis, attention turns to two possible mechanisms:

1. Drug-induced oxidation of hemoglobin in RBCs with intrinsic defects increasing the susceptibility of hemoglobin to oxidation.
2. Drug-induced immune hemolysis.

Drug-Induced Oxidation of Hemoglobin

Phenylhydrazine, a drug no longer used clinically, will oxidize hemoglobin in normal RBCs. Other oxidant drugs—certain antimalarials, a number of sulfa preparations, acetanilid, nitrofurantoin—are not powerful enough to oxidize hemoglobin in normal RBCs but will oxidize hemoglobin in RBCs with one of two types of hereditary intrinsic defects:

1. A limited supply of reduced glutathione (GSH), which is needed to reduce hydrogen peroxide (H_2O_2) in RBCs and thus protect hemoglobin from oxidation. The common cause is G6PD deficiency (see Chapter 7).
2. An unstable hemoglobin (see Chapter 5), in which an amino acid substitution in either an α or β chain close to the attachment of the heme group increases the susceptibility of the hemoglobin molecule to oxidation.

The following clinical screening tests are used to look for these abnormalities:

1. Incubation of RBCs with certain dyes (for example, crystal violet, brilliant cresyl blue) which will stain inclusion bodies of oxidized hemoglobin (Heinz bodies) in the RBC.
2. A screening test for G6PD deficiency (see Chapter 7).
3. An isopropanol precipitation test for an unstable hemoglobin.

Drug-Induced Immune Hemolysis

DRUG ADSORPTION TYPE

In this type of drug-induced hemolysis, a drug or a drug metabolite induces production of an antibody. The drug or the metabolite also binds firmly to the RBC membrane. The antibody, which is of the IgG class, reacts with the drug or the metabolite on the RBC membrane. Hemolysis results usually from the accelerated removal of IgG coated RBCs by phagocytosis, primarily in the spleen.

Penicillin is the most common cause of this type of hemolysis. The clinical and laboratory findings in penicillin-induced hemolytic anemia are:

1. The patient is receiving a large dose of penicillin, for example, 20,000,000 units per day, or is receiving a lesser dose but has impaired renal function with a resultant high plasma concentration of penicillin. Because of the high plasma concentration, penicillin binds to the RBC membrane.
2. Hemolysis begins subacutely. The RBC count starts to fall, despite an increasing reticulocyte count and no evidence of blood loss. If the process goes unrecognized, the anemia worsens and may become severe. Spherocytes can usually be seen on the pe-

ripheral blood smear. The level of indirect reacting bilirubin rises. One does not find evidence of intravascular hemolysis, that is, of hemoglobinemia or hemoglobinuria.
3. Serologic studies reveal:
   a. A positive direct Coombs' test with a broad-spectrum antiserum. The test remains positive when an IgG-specific antiglobulin antiserum is used (see Chapter 9).
   b. A negative indirect Coombs' test with normal RBCs.
   c. A positive indirect Coombs' test with penicillin-coated normal RBCs.

These test results establish that the patient's cells are coated by an IgG antibody present in the serum which will only attach to the RBC membrane when penicillin is bound to the membrane.

IMMUNE COMPLEX TYPE

In this type of drug-induced hemolysis, a drug or a drug metabolite binds to a plasma protein to form an immunogen inducing antibody synthesis. The antibody may be IgM, IgG, or both. The drug or its metabolite does not bind firmly to the RBC surface. However, a drug (or drug metabolite)-plasma protein-antigen combines with the plasma antibody, and the resultant antigen-antibody complex comes down briefly onto the RBC. The mechanism of attachment is unknown but may involve binding to a membrane antigen of the blood group systems, for example, the I antigen (see Chapter 9), that functions as a receptor for the immune complex.

The antigen-antibody complex brings complement components along with it down onto the RBC. The complement components stick to the RBC membrane, whereas the antigen-antibody complex leaves the cell and is then free to bring complement components down onto other RBCs. (Thus, a small amount of drug may precipitate extensive hemolysis.) The complement activation reactions proceed to completion on the RBC membrane with resultant severe membrane damage and intravascular hemolysis.

Drugs in use in the United States that have induced the reaction in rare patients include: quinidine, quinine, triamterene, tetracycline, sodium thiopental, and phenacetin. Clinical and laboratory manifestations are:

1. The dose of the offending drug is not large. Occasionally, the first dose of a second or subsequent course of a drug has triggered the reaction.

2. Hemolysis begins abruptly. The patient suddenly becomes very ill—often experiencing chills, vomiting, tightness in the chest, and diarrhea. Brisk intravascular hemolysis results in both hemoglobinemia and hemoglobinuria and frequently precipitates acute, oliguric renal failure.

3. Serologic studies may reveal:

    a. A positive direct Coombs' test with broad-spectrum Coombs' serum, which recognizes complement on the RBC membrane, but not with antiglobulin antiserum specific for IgG.

    b. Inability of normal RBCs first incubated in vitro with the drug and then added to the patient's serum to give a positive indirect Coombs' test. Thus, one cannot demonstrate direct binding of the drug to the RBC membrane.

    c. A positive indirect Coombs' test with broad-spectrum antiglobulin antiserum when normal RBCs are incubated with patient's serum plus a solution of the drug. In some patients, a metabolite of the drug must be used to obtain a positive test result. (Serum or urine from a normal volunteer who has taken a dose of the drug is the source of the metabolite.) This test result indicates that the patient's serum contains an antibody that, in the presence of the drug or a drug metabolite, can cause complement components to come down onto normal RBCs.

    d. Lysis of enzyme-treated normal RBCs after incubation with the patient's serum, a source of fresh complement, and the drug or a metabolite of the drug.

One must be aware, however, that some patients with acute drug-induced immune intravascular hemolysis have had serologic test results that differ from the above. Findings have been suggestive of a mixed mechanism involving both drug adsorption and immune complexes.

AUTOIMMUNE TYPE

In the preceding types of drug-induced immune hemolysis, the antibody fails to react unless the drug or a metabolite of the drug is present. In drug-induced autoimmune hemolytic anemia, a drug inhibits the function of T supressor lymphocytes and this allows antibodies to be formed to an Rh antigen common to almost all RBCs. Thus, hemolysis and a positive direct Coombs' test are independent of the drug itself and may persist for days or weeks after the drug has been discontinued. The clinical and laboratory findings do not differ from those of an idiopathic autoimmune hemolytic anemia of the warm reactive type (see Chapter 9) except for the history of exposure to the drug.

Drugs implicated in the pathogenesis of this type of hemolytic anemia are: alpha methyldopa (Aldomet), L-dopa, mefanemic acid, and procainamide. Many patients given alpha methyldopa develop a positive direct Coombs' test, yet only a few develop hemolytic anemia. This apparently reflects a second effect of alpha methyldopa—its ability to depress the function of mononuclear phagocytes. As a result, the mononuclear phagocytic system fails to remove the immunoglobulin-coated RBCs and the patient does not become anemic.

REACTIONS PRIMARILY AFFECTING GRANULOCYTES

Agranulocytosis

Certain drugs may produce a profound leukopenia caused by a marked reduction or disappearance of neutrophilic granulocytes from the peripheral blood. Monocytes may or may not also disappear from the blood. The RBCs and thrombocytes are unaffected (except in the special case of phenothiazine-induced agranulocytosis [see below]).

The drugs that may cause agranulocytosis can be divided into the following categories:

1. The *antithyroid drugs*—propylthiouracil, methimazole (Tapazole), carbimazole.
2. *Phenothiazines*—chlorpromazine (Thorazine), prochlorperazine (Compazine), promazine (Sparine), mepazine (Pacatal), and thioridazine (Mellaril).
3. *Sulfanilamides*—trimethoprim-sulfamethoxazole (Bactrim, Septra), sulfasalazine (Azulfidine).
4. *Antibiotics*—usually a semisynthetic penicillin derivative or a cephalosporin but rarely an aminoglycoside.
5. A variety of *cardiovascular agents*—procainamide, quinidine, hydralazine, captopril.
6. *Antiepileptic drugs*—phenytoin (Dilantin), carbamazepine (Tegretol).
7. *Anti-inflammatory and anti-arthritic agents*—phenylbutazone

(Butazolidin), oxyphenbutazone (Tandearil), indomethacin (Indocin), colchicine, gold salts, penicillamine.
8. A miscellaneous group of widely used drugs in which rare instances of agranulocytosis have been reported—cimetidine (Tagamet), hydrochlorothiazide, oral antidiabetic agents.

In addition, analgesics containing amidopyrone or dipyrone are a major cause for agranulocytosis in countries still permitting their sale.

Agranulocytosis may result from one of two mechanisms:

1. *Immunologic mechanism.* Most instances of agranulocytosis result from drug-induced antibodies which, in the presence of the drug, react with granulocytes, their bone marrow precursors, or both. The agranulocytosis is characterized by:
   a. An abrupt onset usually 1 to 3 weeks after beginning the first use of the drug and frequently with severe systemic symptoms and signs—chills, fever, extreme malaise, and sometimes a skin rash. Within a day or two, the patient also usually develops a severe sore throat.
   b. After recovery, an abrupt recurrence of these abnormalities if the patient is given the drug again.
   c. A bone marrow examination which, if done early, reveals a marked depletion of granulocytes and granulocyte precursors but adequate numbers of erythroid precursors and megakaryocytes. If done after recovery has begun, the marrow may contain very large numbers of promyelocytes and early myelocytes with prominent azurophilic granules and therefore may resemble the marrow of a granulocytic leukemia.
   d. Antibodies in the serum that in the presence of the drug:
      (1) May react with mature granulocytes in agglutination or other test systems.
      (2) May inhibit growth of granulocyte colonies in in vitro bone marrow cultures.
2. *Toxic depression of hematopoiesis.* The phenothiazines produce agranulocytosis by a mechanism involving suppression of differentiation of committed progenitor cells of all three marrow lines (myeloid, erythroid, and megakaryocytic). However, because of the short intravascular residence time of granulocytes, the disorder presents as agranulocytosis with only mild or minimal anemia and thrombocytopenia. This type of agranulocytosis is characterized by:
   a. An insidious onset in a psychiatric patient, most often an

older woman, who has been receiving the drug for at least 2 to 15 weeks. The agranulocytosis is discovered because of a routine blood count in an asymptomatic patient or because of a blood count prompted by evidence of infection.

   b. A slowly developing recurrence over days when the offending drug or a different phenothiazine is readministered.

   c. A markedly hypocellular bone marrow resembling that found in aplastic anemia. However, unlike aplastic anemia, which results from destruction or suppression of multipotential stem cells, the toxic depression of committed progenitor cells induced by phenothiazines is rapidly reversed when the drug is stopped. Within a few days, many small cells resembling lymphocytes (stem cells?) are found in the bone marrow, and shortly thereafter hematopoietic cells reappear in large numbers.

   d. No evidence of drug-induced serum antibodies.

Important *therapeutic points* in the management of all patients with agranulocytosis are:

   1. Immediate recognition and removal of the drug. Unexplained fever, rash, or sore throat in a patient receiving one of the drugs listed above calls for obtaining a blood count *at once* and for stopping the drug if the level of granulocytes is depressed.

   2. Administration of antibiotics to combat infection, isolation of the patient, and meticulous nursing care. The administration of adrenal steroids does not seem to hasten recovery and may further impair resistance to infection.

Granulocytes reappear in the peripheral blood after 7 to 14 days. If the patients survives the acute episode, he or she recovers completely without residual marrow damage. Obviously, the offending agent must never be given again. Related drugs should also be avoided, for example, a hyperthyroid patient who develops agranulocytosis after taking methimazole should not later be given propylthiouracil. One should not attempt to confirm the identity of the offending drug by giving a test dose after recovery, because this may precipitate a serious second reaction.

However, if a patient develops agranulocytosis while taking multiple drugs and if techniques are available for testing for antibodies against granulocytes or their bone marrow precursors, then serum obtained during the acute episode should be stored frozen. After the patient has recovered it can be used in test systems with the patient's granulocytes or bone marrow cells to attempt to identify the offending drug.

Neutropenia

Many of the drugs that produce agranulocytosis in an infrequent patient—phenytoin, phenothiazines, trimethoprim-sulfmethoxazole—may cause a moderate neutropenia in a considerably larger group of patients. These moderate neutropenias usually do not progress to agranulocytosis and sometimes disappear even though the drug is continued. Therefore, if a strong indication exists (for example, an epileptic under good control with phenytoin) and the total granulocyte count does not fall below 1500 per μL, the drug often is continued. Clearly, however, such patients must be watched carefully for evidence of fever or infection and must have frequent total and differential WBC counts to ensure that the granulocytes do not fall to unsafe levels.

DRUG-INDUCED THROMBOCYTOPENIC PURPURA

Drug-induced antibodies reacting with platelets may cause thrombocytopenic purpura as a consequence of the rapid removal of antibody-coated platelets by the mononuclear phagocytic system. The onset is sudden. Examination may be negative except for petechiae and scattered small ecchymoses. The spleen is not enlarged. The RBCs and WBCs are normal. Thrombocytopenia is usually profound. Megakaryocytes are found in normal to increased numbers in the bone marrow with an increase in young megakaryocytes.

These findings are distinguished from idiopathic thrombocytopenic purpura (see Chapter 25) only by the history of drug ingestion. Quinidine is the most common drug causing thrombocytopenia by this mechanism. Other drugs include antibacterial and nonantibacterial sulfonamide derivatives (for example, oral diuretics), quinine, and gold compounds.

Treatment consists of the identification and removal of the offending agent and the use of adrenal steroids. Thrombocytes usually return to normal within 2 to 3 weeks. A single dose of the offending drug may precipitate a second attack.

Heparin-induced thrombocytopenia (see Chapter 29) probably represents a second, different type of antibody-induced thrombocytopenia. In this unusual disorder, antibody-damaged platelets apparently are not removed by the mononuclear phagocytic system but instead are deposited upon vessel walls, usually at sites of atherosclerotic vessel wall damage. Despite the anticoagulant effect of the heparin, platelet-fibrin thrombi may form with a resultant high risk for serious thromboembolic complications.

OTHER HYPERSENSITIVITY REACTIONS

Lymphadenopathy and Circulating Activated Lymphocytes

Phenytoin and occasionally other drugs (para-aminosalicylic acid, sulfa drugs) may cause a severe hypersensitivity reaction with the following characteristics:

1. *Clinical findings.*
   a. Lymphadenopathy, frequently generalized. The nodes may be tender.
   b. Fever, which may be high.
   c. An erythematous, pruritic skin eruption which may desquamate.
   d. Pharyngitis.
   e. Hepatomegaly and sometimes jaundice. The liver may be tender.
   f. Miscellaneous findings attributable to other organ involvement.
2. *Laboratory findings.*
   a. The WBC count may be normal or elevated. The smear reveals a *characteristic pattern*: activated lymphocytes resembling the lymphocytes of infectious mononucleosis, occasional plasma cells, and increased numbers of eosinophils.
   b. Liver function tests indicative of hepatocellular damage.
   c. A lymph node biopsy (only rarely done now that the syndrome is better recognized) that shows marked hyperplasia that can be confused with a malignant lymphoma.

The drug must be stopped immediately and never given again. Fatal cases, with death from liver insufficiency, meningoencephalitis, or progressive vasculitis, have occurred.

Lupus-Like Reaction

A reaction resembling systemic lupus erythematosus—with arthralgia, fever, a varying incidence of signs and symptoms of other organ involvement, and a positive test for antinuclear factor—has been seen in patients given procainamide, hydralazine, isoniazid, or phenytoin.

Eosinophilia

Drug reactions are one cause for eosinophilia (see Chapter 21). Slight eosinophilia accompanies many drug hypersensitivity reactions of the type producing skin rashes, urticaria, or fever. Prominent eosinophilia may occasionally accompany hypersensitivity reactions to penicillin, phenytoin, or iodides.

SELECTED READING

1. Holland P, and Mauer AM: Diphenylhydantoin-induced hypersensitivity reaction. J Pediatr 66:322, 1965.
2. Inman WHW: Study of fatal bone marrow depression with special reference to phenylbutazone and oxyphenbutazone. Br Med J 1:1500, 1977.
3. Petz LD: Drug-induced immune haemolytic anemia. Clin Haematol 9:455, 1980.
4. Salama A, and Mueller-Eckhardt C: The role of metabolite-specific antibodies in nomifensine-dependent immune hemolytic anemia. N Engl J Med 313:469, 1985.
5. Young GAR, and Vincent PC: Drug-induced agranulocytosis. Clin Haematol 9:483, 1980.

23

Hemostatic Mechanisms

STEPS IN HEMOSTASIS

The hemostatic process may be divided into three overlapping steps:

1. *Formation of primary platelet hemostatic plugs.* These are masses of platelets that accumulate at the site of vessel wall injury as the result of platelets sticking first to collagen in exposed subendothelial tissue (adhesion) and then to each other (cohesion or aggregation). Collagen and the first traces of thrombin formed at the injury site stimulate the platelet responses leading to cohesion. Primary plugs are unstable and easily swept away.

2. *Conversion of primary plugs into stable permanent plugs reinforced by a supporting fibrin clot.* As the thrombin concentration at the injury site increases, the loosely adherent platelets of the primary plugs are consolidated into stable plugs. An inwardly oriented contraction of the platelet mass compacts the platelets, which appear to lose their distinct borders. The platelet granules disappear as their contents are secreted. Fibrin forms, first at the surface of the aggregated platelets and then as an outwardly spreading network that reinforces the plugs and adds to the bulk of the hemostatic seal. These events require generation of effective amounts of thrombin in the blood coagulation reactions.

3. *Lysis of fibrin.* As the fibrin clot grows, reactions are initiated to dissolve fibrin and confine the clot to the area of vessel wall injury. In these fibrinolytic reactions, the plasma proenzyme,

plasminogen, binds to fibrin and is then activated to plasmin by an activator released from endothelial cells.

When hemostasis is defective, a patient may start to bleed again as late as 7 to 10 days after a procedure such as dental extraction. Giving an antifibrinolytic agent may prevent such late bleeding. One infers, therefore, that balanced deposition and lysis of fibrin normally continues for about 10 days following vessel wall injury—maintaining and remolding the hemostatic seal while the vessel wall heals.

SUPPRESION OF HEMOSTASIS BY NORMAL ENDOTHELIUM

Although essential to stem bleeding after vessel wall injury, the hemostatic reactions are harmful when they occur intralumenally to form a clot (thrombus) that blocks blood flow to or from a tissue. The endothelial cells lining the lumen of blood vessels suppress hemostatic reactions in the absence of vessel wall injury by:

1. Physically separating the blood from materials in the underlying vessel wall that can activate platelets and initiate blood coagulation.
2. Synthesizing and releasing prostacyclin (PGI_2), a prostaglandin that diminishes platelet responsiveness to activating stimuli.
3. Providing surface binding sites essential for reactions that turn off blood coagulation. These surface sites include:
   a. *Thrombomodulin*, a high affinity binding site for thrombin. Binding to thrombomodulin alters thrombin's enzymatic specificity so that it acquires the ability to activate a vitamin K-dependent hemostatic factor, protein C, that has a key anticoagulant function (see later).
   b. *Binding sites for antithrombin III.* Two types of proteoglycans (proteins that contain long polysaccharide side chains called glycosaminoglycans) have been identified on the luminal surface of endothelial cells. The glycosaminoglycan chains on one of these proteins behave like heparin (see Chapter 29) in that they contain four to eight tetrasaccharides (a sequence of four sugar residues) per chain possessing a critical arrangement of sulfate groups that permits the binding of antithrombin III. Binding of antithrombin III to these sites markedly enhances the ability of antithrombin III to neutralize thrombin and other enzymes of blood coagulation.

PROPERTIES OF PLATELETS

Knowledge of platelet ultrastructure, metabolism, and contractile mechanisms is needed to understand how platelets function in hemostasis.

Platelet Ultrastructure

The unstimulated platelet (Fig. 23-1) circulates as a flattened disc. Hollow, tube-like structures, called microtubules, encircle the platelet just beneath its surface membrane and help maintain this shape. Microtubules are polymers of a noncontractile protein called tubulin.

SURFACE MEMBRANE

The platelet surface membrane consists of an outer amorphous coat (glycocalyx) containing carbohydrate-rich proteins (glycoproteins) and an underlying unit membrane made up of a bilayer of phospholipids. As in other cell membranes, the polar groups of the outer layer of phospholipids are oriented toward the cell exterior and the polar groups of the inner layer are oriented toward the platelet cytoplasm. The carbohydrate chains of the glycoproteins are confined to the glycocalyx; the polypeptide chains of the glycoproteins penetrate varying distances into the lipid bilayer. Cholesterol and small amounts of glycolipids are also embedded in the phospholipid bilayer.

The glycoproteins can be extracted from the membrane and separated according to size by sodium dodecyl sulfate polyacrylamide gel electrophoresis. Three glycoprotein peaks of decreasing molecular weight were initially recognized—GP (glycoprotein) I, II, and III. Additional proteins were identified later, both within the originally described peaks (and therefore named by adding a letter to the original Roman numeral, for example, GP Ib) and in new peaks of lesser

---

Fig. 23-1. Electron micrographs of an unstimulated platelet (upper micrograph) and of a stimulated platelet (lower micrograph). Note the pseudopods and the central location of the granules in the stimulated platelet. Abbreviations: DB, dense bodies; DTS, dense tubular system; G, granules; Gly, fine glycogen granules; M, mitochondria; MT, microtubules; OCS, open canalicular system; Ps, pseudopods. (Courtesy of Dr. James White, University of Minnesota School of Medicine, Minneapolis, MN)

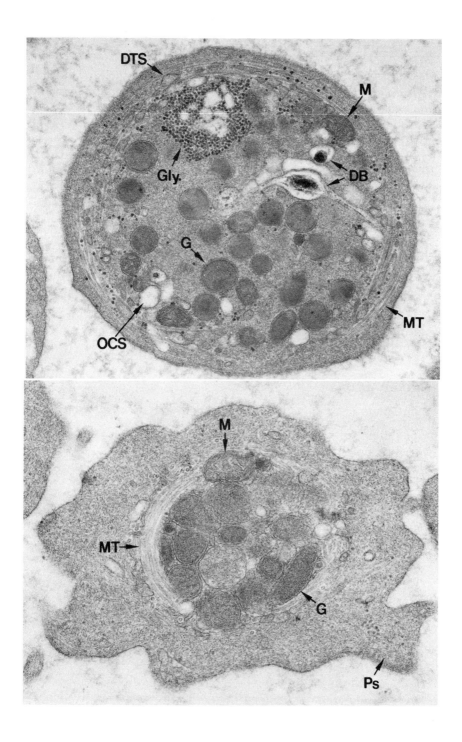

molecular weights, which were given new Roman numeral names, for example, GP V. Two glycoproteins, GP IIb and III, are transmembrane proteins whose polypeptide chains span the lipid bilayer. GP III is thought to provide a site for attachment of actin filaments to the inner surface of the membrane during platelet activation, an association important for orienting the wave of contraction that helps consolidate platelet plugs. Binding sites on the outer surface of the membrane essential for normal platelet function have been identified on GP Ib and on a GP IIb-IIIa complex that forms during platelet activation (see below).

An anionic phospholipid, phosphatidylserine, present in the platelet membrane, possesses procoagulant activity as a cofactor for two of the enzymes of blood coagulation (see later). In the unstimulated platelet, phosphatidylserine is located in the inner layer of the lipid bilayer and so cannot react with plasma coagulation factors. During platelet activation, the membrane is altered and phosphatidylserine becomes available on the outer surface of the membrane and can then react with plasma coagulation factors.

INTERNAL MEMBRANOUS SYSTEMS

The platelet contains two internal membranous systems:

1. The *open canalicular system*, which is made up of multiple, sponge-like invaginations of the platelet surface membrane. During platelet activation, the platelet secretes its granule contents through these channels. The open canalicular system also supplies membrane for the pseudopods platelets form after activation (see Fig. 23-1).
2. The *dense tubular system*, which is made up of remnants of endoplasmic reticulum. This membranous system, which does not communicate with the exterior, serves as an intracellular calcium storage site.

ORGANELLES

Organelles are distributed randomly throughout the unstimulated platelet. These include:

1. Large granules of three types—dense bodies, alpha granules, and lysosomal granules. Dense bodies are recognized as black, electron dense granules; alpha granules and lysosomal granules are morphologically indistinguishable from each other.

2. Fine glycogen granules.
3. Mitochondria.

Platelet Metabolism

Platelets derive energy as ATP from the metabolism of glucose, both by anaerobic glycolysis and by the much more efficient process of mitochondrial oxidative phosphorylation. The unstimulated platelet utilizes ATP to pump sodium out of the cell, to maintain a number of platelet proteins in a phosphorylated state, and to support a continuous basal polymerization-depolymerization of platelet actin. The stimulated platelet generates increased amounts of ATP to provide the added energy for platelet shape change, contraction, and secretion.

Platelet ATP and ADP are found within two pools:

1. A metabolic pool distributed throughout the cytoplasm.
2. A storage pool packaged in the dense bodies for secretion.

The two pools do not readily exchange. In certain pathologic conditions, platelets may be activated to secrete their dense body nucleotides yet still circulate. Such "exhausted" platelets, which apparently cannot replete their dense body ADP stores from the metabolic pool, have permanently impaired hemostatic function.

Platelets can synthesize glycogen and fatty acids but, lacking DNA and RNA, cannot synthesize proteins. Thus, when the enzyme cyclooxygenase is inactivated by acetylation upon exposure of platelets to aspirin, new enzyme cannot be made to replace the inactivated enzyme.

Platelet Contractile System

Platelets contain large amounts of *actin* and small amounts of *myosin*, two proteins that stabilize actin filaments, *actin binding protein*, which crosslinks filaments and α-*actinin*, which helps to anchor filaments to membranes; and *gelsolin*, a protein that both inhibits formation of actin filaments and destabilizes filaments, cutting them between crosslinks. In the unstimulated platelet, actin is found primarily as a small, globular monomer (G actin). When platelets are activated, the contractile system responds in two ways:

1. Large amounts of G actin are polymerized to form double helical filaments called F actin.

2. An increased association of myosin with actin filaments and an activation of myosin ATPase results in the contraction of platelet actomyosin.

The F actin arising during platelet activation forms bundles of microfilaments within the platelet pseudopods and also gives rise to a central filamentous cytoskeletal structure whose strands extend to the platelet membrane. The centripedal contraction of this cytoskeletal structure compacts the aggregated platelets during consolidation of a hemostatic plug.

PLATELET ADHESION TO SUBENDOTHELIUM

This first step in forming hemostatic plugs (Fig. 23-2) involves an initial adherence of platelets to a subendothelial surface followed by a secondary spreading of the platelets on the surface. Three established requirements for platelet adhesion are:

1. Attachment sites for platelets on collagen fibrils in the subendothelium.
2. The presence in plasma of large multimers of a protein called von Willebrand factor.
3. A binding site for von Willebrand factor on GP Ib of the platelet surface membrane. When GP Ib is missing, as occurs in a rare hereditary platelet disorder called the Bernard-Soulier syndrome, platelets cannot adhere normally to subendothelium.

Additional factors may participate in platelet adhesion but their roles are less certain. For example, interactions between thrombospondin (a protein secreted from the alpha granules of activated platelets), fibronectin (a large adhesive protein of plasma, cell surfaces, and extracelluler matrix), and collagen may strengthen the adhesion of platelets to subendothelium during their secondary spreading.

Endothelial cells make von Willebrand factor. It is synthesized as a 220,000 dalton protein from which a peptide is cleaved to form a 200,000 dalton molecule called a protomer. Within the endothelial cells, protomers bind by disulfide bonds to form dimers or tetramers, and these combine, by an unknown mechanism, to form large multimers of up to 14,000,000 daltons. Endothelial cells secrete von Willebrand factor into the plasma and also into the vessel wall, where it is deposited in a thin layer just below the endothelial cells.

On gel electrophoresis of plasma, one finds a series of von Willebrand factor multimers of decreasing size from 14,000,000 to 800,000 daltons (see Fig. 26-5). This presumably reflects a progressive

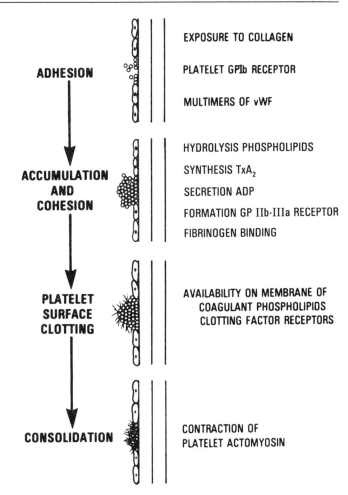

ADHESION

EXPOSURE TO COLLAGEN

PLATELET GPIb RECEPTOR

MULTIMERS OF vWF

ACCUMULATION AND COHESION

HYDROLYSIS PHOSPHOLIPIDS

SYNTHESIS TxA$_2$

SECRETION ADP

FORMATION GP IIb-IIIa RECEPTOR

FIBRINOGEN BINDING

PLATELET SURFACE CLOTTING

AVAILABILITY ON MEMBRANE OF COAGULANT PHOSPHOLIPIDS CLOTTING FACTOR RECEPTORS

CONSOLIDATION

CONTRACTION OF PLATELET ACTOMYOSIN

Fig. 23-2. The formation of a hemostatic plug. Abbreviations: TxA$_2$, thromboxane A$_2$; vWF, von Willebrand factor. (Modified from Rapaport SI. In West JB [ed]: Best and Taylor's Physiologic Basis of Medical Practice, 11th ed. Baltimore, Williams & Wilkins, 1984)

degradation in the circulation of the large multimers secreted by the endothelial cells. The large multimers are essential for normal platelet adhesion. Thus, abnormal bleeding occurs in patients who have variants of von Willebrand's disease (see Chapter 26) in which total plasma von Willebrand factor concentration may be normal but the large multimers are missing.

Megakaryocytes also make von Willebrand factor. This von Willebrand factor remains within the alpha granules of the platelets until it is secreted during platelet activation. The physiologic function of platelet von Willebrand factor is not yet known.

PLATELET ACTIVATION

Stimuli Activating Platelets During Hemostasis

As platelets adhere to subendothelium at an injury site, they begin to activate as a result of exposure to collagen and to the first thrombin formed. New platelets then stick to these activated platelets and are themselves activated. As they do so, they release materials that amplify further platelet activation. These include:

1. Products of oxidation of arachidonic acid by the cyclooxygenase pathway—an endoperoxide called PGH_2 and its metabolic product within the platelet, thromboxane A_2 (Fig. 23-3).
2. Acetyl glceryol ether phosphorylcholine, a lipid inducer of activation also known as platelet activating factor or PAF.
3. Adenosine diphosphate (ADP).

Thus, as the concentration of thrombin increases at the injury site, as PGH_2 becomes available to serve as a cofactor markedly enhancing collagen's ability to stimulate platelets (see below), and as the additional platelet-derived amplifiers of activation mentioned above also become available, the platelet aggregates grow and are molded into effective hemostatic plugs (see Fig. 23-2).

A pharmacologic observation—the effect of aspirin upon the bleeding time (a test that measures the rate of formation of hemostatic plugs, see Chapter 24)—dramatically illustrates the dual roles of thrombin and collagen in initiating platelet activation. As mentioned, collagen by itself is a weak inducer of platelet activation but becomes a powerful inducer of platelet activation in the presence of PGH_2. Aspirin, which inactivates the enzyme cyclooxygenase, prevents the synthesis of platelet PGH_2 (see Fig. 23-3) and so limits collagen's ability to activate platelets. Yet, in a normal person, taking aspirin prolongs the bleeding time only slightly because the normal generation of thrombin suffices to initiate platelet activation (Fig. 23-4). Conversely, although a hemophilic patient cannot generate normal amounts of thrombin at a site of vessel wall damage, his bleeding time is normal or only slightly prolonged. Collagen, with its cofactor

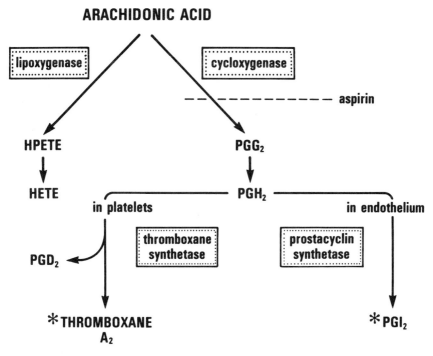

Fig. 23-3. Pathways of arachidonic acid oxidation in the platelet and the products generated. The endoperoxide PGH_2 is shown as a common substrate for the formation of thromboxane A_2 in the platelet and PGI_2 (prostacyclin) in the endothelial cell. (Rapaport SI. In West JB [ed]: Best and Taylor's Physiologic Basis of Medical Practice, 11th ed. Baltimore, Williams & Wilkins, 1984)

PGH_2, suffices to initiate platelet activation. However, if both thrombin-induced activation and collagen-induced activation are impaired, as when a severely hemophilic patient or a patient receiving the anticoagulant heparin is given aspirin, then initation of platelet activation is "paralyzed". The bleeding time may lengthen strikingly, and the patient's risk of serious bleeding is substantially increased.

Stimulus-Response Coupling During Platelet Activation

TURNOVER OF MEMBRANE INOSITOL PHOSPHOLIPIDS

Thrombin and collagen bind to different, as yet poorly delineated, receptors on the platelet surface. By an unknown mechanism or mechanisms, this binding activtates an enzyme, phospholipase C, which hydrolyzes specific phospholipids, called inositol phospho-

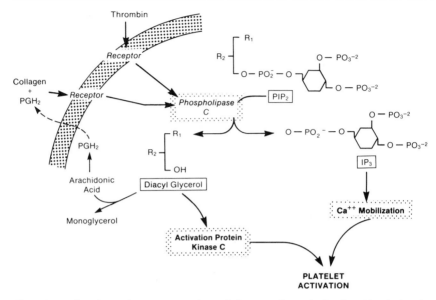

Fig. 23-4. A schematic representation of the coupling of platelet stimulation by thrombin and collagen to platelet activation through the hydrolysis of phosphatidyl inositol diphosphate (PIP$_2$). This generates diacyl glycerol, with resultant activation of protein kinase C, and also generates inositol triphosphate (IP$_3$), with resultant mobilization of calcium ions. PGH$_2$ is an endoperoxide formed from oxidation of arachidonic acid (see Fig. 23-3) that markedly enhances the ability of collagen to stimulate platelets.

lipids, in the platelet membrane. The inositol group is split off and a compound called *diacyl glycerol* is formed (see Fig. 23-4). The hydrolysis of an inositol phospholipid that has two added phosphate groups on the inositol (phosphatidylinositol biphosphate, see Fig. 23-4) is particularly important because its hydrolysis results in the formation of both diacyl glycerol and a second key inducer of platelet activation, *inositol triphosphate (IP$_3$)*.

Diacyl glycerol and IP$_3$ act synergistically to evoke the cellular responses of platelet activation. Diacyl glycerol activates an enzyme called protein kinase C, which catalyzes the phosphorylation of certain platelet proteins, including a 40,000 molecular weight protein whose phosphorylation is required for initiating secretion from platelet granules. IP$_3$ acts as a calcium ionophore, causing intracellular calcium concentration to rise as calcium flows into the cytosol both from the dense tubular system and from the platelet exterior. As the calcium concentration rises, calcium binds to a protein called calmodulin. The calcium-calmodulin complex then catalyzes phosphorylation of the light chain of platelet myosin, a reaction also required for platelet secretion and for other responses dependent upon the contraction of platelet actomyosin. The increased calcium concentration also activates phospholipases, called phospholipase A_2, which split arachidonic acid from the second carbon of the glycerol backbone of phospholipids and so initiate the reactions of arachidonic acid oxidation (see below).

Thus, the breakdown of membrane inositol phospholipids, with generation of both diacyl glycerol and IP_3, is thought to be the key event initiating platelet activation. (This mechanism for transducing extracellular informational signals into cells is also thought important for other cell systems, for example, cells of nervous tissue.)

MODULATION OF PLATELET SENSITIVITY TO STIMULI

An increase in platelet cyclic AMP, through activation of a different protein kinase, protein kinase A, decreases the sensitivity of platelets to activating stimuli. The mechanism is not established but may involve activation of a calcium pump that reduces calcium ion concentration in the platelet cytosol. Thus, one may view platelet responsiveness to activation as regulated by the opposing activity of two protein kinases—protein kinase C, which promotes activation, and protein kinase A, which inhibits activation.

Two mechanisms for increasing platelet cyclic AMP levels are:

1. *Activation of adenyl cyclase*, the enzyme catalyzing formation of cyclic AMP. Prostacyclin, the prostaglandin secreted by endothelial cells that inhibits platelet aggregation, suppresses activation of platelets by this mechanism.
2. *Inhibition of phosphodiesterase*, the enzyme that breaks down cyclic AMP. The drug dipyridamole (Persantin), which is sometimes given to patients to impede platelet activation in thrombotic disorders, acts by this mechanism.

Changes in the lipid composition of the platelet membrane also affect the activatability of platelets. These include alterations in:

1. Platelet membrane cholesterol, which increases when plasma-free cholesterol increases. This heightens platelet sensitivity to activation.
2. The arachidonic acid content of platelet membrane phospholipids. Eating a diet containing large quantities of unsaturated fatty acids reduces platelet membrane arachidonic acid and decreases platelet sensitivity to activation.

Platelet Responses During Activation

A series of progressive, overlapping events occur during platelet activation:

1. Platelet shape change.
2. Platelet cohesion (aggregation).
3. Generation of lipid products both amplifying and dampening activation.
4. Secretion of platelet granule contents.
5. A reorganization of the platelet membrane making phosphatidylserine available to interact with clotting factors and allowing clotting factors to bind to and generate thrombin on the platelet surface.
6. An oriented, centripedal contraction of actomyosin that compacts the aggregated platelets and so consolidates the platelet hemostatic plug.

The first four of these events are discussed in the following sections. The role of platelets in blood coagulation is described further later in the chapter.

PLATELET SHAPE CHANGE

Platelets change shape from flattened discs to spheres with multiple pseudopods within seconds of stimulation. The submembranous bundle of microtubules dissolves, the granules move to the center of the platelet, and the microtubules reform centrally, surrounding the granules (see Fig. 23-1). These structural changes markedly increase the platelet surface area for adhesion and cohesion and also prepare the platelet for secretion of its granules. However, the structural changes are completely reversible. Platelets may escape from the edges of an enlarging hemostatic plug, re-enter the circulation and revert to their original, unstimulated appearance.

PLATELET COHESION

Platelet cohesion, the adherence of platelets to each other, is obviously essential for forming the mass of the hemostatic plug. It has two known requirements:

1. Assembly on the platelet surface membrane of a receptor formed by a complex of GP IIb-IIIa that recognizes a specific

binding sequence of amino acid residues (Arg-Gly-Asp) present on fibrinogen (and certain other adhesive proteins, for example, fibronectin and vitronectin).
2. Binding of fibrinogen to this receptor.

Patients with a rare hereditary disorder called thrombasthenia (Glanzmann's disease) lack the GP IIb-IIIa receptor on their platelets. They bleed seriously, particularly from mucosal surfaces. This clinical observation establishes that assembly of the GP IIb-IIIa receptor during platelet activation is essential for forming normal hemostatic plugs.

Soon after beginning to adhere to each other, the platelets start to release their granule contents. A 400,000 molecular weight protein, *thrombospondin*, released from alpha granules, binds both to the platelet surface membrane and to fibrinogen (as well as to other materials such as fibronectin and collagen). It is possible, although not proved, that thrombospondin forms an important second component of the glue that holds aggregated platelets together.

GENERATION OF LIPID PRODUCTS AFFECTING ACTIVATION

Arachidonic acid, released as described earlier during initiation of platelet activation, is oxidized within the platelet by two pathways—the lipoxygenase pathway and the cyclooxygenase pathway (see Fig. 23-3). The lipoxygenase pathway yields HPETE (12-hydroperoxy-eicosatetraenoic acid), which is reduced to HETE (12-hydroxy-eicosatetraenoic acid). Their physiologic functions are not clear. (Related compounds formed by oxidation of arachidonic acid in WBC serve as precursors of the leukotrienes, potent mediators of delayed hypersensitivity and inflammatory responses.)

The cyclooxygenase pathway yields PGG_2, which is rapidly reduced to PGH_2. As emphasized earlier, PGH_2 functions in an important feedback reaction (see Fig. 23-4) as a cofactor for collagen-induced stimulation of platelet activation. PGH_2 also serves as the precursor of:

1. A minor, nonenzymatic breakdown product, PGD_2, a prostaglandin that can inhibit platelet activation. Because only small amounts are formed, the physiologic significance of PGD_2 is questionable.
2. A major enzymatic product, *thromboxane A_2*, which functions as a potent inducer of vasoconstriction and platelet aggregation. Like thrombin and collagen, thromboxane A_2 is thought to bind

to a platelet surface receptor with consequent activation of phospholipase C and generation of diacyl glycerol and IP_3.

In endothelial cells, liberation of arachidonic acid and its oxidation by cyclooxygenase also yields PGH_2 but the PGH_2 is then further metabolized to prostacyclin (PGI_2), an inducer of vasodilatation and an inhibitor of platelet aggregation. Damage to endothelial cells at a site of vessel wall injury stimulates production of PGI_2. Furthermore, PGH_2 generated within activated platelets may be released from the platelet and be taken up by endothelial cells as additional substrate for PGI_2. PGI_2 formed within endothelial cells counteracts thromboxane A_2 formed within platelets. A balance between the synthesis of these opposing materials has been postulated to regulate growth of platelet hemostatic plugs at a site of vascular injury.

Activated WBCs generate a potent lipid mediator of inflammation whose effects include activation of platelets. Called initially platelet activating factor (PAF), this material has now been identified as *acetyl glycerol ether phosphorylcholine*. Moreover, it is now known that PAF is also generated within stimulated platelets. Exposure of platelets to PAF in vitro induces shape change, cohesion, and secretion. It also induces oxidation of arachidonic acid, but whether this is the primary mechanism of the effect of PAF on platelets is not clear. Nor is the overall importance of PAF for platelet activation presently understood.

PLATELET SECRETION

Soon after platelets form primary hemostatic plugs, they begin to secrete their granule contents—first from the alpha granules and the dense bodies and, later, as the platelets appear to breakdown and fuse, from the lysosomal granules. As mentioned, phosphorylation of the light chain of platelet myosin and of another 40,000 molecular weight protein is required to initiate platelet secretion.

Secretion of Alpha Granule Contents. The contents of the alpha granules may be divided into two categories:

1. *Proteins that are also plasma proteins.* These include albumin, IgG, fibrinogen, fibronectin, von Willebrand factor, high molecular weight kininogen, and factor V. Several of these proteins bind to the surface of activated platelets during hemostasis, and their secretion from platelets seems well designed to facilitate such binding. Nevertheless, no evidence exists yet for the physiologic

importance of their secretion during hemostasis except for factor V. A patient with a severe hereditary bleeding disorder has recently been described in whom platelet factor V, but not plasma factor V, is markedly reduced. The serious bleeding of this patient suggests that secretion of factor V from the alpha granule may be essential for normal generation of thrombin on the platelet surface.

2. *Proteins found only within the alpha granules until platelet activation.* These include:
   a. Proteins that become expressed on the platelet surface membrane after their secretion from the alpha granules:
      (1) Thrombospondin, whose possible roles in platelet adhesion and cohesion have already been mentioned.
      (2) Platelet glycoprotein IIa, a membrane glycoprotein of as yet unknown physiologic function not demonstrable on the surface membrane before platelet activation.
   b. Three cationic proteins—platelet-derived growth factor, platelet factor 4, and β-thromboglobulin.

Platelet-derived growth factor (PDGF) is a low molecular weight, two polypeptide chain, basic protein; one of its chains is homologous to the product of the cellular oncogene, c-*sis*. PGDF stimulates the proliferation of cells of mesenchymal origin and, therefore, smooth muscle cells and fibroblasts of a vessel wall. Its release from activated platelets at a site of vessel wall injury promotes vessel wall repair.

Platelet factor 4 (PF4) is a second low molecular weight, basic protein, which was initially recognized as a platelet-derived material capable of neutralizing the anticoagulant activity of heparin. Within the platelet, PF4 is associated with a larger molecular weight protein. After its secretion, PF4 separates from this larger protein and is rapidly bound to endothelium, apparently competing with antithrombin III for sites on endothelial heparin chains. Both platelet-derived growth factor and PF4 have also recently been shown to function as chemoattractants for granulocytes. β-*thromboglobulin* is a larger molecule with some amino acid homology with PF4 and weak antiheparin activity. It does not bind to endothelium. The physiologic function of β-thromboglobulin is unknown.

Secretion of Dense Body Contents. The dense bodies contain ATP, ADP, serotonin, and calcium ions. *ADP* can initiate platelet activation, and its secretion from the dense bodies helps recruit new platelets into the hemostatic plugs. This amplifying effect of released ADP is physiologically significant, since patients with disorders in which the dense granules are deficient in ADP (storage pool diseases) have a mild to moderate bleeding disorder resulting from impaired formation of hemostatic plugs.

Serotonin is produced in the argentaffin cells of the gastrointestinal tract; secreted into the plasma; taken up by the platelets; and stored within the dense bodies. The physiologic significance of its release from activated platelets at a site of vessel wall damage is unknown. Although serotonin is a potent vasoconstrictor, depleting platelets of serotonin by giving rabbits the drug reserpine has no apparent effect upon hemostasis.

STABILIZATION OF HEMOSTATIC PLUGS

During hemostasis, the unstable primary plugs of loosely aggregated platelets must be consolidated into stable plugs. As already mentioned, an inwardly oriented contraction of platelet actomyosin crushes the platelets together, causing individual platelets to lose their distinct borders and appear to fuse. Adding increasing amounts of thrombin to platelets in vitro will produce these changes. Therefore, the generation of increasing amounts of thrombin in the plasma atmosphere around the primary plugs is thought to mediate the process in vivo. Thrombin also clots fibrinogen on the platelet surface, which further stabilizes the plugs. Moreover, as increasing amounts of fibrin are laid down in the surrounding plasma and extracellular fluid, a scaffolding of fibrin is formed to which the fused masses of platelets can adhere.

Thus, although unstable primary hemostatic plugs can form in patients with an impaired ability to generate thrombin, the stable hemostatic plugs needed for a hemostatic seal to hold require the effective generation of thrombin in the blood coagulation reactions.

THE BLOOD COAGULATION REACTIONS

Blood clotting may be viewed as taking place in three steps:

1. An initial sequence of reactions that generate an activator of prothrombin.
2. A second step in which the prothrombin activator converts prothrombin to thrombin.

3. A third step in which thrombin cleaves fibrinopeptides from fibrinogen and activates factor XIII, with resultant deposition
and crosslinking of fibrin.

Nomenclature and Classification of the Clotting Factors

Some years ago, an international committee assigned Roman numerals to all factors then recognized as participating in blood coagulation.
This nomenclature has been accepted for most but not all factors, for
example, calcium is never called factor IV and fibrinogen is rarely
referred to as factor I. When a clotting factor with a Roman numeral
name is activated, the lower case letter a is added to its name, for
example, the activated form of factor X is written factor Xa or simply
Xa. Four plasma factors, recognized more recently, do not have Roman
numeral names. The names of two, prekallikrein and high molecular
weight kininogen (HMW kininogen), reflect their recognition as par-
ticipants in the generation of kinins before their recognition as par-
ticipants in blood coagulation. The other two are recently identified
vitamin K-dependent plasma proteins, which were named protein C
and protein S by their discoverers.

The international committee also assigned Arabic numerals to
coagulant activities associated with platelets. However, what was
once called platelet factor 1 is today recognized as platelet factor V
and what was once called platelet factor 2 is platelet fibrinogen.
Platelet phospholipid procoagulant activity was given the name platelet factor 3, but this term is falling into increasing disuse. Only the
name platelet factor 4 (PF4) persists as the name for the alpha granule
protein that neutralizes the anticoagulant activity of heparin (discussed earlier).

The nomenclature used in this book is summarized in Table 23-
1. In this table, the blood clotting factors have been divided into
functional groups. The first group is the *contact activation factors*.
These are the proteins that initiate clotting when blood is exposed in
vitro to a negatively charged activating surface such as glass. They
consist of three serine protease proenzymes, factor XII, prekallikrein,
and factor XI, and a fourth protein, HMW kininogen, which forms
complexes in plasma with prekallikrein and factor XI.

The second group is the *vitamin K-dependent proenzymes*. These
are 50,000 to 70,000 dalton serine protease proenzymes possessing
residues of a unique amino acid, γ-carboxyglutamic acid (Gla). Vitamin K acts as a cofactor in a posttranslational reaction that adds a
second carboxy group to the γ-carbon of selected glutamic acid resi-

Table 23-1. The Blood Coagulation Factors

CATEGORY AND NAME	HEMOSTATIC FUNCTION	PLASMA CONCENTRATION (μg/mL)
CONTACT ACTIVATION FACTORS		
F.XII (Hageman factor)	Activate F.XI and PK	30
HMW kininogen	Bring F.XI and PK to a surface	70
Prekallikrein	Activate F.XII	45
F.XI (PTA)	Activate F.IX	4
VITAMIN K-DEPENDENT PROENZYMES		
Prothrombin (F. II)	Precursor of thrombin	150
F.X (Stuart-Prower factor)	Activate prothrombin	8
F.IX (Christmas factor)	Activate F.X	4
F.VII (proconvertin)	Activate F.IX and F.X	0.5
Protein C	Inactivate VIII$_a$ and V$_a$	3.5
COFACTORS		
Tissue factor (F.III)	Cofactor for F.VII and VII$_a$	—
Platelet procoagulant phospholipid (PF 3)	Cofactor for F.IX$_a$ and F.X$_a$	—
F.VIII (antihemophilic factor)	Cofactor for F.IX$_a$	0.1
F.V (proaccelerin)	Cofactor for F.X$_a$	7
Protein S	Cofactor for activated protein C	35
FACTORS OF FIBRIN DEPOSITION		
Fibrinogen (F.I)	Precursor of fibrin	2,500
F.XIII (fibrin stabilizing factor)	Crosslink fibrin	8

Abbreviations are: F, factor; PK, prekallikrein; HMW, high molecular weight; PTA, plasma thromboplastin antecedent; PF, platelet factor.

dues in the NH$_2$-terminal segment of these proteins (Fig. 23-5). The Gla residues so formed create strong calcium binding sites. Binding of calcium to these sites confers on the vitamin K-dependent proenzymes the tertiary structural conformation they need for hemostatic function.

Factor VII is thought to have slight enzymatic activity in its "proenzyme" form; prothrombin, factor IX, and factor X are inert in their proenzyme form. During blood coagulation, each of these factors is activated by cleavage of only one or two peptide bonds in the molecule to form potent serine proteases. Factors VIIa, IXa, Xa, and thrombin are *procoagulant* serine proteases. Activated protein C is an *anticoagulant* serine protease.

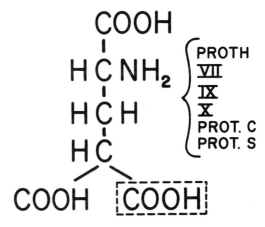

Fig. 23-5. The structure of γ-carboxyglutamic acid, a unique amino acid found in the vitamin K-dependent clotting proteins. Vitamin K is required to add a second carboxyl group, shown within the dotted lines, to the γ-carbon of glutamic acid.

The third group listed in Table 23-1 is the *cofactors*. These are required to form enzyme-cofactor complexes, which provide specificity and kinetic efficiency for several of the enzymatic reactions of blood coagulation (see below) and which also localize these reactions to the surface of cells. Cofactors may be divided into two groups:

1. Structural components of cell membranes. These are:
   a. Tissue factor (tissue thromboplastin) a lipoprotein activity that is normally present on the surface of certain cells and induced after injury on the surface of other cells. It is made up of a 43,000 dalton protein component and a phospholipid component. Tissue factor serves as the cofactor for factor VII.
   b. Phospholipid activity (primarily phophatidylserine) that becomes manifest on the surface of activated platelets and that is also present in apparently lesser amounts on endothelial cells and other cell surfaces. It is one component of a trimolecular factor IX enzyme-cofactor complex and also of a trimolecular factor Xa enzyme-cofactor complex arising during blood clotting.
2. Soluble protein factors, which include:
   a. Factor VIII and factor V. These are high molecular weight, single chain plasma proteins with areas of amino acid homology indicating that a segment of these molecules shared a common ancestral gene. Each is inert in its native state; proteolysis by trace amounts of thrombin or factor Xa can convert each into an activated form with cofactor function. Factor

VIIIa is part of the factor IXa enzyme-cofactor complex and factor Va is part of the factor Xa enzyme-cofactor complex.

b. Protein S. This vitamin K-dependent protein differs from the vitamin K-dependent proteins mentioned earlier in that it is not a serine protease proenzyme. It circulates in plasma partly bound to the C4b binding protein of the complement system and partly free. The function of the bound protein S is not known. The free protein S apparently functions as a cofactor required for the binding of activated protein C to the surface of platelets and other cells (see later).

The fourth group of Table 23-1 is the *factors of fibrin deposition.* These are fibrinogen and factor XIII, a transpeptidase that strengthens the fibrin clot by catalyzing formation of covalent bonds between fibrin molecules.

The Reactions Leading to the Generation of Thrombin

THE SEQUENCE OF ENZYMATIC ACTIVATIONS

Figure 23-6 shows the sequence of activation of the enzymes of blood coagulation. It is incomplete in that the contact activation reactions leading to formation of factor XIa when plasma is exposed to

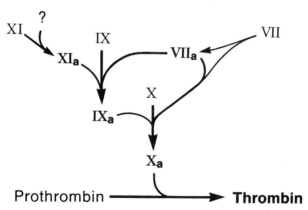

Fig. 23-6. The sequence of activation of the serine protease enzymes of blood coagulation. Note the dual mechanisms for activating factor IX and factor X. Mechanisms of activation of factor VII and factor XI are not shown (see text).

a negatively charged surface in vitro have been left out. However, as discussed later, these reactions seem not to be required for generation of factor XIa in vivo, and other as yet unknown reactions apparently activate factor XI in vivo during hemostasis. Native factor VII is shown to have minimal enzymatic activity capable of initiating the activation of factor X. The importance of this reaction will also be discussed later.

As seen in Figure 23-6, two enzymes, VIIa and XIa, activate factor IX; and two enzymes, VIIa and IXa, activate factor X. A single enzyme, Xa, activates prothrombin. *Amplification* occurs during the activation sequence. Generation of only a few molecules of the initial serine proteases culminates in the conversion to thrombin of many molecules of prothrombin—whose molar concentration in plasma is 80-fold higher than that of factor XI and 400-fold higher than that of factor VII.

As mentioned, calcium ions are required for the function of the vitamin K-dependent proteins shown in Figure 23-6. Cofactors are also needed for each of the reactions of Figure 23-6, except the activation of factor IX by factor XIa.

In Figure 23-7, the enzymatic skeleton of Figure 23-6 has been "fleshed out" by adding:

1. The participation of cofactors to form the enzyme-cofactor complexes essential for the enzymes to function physiologically.
2. Key feedback reactions triggered by Xa and thrombin. (These are represented by dashed lines in the figure.)

Note in Figure 23-7 that tissue factor is a cofactor only for factor VII(a), which is physiologically inert in its absence. The pathway of blood coagulation independent of factor VII, that is, the reactions mediated by generation of factor XIa, proceed unimpeded in the absence of tissue factor.

As already mentioned, factor IXa requires two cofactors for its physiologic function—factor VIIIa and the phospholipid procoagulant activity that becomes available on activated platelets (and is present on endothelial and other cell surfaces). Factor Xa has analogous cofactor requirements—factor Va (in place of factor VIIIa) and the phospholipid procoagulant activity. Native factors VIII and V are inert and must be activated by proteolysis to factors VIIIa and Va before they can function effectively in these cofactor complexes. A protease from platelets possibly initiates activation of platelet factor V. Plasma factors V and VIII are activated as described below.

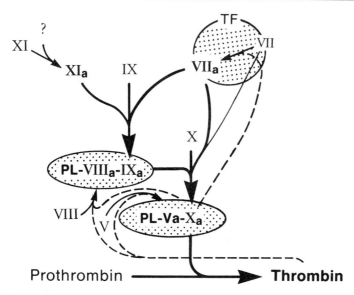

Fig. 23-7. The known blood coagulation reactions that lead to generation of thrombin during hemostasis. The reactions of Fig. 23-6 have been expanded to show the enzyme-cofactor complexes and also to show the feedback reactions. The latter are indicated by dashed lines. The reactions that lead to activation of factor XI when plasma is exposed in vitro to a negatively charged surface (contact activation reactions) are not shown (see text).

FEEDBACK REACTIONS

The reactions of blood coagulation not only go forward; some go backward in important feedback reactions that shift the process into high gear. Factor Xa and thrombin play key roles in these feedback reactions:

1. Factor Xa, in trace amounts, in the presence of calcium and procoagulant phospholipid, rapidly activates factor VII to factor VIIa, with a resultant many-fold increase in the enzymatic activity of factor VII. (This does not, however, alter factor VII's requirement for tissue factor as a cofactor.)

2. Thrombin, in trace amounts, initiates:

   a. Limited proteolysis with consequent activation of factors V and VIII. (Factor Xa at a higher concentration can also catalyze proteolysis with consequent activation of factor VIII.)

   b. Activation of platelets with resultant reorientation of the membrane to make procoagulant phosphatidylserine available and secretion of alpha granule factor V.

INITIATION OF BLOOD COAGULATION

In vitro one can initiate blood coagulation in two ways:

1. By exposing blood to a negatively charged surface, for example, the wall of a glass test tube. This leads to activation of XI.
2. By adding tissue factor to blood with resultant formation of a factor VII-tissue factor complex.

Activation of Factor XI. The reactions initiated when blood is exposed to a negatively charged surface are called the *contact activation reactions.* Both factor XII and high molecular weight kininogen will bind to a negatively charged surface. The binding of the latter also brings prekallikrein and factor XI down onto the surface, since these factors circulate in plasma as bimolecular complexes with high molecular weight kininogen. Binding to the surface is thought to induce a conformational change in factor XII, giving it a minimal enzymatic activity that begins the activation of prekallikrein to kallikrein. The kallikrein then catalyzes further activation of factor XII—setting a reciprocal activation sequence in motion. By this process, sufficient factor XIIa forms to activate factor XI to factor XIa rapidly.

The blood of individuals with a hereditary deficiency of factor XII, prekallikrein, or high molecular weight kininogen may take longer to clot in a glass tube than the blood of a patient with severe hemophilia. Yet, in contrast to a hemophilic patient, individuals with factor XII, prekallikrein, or high molecular weight kininogen deficiency do not bleed abnormally. Thus, although essential for initating clotting in a test tube in the absence of tissue factor, the contact activation reactions are not needed for physiologic hemostasis.

Patients with factor XI deficiency have a mild bleeding disorder. They do not bleed excessively into tissues after trauma, but they may experience persistent oozing after dental extraction and more serious bleeding after certain surgical procedures, such as prostatectomy. One may therefore conclude that:

1. Activation of factor XI is required for normal hemostasis in some, but not all, circumstances.
2. An as yet unidentified mechanism must exit in vivo for activating factor XI independent of the presently known roles of factor XII, prekallikrein, and high molecular weight kininogen in the contact activation reactions.

The Tissue Factor Pathway. Although patients with moderate hereditary factor VII deficiency (factor VII levels of 5% to 10% of normal) may have little or no abnormal bleeding, patients with severe hereditary factor VII deficiency (a factor VII level of 1% of normal) may bleed as seriously as patients with severe hemophilia. Since clotting initiated independent of tissue factor does not require factor VII, this clinical observation establishes that the tissue factor pathway for initiating blood coagulation is essential for normal hemostasis.

When blood is exposed to tissue factor, native factor VII binds to the tissue factor. This native factor VII-tissue factor complex is thought to possess minimal enzymatic activity capable of generating a trace amount of factor Xa. As mentioned, the first Xa generated then catalyzes conversion of the factor VII-tissue factor complex to a factor VIIa/tissue factor complex with many-fold increased enzymatic activity. It can activate factor X much more efficiently and can now also activate factor IX.

Since the role of factor IXa is also to activate factor X, direct factor VIIa/tissue factor activation of factor X should theoretically make factor VIIa/tissue factor activation of factor IX physiologically irrelevant (see Fig. 23-7). However, during hemostasis, blood is exposed to only a limited number of cell surface tissue factor sites and the extent of the direct factor VIIa/tissue factor activation of factor X that results is insufficient for normal generation of thrombin. If it were sufficient, neither hemophilia A (factor VIII deficiency) nor hemophilia B (factor IX deficiency) would be bleeding disorders (see Fig. 23-7). Taken with the observation that hereditary factor XI deficiency is a mild bleeding disorder, whereas hereditary factor IX deficiency is a severe bleeding disorder, one concludes that dual activation of factor IX by both XIa and tissue factor-VIIa is required for normal hemostasis.

LOCALIZATION OF BLOOD CLOTTING TO CELL SURFACES

Tissue factor localizes the factor VIIa/tissue factor activation of factors IX and X to the surface of tissue cells (for example, injured endothelial cells, smooth muscle cells, fibroblasts, activated monocytes). Factors IXa and Xa then form surface bound IXa/VIIIa/phospholipid and Xa/Va/phospholipid complexes.

Formation of a Xa/Va/phospholipid complex on the platelet surface has been extensively studied. Opinion differs, but many believe that the platelet procoagulant phospholipid activity that becomes available on the surface of activated platelets serves as a platelet binding site for Va. Va so bound then functions as a platelet surface binding site for Xa. An analagous binding sequence is assumed to result in formation of a IXa/VIIIa/phospholipid complex on the platelet surface, but direct experimental evidence of this is still lacking.

Complexes of IXa/VIIIa/phospholipid and Xa/Va/phospholipid form, not just on the platelet surface, but also on the surface of other cells, for example, endothelial cells, smooth muscle cells, and fibroblasts at the site of a vessel wall injury. These cells have phospholipid surface moieties presumably capable of functioning as binding sites for Va and VIIIa.

Whereas the reactions generating thrombin are localized to cell surfaces, thrombin diffuses from cell surfaces and can act on fibrinogen in the fluid phase. Thus, although fibrin first begins to form on the surface of aggregated platelets in hemostatic plugs, its strands rapidly extend outward into the surrounding extracellular fluid and plasma.

Formation of Fibrin

Fibrinogen is a dimeric molecule made up of two pairs of three different polypeptide chains called α, β, and γ chains. It has a trinodular structure. The central nodule is made up of the NH_2-terminal ends of all six chains; each distal nodule is made up of the carboxy-terminal segments of one pair of the three chains.

Thrombin catalyzes two reactions that lead to the formation and stabilization of fibrin (Fig. 23-8):

1. Cleavage of small peptides from the NH_2-terminal segment of the α (fibrinopeptide A) and β (fibrinopeptide B) chains.
2. Cleavage of a peptide from factor XIII, following which calcium ions induce a conformational change in the molecule that activates factor XIII.

Cleavage of the fibrinopeptides from fibrinogen gives rise to a minimally altered molecule called *fibrin monomer.* New sites are exposed in the central nodule that can form noncovalent bonds with sites present in the distal nodule of other molecules. This causes fibrin monomer molecules to polymerize and form insoluble strands of fibrin.

Factor XIIIa functions as a transglutaminase. It catalyzes formation of amide bonds between a γ carboxyl group of a glutamine residue on one fibrin molecule and an ϵ amino group of a lysine residue on another fibrin molecule. These covalent bonds stabilize the fibrin polymers. In addition, factor XIIIa crosslinks fibrin to fibronectin and also crosslinks fibronectin to collagen. In this way, factor XIIIa brings about the binding of fibrin to collagen. Moreover, factor XIIIa links

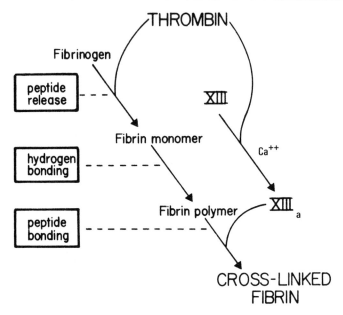

Fig. 23-8. Formation and stabilization of fibrin.

the alpha$_2$ plasmin inhibitor (see below) to fibrin, which may be important in limiting the lysis of fibrin during the several days in which the hemostatic seal must hold.

These reactions initiated by factor XIIIa are essential for normal hemostasis and also for normal wound healing. Patients with a hereditary deficiency of factor XIII not only experience serious bleeding; they also form fine, tissue paper-like scars after tissue abrasion, indicative of impaired wound healing.

Regulation of Coagulation

Blood does not clot as it circulates because it is not normally exposed to material capable of initiating clotting. However, in certain pathologic conditions, materials capable of triggering coagulation do gain access to the circulation. If in large amounts (for example, after premature separation of the placenta), then extensive intravascular coagulation may occur with resultant depletion of fibrinogen, other clotting factors, and platelets (acute defibrination). If in small amounts, then only small amounts of active clotting intermediates are formed. These are usually quickly removed by cellular clearance, particularly as blood flows through the liver.

However, when small amounts of clotting intermediates are trapped in an area of stasis, the clotting reactions may continue to completion in that area with the formation of a small thrombus. External counting of radioactivity over the legs after the intravenous injection of radioactive fibrinogen reveals a surprisingly high prevalence of "hot spots" indicative of such small thrombi in the deep veins of the legs of older patients after surgery. Fortunately, only a small fraction of such thrombi grow into larger, clinically significant thrombi because:

1. Coagulant serine proteases that may continue to be formed in the static blood are inactivated by protease inhibitors, primarily antithrombin III.
2. Thrombin is also partially inactivated by its absorption onto fibrin. Moreover, thrombin binds to thrombomodulin, which decreases the ability of thrombin to clot fibrinogen and activate factors V and VIII while conferring on thrombin the ability to activate protein C.
3. Factors VIIIa and Va rapidly lose their coagulant activity because of inactivation by activated protein C.
4. Fibrinolytic reactions are initiated to dissolve the thrombus.

When these mechanisms fail to check its growth, a thrombus may continue to enlarge over hours to days. If it obstructs blood flow in major veins, the patient may develop a painful, swollen leg. Moreover, as it grows, pieces of a thrombus may break off and be carried to the lungs. Such pulmonary emboli obstruct blood flow in branches of the pulmonary artery, and, if very large, may be fatal.

ANTITHROMBIN III AND OTHER PLASMA PROTEASE INHIBITORS

Serine proteases are formed in four plasma proteolytic systems: coagulation, fibrinolysis, complement activation, and generation of kinins. Plasma protease inhibitors inactivate these proteases and also proteases liberated from WBC during the inflammatory response. A given protease inhibitor may neutralize several serine proteases, including proteases from different proteolytic systems; conversely, several protease inhibitors may neutralize a given serine protease. Kinetic studies with different inhibitors must be carried out for each serine protease in order to identify its primary inhibitor. Protease inhibitors neutralizing the serine proteases of blood coagulation and fibrinolysis are listed in Table 23-2.

Antithrombin III, which is the primary inhibitor of thrombin, Xa, and IXa, is the most important of the protease inhibitors of coagulation

Table 23-2. Inhibitors of the Serine Proteases of Hemostasis

INHIBITOR	SERINE PROTEASE INHIBITED	DISORDER CAUSED BY INHIBITOR DEFICIENCY
Antithrombin III	Thrombin X_a IX_a VII_a*	Venous thrombosis
Alpha$_2$ macroglobulin	Thrombin Plasmin	None known
C1 esterase inhibitor	XII_a Kallikrein	Hereditary angioneurotic edema†
Alpha$_1$ antitrypsin (alpha$_1$, protease inhibitor)	XI_a	Pulmonary emphysema‡
Protein Ca inhibitor	Protein Ca	None known
Tissue plasminogen activator inhibitor	Tissue plasminogen activator	None known
Alpha$_2$ antiplasmin	Plasmin	Fibrinolytic bleeding

* Antithrombin III inhibits VII_a only when VII_a is bound to tissue factor and then only slowly. The physiologic mechanism for inhibition of the enzymatic activity of the tissue factor-factor VII_a complex is not yet known.
† Due to effects of activated complement proteases and kallikrein on blood vessels.
‡ Due to effects of elastases from granulocytes upon pulmonary alveolar membranes.

and the only one whose deficiency state is associated with a known increased risk of thrombosis. Many families have now been described in whom heterozygotes for hereditary antithrombin III deficiency, with plasma antithrombin III activity of about 50% of normal, have experienced venous thrombotic disease. A homozygote has never been identified, presumably because homozygosity for antithrombin III deficiency is lethal in utero.

Antithrombin III neutralizes serine proteases in a 1:1 stoichiometric reaction in which the active serine of the enzyme binds covalently to an arginine group at the reaction site of the inhibitor. The reaction is slow in solution in vitro but becomes almost instantaneous if heparin is added to the reaction mixture. As discussed earlier, antithrombin III binds to tetrasaccharides on heparin chains on endothelium, and this binding enables antithrombin III to function as a physiologic inhibitor of blood coagulation. However, antithrombin

III must compete with platelet factor 4 secreted from activated platelets, with a plasma protein known as histidine-rich glycoprotein, and possibly with other plasma proteins for these tetrasaccharide binding sites. This competition for binding to endothelial heparin chains probably explains why a 50% reduction in antithrombin III concentration—whose normal plasma concentration of 2.5μM modestly exceeds the 2.0 μM concentration of prothrombin and far exceeds the plasma concentrations of factor X and factor IX—is enough to increase an individual's risk for thrombotic disease.

Alpha₂ macroglobulin is a plasma protease inhibitor that binds several plasma serine proteases, including thrombin and plasmin, by a unique mechanism, that inhibits their activity against protein substrates without inhibiting their ability to hydrolyze small synthetic esters. Alpha₂ macroglobulin appears to be concentrated at cell surfaces, including the luminal surface of endothelium. A specific regulatory role for alpha₂ macroglobulin in hemostasis has yet to be identified.

PROTEIN C AND PROTEIN S

When activated by thrombin bound to thrombomodulin, the vitamin K-dependent protein, protein C, functions as an anticoagulant. It may also enhance the induction of fibrinolysis. Activated protein C requires protein S, phospholipid, and calcium ions for its anticoagulant effect (Fig. 23-9). Protein S appears needed for activated protein C to bind to phospholipid on the platelet and other cell surfaces. The activated protein C/phospholipid complex that forms competes with a IXa/phospholipid complex for VIIIa and with a Xa/phospholipid complex for Va. It inactivates by proteolysis the coagulant activity of these cofactors and so turns off further generation of thrombin. Activated protein C may enhance fibrinolytic activity by proteolytic inactivation of an inhibitor of tissue plasminogen activator (see later).

Growing clinical experience confirms the importance of protein C, with its cofactor protein S, as a natural anticoagulant regulating blood coagulation in vivo. Numerous families have now been discovered in which heterozygotes for different forms of protein C or protein S deficiency, with protein C or protein S antigen or activity in the 35% to 50% of normal range, have experienced recurrent episodes of venous thrombosis. Homozygotes for protein C deficiency, who have virtually undetectable protein C antigen in the plasma, die with extensive venous thromboses within the first days or weeks of life

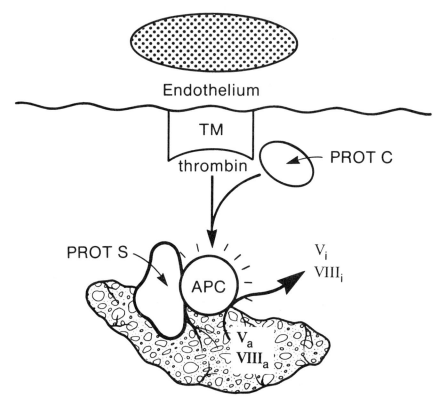

Fig. 23-9. A schematic representation of the activation of protein C and its subsequent inhibition of factors VIIIa and Va. Protein S is shown as a cofactor enabling activated protein C to bind to the platelet surface. The symbols VIII_i and V_i stand for inactivated factor VIII and factor V. TM is thrombomodulin.

(neonatal purpura fulminans). Homozygotes for protein S deficiency apparently have less severe thrombotic disease.

FIBRINOLYSIS

Activation of fibrinolysis is normally a physiologic response to the deposition of fibrin in vivo (Fig. 23-10). Plasminogen, the inert precursor of plasmin, binds to the fibrin. A plasminogen activator released from endothelial cells is also adsorbed onto the fibrin and converts plasminogen to plasmin. Plasmin cleaves a series of peptide bonds in fibrin, degrading the molecule into successively smaller, soluble fibrin degradation products (also called fibrin split products).

Plasminogen

Plasminogen is a single polypeptide chain protein made in the liver and found in plasma in a concentration of about 200μg per mL (2μM). Plasminogen activators split a single peptide bond in the molecule, which converts the inactive single chain proenzyme into an active two-chain serine protease.

Plasminogen contains binding sites for the amino acid lysine. Through these lysine binding sites, plasminogen can bind to at least four plasma proteins:

1. Fibrinogen and fibrin. Plasminogen binds only loosely to fibrinogen but tightly to a site or sites that becomes available when fibrinogen is converted to fibrin. This increased affinity of plasminogen for fibrin is important in localizing fibrinolysis to fibrin surfaces.
2. Histidine-rich glycoprotein. About 50% of the plasminogen in plasma circulates as a complex with histidine-rich glycoprotein.
3. Alpha$_2$ antiplasmin. Although this protease inhibitor binds only weakly to plasminogen (in contrast to the stable complex that it

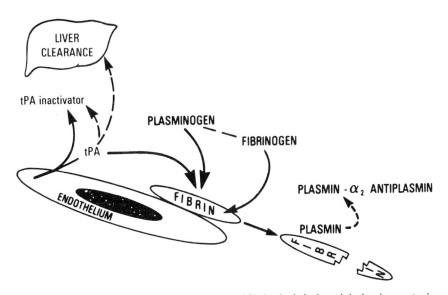

Fig. 23-10. A representation of the reactions of fibrinolysis induced during hemostasis by the release of tissue plasminogen activator (tPA) from endothelial cells. (Modified from Rapaport SI. In West JB [ed]: Best and Taylor's Physiologic Basis of Medical Practice, 11th ed. Baltimore, Williams & Wilkins, 1984)

forms with plasmin, see below), about 15% of plasminogen circulates in a complex with alpha$_2$ antiplasmin.

4. Thrombospondin released from the platelet alpha granules.

Competition between these proteins for the lysine binding site of plasminogen affects fibrinolyis, primarily by reducing the number of plasminogen molecules with a free lysine binding site available for binding to lysine on fibrin. Analogues of lysine, for example, 6-aminohexanoic acid (epsilon aminocaproic acid or EACA) are sometimes given to patients as an antifibrinolytic agent. By occupying free lysine binding sites, these compounds prevent plasminogen from binding to fibrin and so block its subsequent activation on fibrin to plasmin.

Plasmin cleaves many other plasma proteins besides fibrinogen and fibrin, including its own precursor, plasminogen. Plasmin splits a small peptide from the NH$_2$-terminal end of plasminogen, converting native plasminogen, which has glutamic acid as its NH$_2$-terminal amino acid (glu-plasminogen), to a molecule which has lysine as its NH$_2$-terminal amino acid (lys-plasminogen). This reaction may facilitate plasminogen activation during fibrinolysis, since one of the plasminogen activators, urokinase (see below), has been shown to activate lys-plasminogen about 20-fold faster than it activates glu-plasminogen.

Plasminogen Activators

Cells release two physiologically important plasminogen activators:

1. *Tissue plasminogen activator* (t-PA), a serine protease released from vascular endothelium that functions as a key activator of fibrinolysis when fibrin is laid down within vessels.

2. *Urokinase*, a serine protease so named because it was first recognized in urine. Urokinase is released from epithelial cells lining channels that must be kept free of fibrin to allow the flow of secreted fluids (for example, the renal tubules, the ducts of the salivary and mammary glands). It is also released from vascular endothelium and from activated macrophages. Urokinase from macrophages, which may be secreted as a soluble activator or remain bound to the surface of the macrophage, functions to initiate fibrinolysis during tissue remodeling after injury or inflammation.

Tissue plasminogen activator is a poor activator of plasminogen in solution but acquires a much higher affinity for plasminogen, and therefore becomes a very powerful activator of plasminogen, when both t-PA and plasminogen are bound to a fibrin surface. This fits teleologically with a primary role for tissue plasminogen activator in initiating fibrinolysis within blood vessels, where lysis of circulating fibrinogen as a consequence of activation of circulating plasminogen would produce a systemic hemostatic defect.

Urokinase is a two polypeptide chain molecule. Two-chain urokinase is an equally potent activator of plasminogen in solution and plasminogen bound to fibrin (which fits teleologically with a role for urokinase in keeping excretory ducts open). A single polypeptide chain form of urokinase has also been identified. It was originally called pro-urokinase but was recently renamed single chain urokinase-type plasminogen activator or scu-PA. Plasmin, and possibly other proteolytic enzymes, cleave scu-PA to form urokinase. Unlike urokinase, scu-PA fails to activate circulating plasminogen efficiently; however, it can readily activate plasminogen bound to fibrin, apparently because a competitive inhibitor of scu-PA in plasma does not inhibit scu-PA in the presence of fibrin. Thus, although for different reasons, both scu-PA and t-PA can preferentially trigger lysis of fibrin as contrasted to circulating fibrinogen.

Other plasminogen activators have also been identified. Each of the serine proteases arising during the contact activation reactions— factor XIIa, kallikrein, and factor XIa—can activate plasminogen. However, these so-called intrinsic plasminogen activators are weak activators of little-recognized physiologic significance.

Traces of plasminogen activator are normally detectable in blood. This reflects a balance between a basal release from vascular endothelium of tissue plasminogen activator and its:

1. Inactivation by a tissue plasminogen inactivator that is released from vascular endothelium and also from activated platelets.
2. Rapid clearance from blood as its circulates through the liver.

Stress increases blood fibrinolytic activity, possibly because a hypothalamic neurohumoral agent stimulates activator release from endothelium. Vasodilatation (for example, as occurs after vigorous exercise, venous occlusion, or injection of nicotinic acid) also stimulates release of activator from endothelial cells. Why an increased release of activator follows the deposition of fibrin in blood vessels is not yet understood. It may be related to the generation of thrombin, which, when added to endothelial cells in culture, causes plasminogen activator release after a delay of several hours. As mentioned earlier, activation of protein C by thrombin may also cause blood to acquire increased plasminogen activator activity.

Control of Fibrinolysis

Intravascular fibrinolysis is normally limited to the lysis of fibrin without accompanying proteolysis of circulating fibrinogen because:

1. Plasminogen binds preferentially to fibrin due to the greater affinity of the lysine binding sites of plasminogen for fibrin than for fibrinogen.
2. Tissue plasminogen activator and urokinase have short intravascular half-times because of their rapid inactivation by plasminogen activator inhibitor and their rapid clearance from blood as it flows through the liver.
3. The activity of tissue plasminogen activator is markedly enhanced when it and plasminogen are adsorbed together onto a fibrin surface.
4. The plasmin inhibitor, alpha$_2$ antiplasmin, inactivates plasmin escaping from a fibrin surface almost instantaneously. *Alpha$_2$antiplasmin* functions as a key regulator of fibrinolysis. It inactivates free plasmin within a millisecond in a reaction in which the inhibitor combines with both the active serine site and the lysine binding site of plasmin. Moreover, even though both of these sites are temporarily occupied while plasmin is degrading fibrin, alpha$_2$ antiplasmin can inactivate plasmin bound to fibrin within about 10 seconds.

Alpha$_2$ macroglobulin can also inhibit plasmin in solution, but alpha$_2$ macroglobulin cannot inhibit plasmin bound to fibrin. Therefore, alpha$_2$ macroglobulin cannot substitute for alpha$_2$ antiplasmin in the regulation of fibrinolysis.

The plasma concentration of plasminogen (2μM) exceeds the plasma concentration of alpha$_2$ antiplasmin (1μM). Thus, since alpha$_2$ antiplasmin inactivates plasmin in a 1:1 stoichiometric reaction, even a moderate fall in plasma alpha$_2$ antiplasmin concentration probably impairs the regulation of fibrinolysis. Rare patients have been discovered with a hereditary deficiency of alpha$_2$ antiplasmin and virtually undetectable levels of the inhibitor in plasma. These patients may bleed extensively into their tissues because of uncontrolled fibrinolysis set off by the hemostatic response to minor tissue trauma.

Increased Fibrinolysis in Acquired Disorders

Fibrinolysis following fibrin deposition is often called *secondary fibrinolysis* because fibrin deposition is the primary event. When an episode of disseminated intravascular clotting results in widespread deposition of fibrin in the microcirculation, secondary fibrinolysis may cause large amounts of fibrin degradation products to accumulate in the blood. These degradation products impede hemostasis in at least two ways:

1. By competing with fibrinogen for binding to the GP IIb-IIIa receptor on platelets and so impairing formation of platelet hemostatic plugs.
2. By interfering with the polymerization of fibrin monomer, which weakens the fibrin clot.

Moreover, enough plasmin may be generated after extensive intravascular clotting and secondary fibrinolysis to deplete plasma alpha$_2$ antiplasmin. This then intensifies the fibrinolysis. If the episode of intravascular coagulation has developed after a procedure, such as surgery or childbirth, that leaves multiple severed small blood vessels at a local site sealed by platelets and fibrin, then the intensified fibrinolysis may dissolve the seals and cause renewed bleeding from the site.

Plasminogen activators are sometimes infused intravenously into patients to dissolve thrombi. Unlike tissue plasminogen activator, the agents currently being used—urokinase and a product of the hemolytic streptococcus called streptokinase—are potent activators of circulating plasminogen. Large amounts of circulating plasmin are formed and alpha$_2$ antiplasmin and alpha$_2$ macroglobulin levels fall. Following this, the circulating plasmin can attack the fibrin of the thrombus, but it also can attack circulating fibrinogen and other plasma proteins, such as factors V and VIII. This creates a potentially hazardous bleeding tendency and invasive procedures must be scrupulously avoided in such patients.

Lysis of circulating fibrinogen by plasmin, a phenomenon sometimes called *primary fibrinogenolysis*, may also occur in rare patients due to release of a plasminogen activator from a malignant tumor.

PRODUCTION, DISTRIBUTION, AND LIFE SPAN OF HEMOSTATIC FACTORS

The kinetics of platelet production and destruction are discussed in Chapter 25. Synthesis by hepatocytes is the primary source for all of the plasma coagulation factors except factor VIII. Factor VIII is made in hepatic sinusoidal endothelial cells (but not other endothelial cells) and also in scattered mononuclear cells in the spleen, kidney, alveolar macrophages, and lymph nodes. Humans have limited vitamin K stores and the plasma activity of the vitamin K-dependent clotting proteins falls within a few days when the absorption or metabolism of vitamin K is impaired (see Chapter 29).

As discussed earlier, all endothelial cells can synthesize von Willebrand factor. Both plasma von Willebrand factor and plasma factor VIII levels rise sharply after vigorous muscular exercise, an infusion of adrenalin, or an infusion of an analogue of vasopressin (desmopressin). Their levels do not rise when these stimuli are repeated after only a short interval, which suggests that the initial rise reflects release of limited stores of these proteins into the circulation. Extensive damage to endothelium (for example, to the endothelial cells of the pulmonary capillaries in the acute respiratory distress syndrome) may cause plasma levels of von Willebrand factor to rise to very high levels.

Fibrinogen, von Willebrand factor, and factor VIII are acute phase proteins whose production and release are increased in infection and other inflammatory states. Interleukin 1, a monokine secreted by activated monocytes and macrophages, appears to stimulate this increased synthesis. Factors VII, VIII, X, von Willebrand factor, and fibrinogen levels are elevated in pregnancy and in patients using oral contraceptives.

All hemostatic factors except platelets are found in extravascular fluids. Their levels in thoracic duct lymph are between 25% and 75% of their plasma levels. Levels of the larger proteins—fibrinogen, factor V, and factor VIII—are lower than levels of the vitamin K-dependent clotting factors.

The plasma clotting factors have short intravascular half-times. The factors may be grouped by intravascular half-times as follows:

1. Fibrinogen, factor XIII—5 to 7 days
2. Prothrombin, factors V, IX, X, XI, XII—1 to 3 days
3. Factor VIII—10 hours; protein C—8 to 10 hours; factor VII—5 hours.

Because of such short intravascular half-lives, control of postoperative bleeding in patients with a severe clotting factor deficiency may require repeated daily to twice daily replacement therapy for 7 to 14 days.

SELECTED READING

1. Doolittle RF: Fibrinogen and fibrin. Sci Am 245:126, 1981.
2. Esmon CT: Protein C: biochemistry, physiology, and clinical implication. Blood 62:1155, 1983.
3. McDonagh J: Structure and function of factor XIII. *In* Colman RW, Hirsh J, Marder VJ, and Salzman EW (eds): Hemostasis and Thrombosis: Basic Principles and Clinical Practice Ed. 2. Philadelphia, JB Lippincott, 1987.
4. Nishizuka Y: Turnover of inositol phospholipids and signal transduction. Science 225:1365, 1984.
5. Rosenberg RD, and Rosenberg JS: Natural anticoagulant mechanisms. J Clin Invest 74:1, 1984.
6. Shattil SJ, and Bennett JS: Platelets and their membranes in hemostasis: physiology and pathophysiology. Ann Intern Med 94:108, 1981.
7. Verstraete M, and Collen D: Thrombolytic therapy in the eighties. Blood 67:1529, 1986.
8. Zur M, and Nemerson Y: Tissue factor pathways of blood coagulation. *In* Bloom AL, and Duncan PT (eds): Hemostasis and Thrombosis, New York, Churchill Livingstone, 1981.

24

Screening Evaluation of Hemostasis

ROUTINE EVALUATION OF THE PREOPERATIVE PATIENT

A screening evaluation of hemostasis before surgery requires that the physician take a history and examine the patient. From this and the nature of the intended surgery, one decides what laboratory tests are needed.

Screening History

A history taken to evaluate hemostasis should answer these questions:

1. Has the patient experienced abnormal bleeding or bruising? If so, are symptoms of recent origin, suggesting an acquired disorder, or do they date back to childhood, suggesting a hereditary disorder?
2. Is there a history of an acquired disorder that could impair hemostasis, for example, chronic liver disease, systemic lupus erythematosus, uremia, a hematologic malignancy?
3. Is the patient taking a drug that could interfere with hemostasis?
4. Have other members of the family bled abnormally?

In questioning a parent about *significant bleeding in a small child*, one should ask specifically about:

470

1. Bleeding from the umbilical stump.
2. Bleeding after circumcision.
3. Bleeding from cuts in the mouth. (The central incisors have erupted by the time an infant is learning to walk, and, therefore, many children fall and cut their mouth at this time.)
4. Frequency and size of hematomas of the scalp.
5. Extent of bruising from minor trauma, for example, falls from swings or bicycles or down steps.
6. Nosebleeds. Nosebleeds that stop within minutes, even if frequent, suggest that hemostasis is normal. Prolonged nosebleeds requiring medical intervention arouse suspicion of impaired hemostasis.

In assessing the bleeding history of an *adult patient*, one evaluates:

1. Abnormal bruising, by asking such specific questions as:
   a. How often do you notice a new bruise on your body?
   b. Do you develop bruises larger than a silver dollar without remembering how you got the bruise? If so, how big was the largest of these bruises?
   c. Do you notice bruises after injections, for example, after a penicillin shot?
2. Excessive bleeding from small cuts, by asking the patient to point out a scar from a small laceration and then asking specifically how the laceration occurred and how long it bled.
3. Bleeding after previous surgery. Although patients readily recall major surgery, they often need prompting to recall minor procedures such as biopsies, which can also bleed abnormally when hemostasis is defective. Late bleeding, for example, bleeding beginning on the second or third postoperative day, arouses particular suspicion of defective hemostasis.
4. Bleeding after dental extractions. Although many adults have escaped prior surgery, few have escaped dental extractions, which are a good test of hemostasis. Bleeding that lasts longer than 24 hours after extraction of a permanent tooth or that starts again after 3 or 4 days is suggestive of a hemostatic abnormality. A history of many extractions without abnormal bleeding makes a hereditary life-long bleeding tendency unlikely.

Drugs that interfere with hemostasis are of two types:

1. Drugs that impair formation of hemostatic plugs, of which the most important is *aspirin*. Taking a single aspirin tablet slightly

prolongs the bleeding time of most normal subjects but may substantially prolong the bleeding time of occasional, otherwise normal individuals. Since aspirin irreversibly inactivates platelet cyclooxygenase (see Chapter 23), the effect of aspirin on the bleeding time may persist for several days. (Therefore, unless it is being used as antithrombotic therapy, aspirin should not be taken for several days before elective surgery.) Other nonsteroidal anti-inflammatory agents that impair prostaglandin synthesis, for example, phenylbutazone, indomethacin, naproxen, also interfere with platelet aggregation, but their effect is transient, disappearing as blood levels fall. (These drugs should be discontinued in most patients 24 hours before elective surgery.)

2. Drugs that interfere with blood coagulation: heparin and oral anticoagulants. Although a routine preoperative patient would not be expected to be receiving therapeutic doses of heparin, preoperative patients will be encountered who are being maintained on long-term oral anticoagulant therapy, for example, a patient with a prosthetic heart valve. Planning when and how to stop and resume oral anticoagulants is a key part of such a patient's surgical management.

The *family history* must never be neglected in taking a bleeding history. The hemophilias, which are the most common of the severe hereditary bleeding disorders, are transmitted as X-linked genetic abnormalities. Therefore, a history suggestive of abnormal bleeding in a male member of the mother's side of the family deserves particular attention.

Physical Examination

On physical examination one looks particularly for:

1. Evidence of abnormal bleeding into the skin. Large ecchymoses (bruises) will be apparent on even cursory examination; their presence arouses concern for defective blood coagulation or excessive fibrinolysis. Petechiae (multiple bleeding spots the size of freckles) require a more careful search, particularly of the lower legs and ankles where the capillaries must withstand the greatest hydrostatic pressure. Petechiae suggest increased vascular fragility secondary to thrombocytopenia. Small purpuric spots with a firm center (so-called palpable purpura) suggest a vasculitis of small vessels as occurs in disorders such as Schönlein-Henoch purpura or mixed cryoglobulinemia. Hospi-

talized patients often receive multiple venipunctures and parenteral injections; these sites deserve particular scrutiny for suspicious ecchymoses or hematomas.

2. Abnormal elasticity of the skin and hyperextensibility of joints as evidence of a hereditary connective disorder associated with vascular bleeding.

3. Stigmatas of chronic liver disease: spider angiomas, palmar erythema, dilated abdominal veins, an enlarged liver and spleen.

Laboratory Tests

If the history and physical examination are negative, only two laboratory tests are usually needed:

1. A platelet count, which should be readily available in virtually all hospitals in the United States since the advent of electronic blood counting. A moderately depressed platelet count, in the 50,000 to 100,000 per μL range, will be discovered just often enough in a patient with a negative history and physical examination to justify counting platelets in all patients before major surgery.

2. An activated partial thromboplastin time (APTT or, as sometimes abbreviated, PTT). The APTT is recommended because:

    a. A slightly prolonged APTT may provide the first clue to mild hemophilia if a subtle history of abnormal bleeding has been missed, either because the physician has not questioned the patient adequately or because the patient may not have been aware that past bleeding he has experienced has been excessive. Such a patient may bleed seriously after many types of major surgery.

    b. A markedly prolonged APTT may be discovered in a patient with hereditary factor XI deficiency, who may not have bled abnormally after past surgery yet, nevertheless, could bleed excessively after the next surgical procedure. Because of the high gene frequently for factor XI deficiency in Ashkenazic Jews (Jews from eastern Europe), a routine preoperative APTT is particularly important in communities with a large Jewish population.

    c. A prolonged APTT may uncover the presence of the lupus anticoagulant. Although patients with the lupus anticoagulant rarely bleed abnormally after surgery (see Chapter 28), they have a paradoxically increased risk of thrombosis and, there-

fore, may be candidates for prophylactic perioperative administration of low-dose heparin (see Chapter 29).
   d. An abnormally short APTT may be found. This can stem either from an elevated level of factor VIII, which is an acute phase protein, or from the presence of activated clotting factors arising in an ongoing thrombotic process. The former may be another indication for prophylactic perioperative heparin; the possibility of the latter clearly should be assessed before proceeding with elective surgery.

In performing only a platelet count and APTT as preoperative screening tests, one accepts not routinely testing for abnormalities of platelet function that could impair formation of hemostatic plugs. One relies instead on the absence of a history of abnormal bleeding and on the absence of evidence, on general clinical evaluation, of an acquired disorder known to affect platelet function (for example, uremia, a monoclonal gammopathy, a myeloproliferative disorder). However, if the surgical procedure itself can impair platelet function (for example, cardiac surgery utilizing a pump oxygenator) or if the procedure is one in which even minimal postoperative bleeding could be hazardous (for example, brain surgery), then, despite other negative findings, one may wish to screen for the adequacy of formation of hemostatic plugs by performing a bleeding time test.

EVALUATION OF THE PATIENT WITH A SUSPECTED HEMOSTATIC ABNORMALITY

Initial Evaluation

When a patient is being assessed because of the question of a systemic hemostatic defect, one may screen for adequacy of the steps of hemostasis as follows:

1. For formation of hemostatic plugs by:
   a. Performing a platelet count.
   b. Examining platelet morphology on a blood smear.
   c. Performing a *bleeding time* by a template method.
2. For generation of thrombin by:
   a. Performing an APTT test, which screens for the reactions initiated by contact activation of plasma.
   b. Performing a prothrombin time test, which screens for the reactions initiated by adding tissue factor to plasma.

3. For the thrombin-fibrinogen reaction and stability of the fibrin clot by:
   a. Performing a thrombin time test.
   b. Examining the stability of plasma clots incubated in physiologic saline and in 5M urea.

In occasional patients, one may also wish to include a plasma protamine paracoagulation test for fibrin monomer and a serologic test for fibrin degradation products as part of the screening evaluation.

Theory and Technique of the Screening Tests

THE BLEEDING TIME

Hemostatic plugs of aggregated platelets stop bleeding from the small vessels cut in a bleeding time test. Although thrombin is an important stimulus for platelet activation (see Chapter 23), hemostatic plugs of sufficient stability form in patients with disorders of thrombin generation (for example, hemophilia) to stop bleeding from the minimal cuts of a bleeding time test in a normal time. Therefore, the bleeding time test screens for the overall adequacy of the reactions leading to formation of hemostatic plugs independent of the blood coagulation reactions.

One should use a bleeding time technique in which a standardized incision is made and in which the hemostatic plugs must hold against a back pressure. In the *template bleeding time*, two incisions, 9 mm long and 1 mm deep, are made on the volar surface of the forearm and back pressure is maintained by inflating a blood pressure cuff on the upper arm to 40 mmHg pressure. (A convenient, disposable spring-loaded bleeding time device is commercially available for making such incisions.) Excess blood is blotted away every 30 seconds with filter paper, with care not to disturb the wound edge. Bleeding will stop within 7 minutes in a normal individual who has not been taking aspirin or other drugs impairing platelet function. As discussed later, one occasionally repeats the test after giving a patient aspirin. The test may leave fine scars, and the patient should be told this.

THE ACTIVATED PARTIAL THROMBOPLASTIN TIME

In this test, a reagent supplying a phospholipid substitute for platelet procoagulant phospholipid activity and also supplying a surface activator (for example, kaolin powder) is added to plasma, the plasma is recalcified, and the clotting time is noted. The test is called an activated partial thromboplastin time (APTT) because the surface activator initiates a standardized contact activation of the plasma and the phospholipid provides a "partial thromboplastin" activity equivalent to that of the lipid component of complete tissue thromboplastin (tissue factor). With the rare exceptions mentioned later, a normal test rules out a significant abnormality of the plasma clotting factors shown on the left side of the vertical arrow in Figure 24-1. These include the factors deficient in the two forms of hemophilia, hemophilia A (factor VIII deficiency) and hemophilia B (factor IX deficiency).

Because commercial reagents and coagulation instrumentation vary, each laboratory should determine its own normal range for the APTT by performing the test on a group of normal subjects. Since the activity of a clotting factor must fall to 30% to 40% of normal before the APTT lengthens beyond the normal range, values only slightly longer than the upper limit of normal cannot be ignored (for example, a value of 40 seconds when the upper limit of normal is 36 seconds).

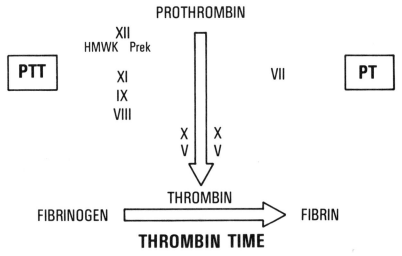

Fig. 24-1. A diagram illustrating the plasma clotting factors that influence the different screening tests of blood coagulation. Note that factors V and X, prothrombin, and fibrinogen affect both the APTT and the prothrombin time. The contact activation factors and the factors deficient in the two forms of hemophilia affect only the APTT. Factor VII affects only the prothrombin time. Note also that the thrombin time tests for the last step in coagulation independent of reactions involved in the generation of thrombin. Abbreviations: PTT, activated partial thromboplastin time; HMWK, high-molecular-weight kininogen; PK, prekallikrein; PT, prothrombin time.

THE PROTHROMBIN TIME

In this test, a potent tissue factor preparation (tissue thromboplastin) is added to plasma, the plasma is recalcified, and the clotting time is noted. The test was called a prothrombin time when first described in 1935 because the factors other than prothrombin (and fibrinogen) that can affect the test result were then unknown. The name has persisted, although it is clearly a misnomer since the factors shown on the right side of the vertical arrow in Figure 24-1—factors VII, X, and V—also affect the test result. One of these factors, factor VII, is unique in being required only for clotting induced by tissue factor.

Clotting induced by a strong concentration of tissue factor in the prothrombin time test differs from clotting induced by exposure of blood to a limited number of tissue factor sites in vivo. As discussed in Chapter 23, the tissue factor-factor VII activation of factor IX may play an important role in initiating physiologic hemostasis. However, in the prothrombin time test, an unphysiologically high concentration of tissue factor causes the plasma to clot within 10 to 12 seconds as a result of the direct tissue factor-factor VII activation of factor X (see Fig. 23-7). This bypasses the tissue factor-factor VII activation of factor IX and the subsequent IXa-VIIIa-phospholipid activation of factor X. Therefore, the prothrombin time is normal in both forms of hemophilia.

THE THROMBIN TIME

In this test, dilute thrombin is added to the patient's plasma and to a control plasma and the clotting times are compared. Since the plasma is not recalcified, its clotting time is independent of the reactions involved in the generation of thrombin and depends only upon the reactions initiated by adding the weak exogenous thrombin. Clotting with a low concentration of thrombin (for example, a thrombin concentration that clots normal plasma in about 20 seconds) brings out abnormalities in the thrombin-fibrinogen reaction that clotting with stronger, endogenously generated thrombin may mask. Causes of a long thrombin time include:

1. Increased antithrombin activity, as is found when plasma contains heparin.
2. Presence of large fibrin degradation products that interfere with polymerization of fibrin monomer to form visible fibrin.

3. Hypofibrinogenemia, when levels fall below about 80 mg per dL.
4. Qualitatively abnormal fibrinogens, as are found in the hereditary dysfibrinogenemias.

FIBRIN CLOT STABILITY

In this test, 0.2 mL of plasma is clotted with 0.2 mL of calcium chloride solution in each of two glass tubes. Three mL of physiologic saline is added to one tube and 3 mL of 5M urea to the other, and both clots are examined after incubation for 24 hours at 37°C. In a normal individual, both clots are stable. In a patient with excessive systemic fibrinolytic activity, the clot incubated in saline or both clots may dissolve. In hereditary factor XIII deficiency, the clot incubated in saline remains, whereas the clot incubated in 5M urea dissolves. Although simple, unfortunately, this screening procedure is not very sensitive. It fails to detect reduced plasma alpha$_2$ antiplasmin levels until the concentration falls below about 10% of normal.

PLASMA PROTAMINE PARACOAGULATION TEST

If thrombin has formed intravascularly, the blood may contain soluble fibrin monomer complexed with fibrinogen, with fibrin degradation products, or with both. Adding materials called paracoagulants, for example, protamine, to the plasma precipitates the fibrin monomer. In one test, one tenth volume of 1% protamine sulfate is added to plasma and the plasma is examined for visible fibrin after 15 minutes at 37°C. This simple test occasionally proves useful in confirming suspected disseminated intravascular coagulation.

MEASUREMENT OF FIBRIN DEGRADATION PRODUCTS

The patient's blood is clotted in a tube containing a high concentration of thrombin and inhibitors of fibrinolysis. The thrombin is added to make sure that no residual unclotted fibrinogen remains in the serum; the inhibitors of fibrinolysis block fibrinolysis in vitro. Dilutions of the serum are mixed with latex particles coated with an antifibrinogen fragment antiserum. Agglutination of the particles is considered evidence of circulating non-clottable fibrin (or fibrinogen) degradation products.

Normal serum may contains trace amounts of fibrin degradation products that cause a low dilution of serum to agglutinate the particles. Agglutination with higher dilutions of serum—although theoretically possible as a consequence of degradation of either fibrinogen or fibrin—is usually taken to mean that fibrin has been deposited intravascularly with resultant secondary fibrinolysis.

Further Tests When Screening Tests Are Normal

When the screening tests described above are all negative, the chance of overlooking a significant abnormality of hemostasis is small but not absent. Additional tests may be indicated as follows:

1. *If the patient's history still sounds convincing for excessive mucosal bleeding,* then adequacy of formation of hemostatic plugs should be investigated further by repeating the bleeding time 2 hours after giving the patient two aspirin tablets. Aspirin slightly prolongs the bleeding time of most normal individuals and the upper limit of normal for the template bleeding time after aspirin rises to 11 minutes. An occasional patient with mild von Willebrand's disease or a mild qualitative platelet disorder has a normal bleeding time before aspirin but a bleeding time after aspirin that substantially exceeds 11 minutes. (If a patient is bleeding at the time of evaluation or if surgery is urgent, one should not perform an aspirin bleeding time, for it may take several days for a prolonged bleeding time induced by aspirin to return to normal. Instead, one may have to proceed directly to platelet aggregation tests as described in Chapter 26.)
2. *If the patient's history still sounds convincing for increased bleeding after trauma or surgery,* then specific assays for factor VIII and factor IX should be carried out despite a normal APTT. When other coagulation factor levels are elevated, a rare patient with mild hemophilia may have an APTT test result within a laboratory's normal range. This usually happens in a patient with mild hemophilia B, in whom the effect upon the APTT of a factor IX level in the 20% range may be masked by a markedly elevated factor VIII level stemming from an acute phase reaction.
3. *If all tests described thus far are normal but on questioning*

again one still remains suspicious of excessive postoperative bleeding, then a quantitative assay for plasma alpha$_2$ antiplasmin should be carried out. A partial deficiency of this inhibitor (for example, in the 30 to 40% of normal range) will not be picked up in the fibrin clot stability test, yet may be associated with abnormal surgical bleeding if an event, such as an acute hypotensive episode, triggers an unusual degree of fibrinolytic activity after many small blood vessels have been severed.

Further Tests When Screening Tests Are Abnormal

The further study of a patient with an abnormal screening test or tests is guided by:

1. The diagnosis suspected from the history and physical examination.
2. Knowledge of what factors affect each screening test (see Fig. 24-1).
3. Knowledge of the screening test patterns of the common hemorrhagic disorders (Table 24-1).

The following points should also be kept in mind:

1. A long bleeding time in a nonthrombocytopenic patient usually indicates a need to measure von Willebrand factor antigen and activity. One also evaluates the ability of platelets to aggregate after adding different physiologic test materials to the patient's platelet-rich plasma (see Fig. 26-1).
2. A male patient with a life-long bleeding tendency and an isolated prolongation of the APTT has hemophilia (either factor VIII or factor IX deficiency) until proved otherwise.
3. Vitamin K deficiency and chronic hepatocellular disease may produce the same pattern of screening test abnormalities (see Table 24-1) but can be distinguished from each other by repeating the tests 24 hours after the parenteral administration of vitamin K.
4. An APTT, prothrombin time, or both test results may be prolonged either because a clotting factor is lacking or because a circulating anticoagulant, usually an antibody, is interfering with the clotting factor's function. If the former, mixing the patient's plasma with an equal volume of normal plasma will

TABLE 24-1. Screening Test Patterns in Hemorrhagic Disorders

TYPE OF DISORDER	PLATELETS	BLEEDING TIME	PROTHROMBIN TIME	APPT	THROMBIN TIME
HEREDITARY					
von Willebrand's disease	Normal	Long	Normal	Normal or long	Normal
F. VIII (Hemophilia A), F. IX (Hemophilia B) or F. XI deficiency	Normal	Normal	Normal	Long	Normal
F.V, X, or pro-thrombin deficiency	Normal	Normal	Long	Long	Normal
F. VII deficiency	Normal	Normal	Long	Normal	Normal
ACQUIRED					
Thrombocytopenia	Decreased	Long	Normal	Normal	Normal
Vitamin K deficiency (oral anticoagulants)	Normal	Normal	Long	Normal or long	Normal
Chronic liver disease	Normal or moderately decreased	Normal	Long	Long	Normal or slightly long
Acute, massive hepatic necrosis	Decreased	Long	Long	Long	Long
Massive intravascular clotting	Decreased	Long	Long	Long	Long
Lupus anticoagulant	Normal	Normal	Normal or slightly long*	Long†	Normal
F. VIII antibody	Normal	Normal	Normal	Long†	Normal
F. V antibody	Normal	Normal	Long†	Long†	Normal
Heparinemia	Normal	Normal	Normal or long	Long	Long

APPT is the abbreviation for the activated partial thromboplastin time test.
*May be very long if there is an associated severe specific hypoprothrombinemia.
†Failure to correct on mixing equal parts of patient's plasma and normal plasma.

shorten the clotting time almost to normal. If the latter, mixing the patient's plasma with an equal volume of normal plasma will fail to shorten the clotting time significantly.

SELECTED READING

1. Bachmann F: Diagnostic approach to mild bleeding disorders. Semin Hematol 17:292, 1980.

25

Platelets and Thrombocytopenic Purpuras

PLATELET KINETICS

Knowledge of normal platelet production, distribution, life span, and sites of destruction is needed to understand the pathogenesis of the thrombocytopenias.

Production

Platelets (thrombocytes) are formed in the bone marrow from the cytoplasm of large cells called *megakaryocytes*. After its cytoplasm is shed as platelets, the megakaryocyte dies.

STAGES OF THROMBOPOIESIS

A committed progenitor cell specific for megakaryocytes, the *colony forming unit-megakaryocyte (CFU-M)*, exists in the bone marrow. In an in vitro culture, a single CFU-M may divide repeatedly, giving rise to up to 50 megakaryocytes. In the steady state in vivo a new cell from the CFU-M pool in the bone marrow must undergo megakaryocytic differentiation to replace a megakaryocyte that has formed platelets.

A CFU-M differentiates into a *megakaryoblast*, which is the youngest cell morphologically identifiable on conventional staining of a bone marrow smear as belonging to the megakaryocytic series. It is a cell of intermediate size with an immature, oval nucleus and scanty, deeply basophilic cytoplasm. The megakaryoblast cannot divide into daughter cells but instead undergoes *endoreduplication,* that is, replication of its nuclear material without division of its cytoplasm. Cells are formed that contain a multilobulated nucleus and multiples of the original two sets of chromosomes (2n ploidy). The number of mitoses during endoreduplication can be estimated from the degree of nuclear lobulation of a megakaryocyte, each lobule corresponding to about 2n chromosomal material. The extent of endoreduplication determines the amount of cytoplasm that a megakarocyte can support, that is, the number of platelets that will arise from the megakaryocyte. In a normal bone marrow, about two thirds of the megakaryocytes are 16n, that is, have undergone endoreduplication eight times.

Cytoplasmic maturation begins after endoreduplication ceases. Cells with a multilobulated nucleus but a deeply basophilic cytoplasm that has not yet started to mature are called *promegakaryocytes.* With maturation, cytoplasmic basophilia fades, and the cytoplasm becomes filled with reddish-purple granules. At the ultrastructural level, the organelles and precursors of the membranous systems found in the platelet (see Fig. 23-1) become evident.

The mature megakaryocyte is an ameboid cell whose cytoplasmic pseudopods push their way through the endothelial lining cells into the lumen of the marrow sinusoids where they fragment into platelets. The bare nucleus of the megakaryocyte is then engulfed and digested by bone marrow macrophages. The time required to make new platelets, that is, the time required for a cell to progress from a morphologically unrecognizable precursor to a megakaryocyte that has shed its platelets, is about 5 days in humans.

REGULATION OF THROMBOPOIESIS

Thrombopoiesis is regulated by a two-tiered process. A material called *Meg-CSA* (megakaryocytic-colony stimulating activity) regulates the early proliferative phase of megakaryopoiesis. A second material called *thrombopoietin* stimulates megakaryocyte maturation and platelet release. Meg-CSA is assayed in vitro by its ability to increase the number and size of megakaryocyte colonies obtained on culture of bone marrow cells. Thrombopoietin is assayed by its ability, after infusion into an animal, to increase the rate and extent of incorporation of a radiolabel such as ^{35}S into the animal's platelets. The chemical composition of Meg-CSA and of thrombopoietin, their cellular sources, and the sensors triggering their synthesis and release are unknown.

Platelet production increases in thrombocytopenias caused by increased platelet destruction; in chronic states, production may be augmented three- to fivefold over normal. This results from an increase in:

1. Total numbers of megakaryocytes.
2. The number of mitoses individual megakaryoblasts undergo during endoreduplication and, therefore, the number of platelets a single megakaryocyte makes.

When platelet production is increased, large platelets are noted on the peripheral blood smear. They increase the value for mean platelet volume obtained with an electronic blood counter.

Distribution, Life Span, and Destruction

Platelets remain within the vascular system and are not present in extracellular fluids. At any moment, about two thirds of the platelets are circulating and about one third are concentrated within an exchangeable pool in the red pulp of the spleen. If the spleen enlarges, the distribution shifts. Up to 85% of the platelets may be sequestered in a markedly enlarged spleen. The bone marrow does not increase production sufficiently to compensate for this and a moderate thrombocytopenia results (hypersplenic thrombocytopenia).

Platelets have a life span of 8 to 10 days. Mononuclear phagocytes, primarily in the spleen but also in the liver and bone marrow, remove senescent platelets. In thrombocytopenias due to increased platelet consumption, platelets are randomly destroyed, regardless of their age. In immune thrombocytopenias, platelets coated lightly with antibody may be removed primarily by splenic mononuclear phagocytes as blood percolates slowly through the red pulp of the spleen. In contrast, platelets coated heavily with antibody and complement may be removed primarily by hepatic mononuclear phagocytes as a much larger fraction of the cardiac output flows rapidly through the sinusoids of the liver. This partly explains why the platelet count rises after splenectomy in most but not all patients with idiopathic thrombocytopenic purpura (see below).

The bone marrow does not contain a reserve of platelets. If for any reason most of the circulating platelets are destroyed or lost (for example, after a massive hemorrhage with replacement by banked blood, which does not contain viable platelets), the resultant thrombocytopenia persists for several days before enough new platelets can be made to correct it.

Ineffective Thrombopoiesis

Platelet survival times are not routinely measured in the diagnostic evaluation of a thrombocytopenic patient. If they were, an occasional thrombocytopenic patient would be shown to have the following combination of findings:

1. A normal intravascular survival time for radiolabeled *normal* platelets injected into the patient.
2. Bone marrow morphology suggestive of increased platelet production, that is, increased numbers of megakaryocytes and large megakaryocytes containing increased nuclear lobulations.

One may infer from these observations that the patient's megakaryocytes are making platelets, which, unlike the normal platelets, cannot survive normally in the circulation. The patient's thrombopoiesis, therefore, is ineffective. Ineffective thrombopoiesis is a cause for thrombocytopenia in several clinical situations cited later.

RELATION BETWEEN PLATELET LEVELS AND BLEEDING

When the platelet count falls from the normal range of 150,000 to 400,000 per µL to about 60,000 per µL, an individual may have enough thrombocytes to withstand ordinary hemostatic stresses but could bleed excessively after surgery leaving raw surfaces, for example, after a transurethral prostatectomy. When the platelet count drops below about 20,000 per µL, a patient develops a serious bleeding tendency characterized by:

1. Petechiae and small ecchymoses (but not the large tissue hemorrhages of patients with severe blood coagulation disorders or fibrinolytic bleeding).
2. Bleeding from mucosal surfaces (for example, heavy menstrual bleeding, a gastrointestinal hemorrhage).
3. Increased bleeding from severed small blood vessels after any surgical procedure.
4. A threat of CNS bleeding.

Accurate platelet counts are important in managing a severely thrombocytopenic patient. The difference between a platelet count of 5000 and 20,000 per μL represents a real difference in risk of life-threatening bleeding. When the platelet count falls below 5000 per μL, a patient is in imminent peril of fatal CNS bleeding or of massive gastrointestinal hemorrhage.

Patients with platelet counts in the 20,000 to 60,000 range vary in their risk for serious bleeding, according to the functional state of their platelets. Factors affecting the function of the reduced number of circulating platelets include:

1. *The proportion of the circulating platelets that are "young" platelets.* In most, but not all, circumstances (see below), newly made, larger platelets released from a marrow attempting to compensate for thrombocytopenia due to increased destruction are hemostatically more effective than older platelets, which make up a much higher proportion of the circulating platelets in a patient with thrombocytopenia due to impaired platelet production.

2. *Damage to circulating platelets.* In some thrombocytopenias due to increased destruction, the pathologic process also impairs the function of the platelets remaining in the circulation. Then, the patient's risk of bleeding may be greater than expected from the level of the platelet count.

3. *Use of drugs impairing platelet function, particularly aspirin.* Such drugs magnify substantially the risk of bleeding of any thrombocytopenic patient.

If a patient's platelet count is above about 20,000 per μL, then performing a bleeding time test may help one evaluate the extent to which the above factors may have modified the patient's risk of bleeding. However, if the platelet count is less than 20,000 per μL, the bleeding time test will always be substantially prolonged and rarely provides added useful information.

CLASSIFICATION OF THROMBOCYTOPENIAS

Thrombocytopenias may be divided into groups according to mechanism:

1. *Thrombocytopenias caused by failure of production.*
   a. With reduced numbers of megakaryocytes in the marrow.
   (1) Infiltrative disorders of the marrow, for example, acute

leukemia, in which blasts replace normal marrow elements.

(2) Marrow aplasias (idiopathic, drugs, toxins) in which fat, fibrous tissue, or both replace normal marrow elements.

(3) Rare hereditary amegakaryocytic thrombocytopenias in infants.

b. With normal to increased numbers of megakaryocytes in the marrow but ineffective thrombopoiesis.

(1) Thrombocytopenia in megaloblastic anemias.

(2) Alcohol-induced thrombocytopenia. Heavy drinking may induce severe thrombocytopenia stemming from a suppressive effect of alcohol on thrombopoiesis, often compounded by folate deficiency. (After the patient stops drinking, the platelet count may rebound transiently to very high levels.)

(3) Some instances of thrombocytopenia occurring in myelodysplastic disorders (for example, in preleukemia).

(4) Rare hereditary disorders: Wiskott-Aldrich syndrome, May-Hegglin anomaly.

2. *Thrombocytopenias caused by a shift in platelet distribution: the hypersplenic thrombocytopenias.* The characteristic findings are prominent splenomegaly; moderate thrombocytopenia in the range of 30,000 to 100,000 per μL; and normal to increased numbers of megakaryocytes in the bone marrow. Examples include:

a. Thrombocytopenia in cirrhosis with portal hypertension and congestive splenomegaly.

b. Thrombocytopenia in splenic infiltrative diseases, for example, Gaucher's disease.

c. Thrombocytopenia in myelofibrosis with extramedullary myeloid metaplasia. (Ineffective thrombopoiesis also usually contributes to thrombocytopenia in this disorder.)

3. *Thrombocytopenias caused by increased platelet destruction.*

a. *Thrombocytopenias caused by removal of IgG-coated platelets by the mononuclear phagocytic system.* IgG may bind to the platelet surface by three mechanisms (Fig. 25-1). In one, IgG binds by its antigen combining sites (Fab segment) to antigenic determinants that are normal structural components of the platelet surface membrane. In another, IgG binds by its Fab segment to an antigenic determinant formed when a drug binds to a binding site on the platelet surface membrane. In the third, IgG in immune complexes binds by a site on its Fc segment to Fc receptors on the platelet surface. The thrombo-

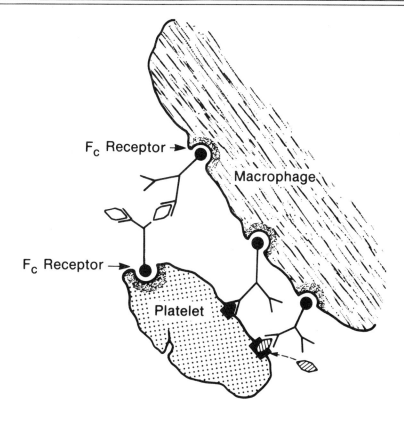

F_C Receptor →

Macrophage

F_C Receptor →

Platelet

● = Site on F_C segment of IgG binding to F_C receptors
▲ = Structural antigenic determinant of the platelet membranes
◇ = antigen of plasma immune complex
◁▨ = drug
▨▨ = drug + platelet surface binding site

Fig. 25-1. An illustration of mechanisms whereby IgG could bind to the platelet surface membrane with resultant removal of the IgG-coated platelet by its binding to the macrophage Fc receptors (see text).

cytopenia resulting from coating of platelets with IgG by any of these mechanisms is frequently severe (for example, below 10,000 per μL). The immune thrombocytopenias include:
(1) Idiopathic (immunologic) thrombocytopenic purpura (ITP). ITP in adults was formerly thought to result almost always from a platelet autoantibody, that is, an antibody against one of the patient's own platelet surface antigens.

However, the increasing incidence of thrombocytopenia now being seen in homosexual men may stem largely from immune complex-induced thrombocytopenia. ITP in small children usually follows a viral infection and results from immune complexes of viral antigen and antibody or from an antibody to a viral antigen bound to the platelet surface.

(2) Secondary immune thrombocytopenia in which platelet autoantibodies develop as a complication of a recognizable disease affecting immune function—systemic lupus erythematosus, lymphoma, or chronic lymphocytic leukemia.

(3) Drug-related immune thrombocytopenias, for example, thrombocytopenia arising in a patient receiving quinidine, which often probably result from an antibody reacting with an antigenic determinant formed when a drug binds to a binding site on the platelet surface. The thrombocytopenia found in an occasional patient receiving heparin (Chapter 29) is also now known to be of immune origin.

(4) Post-transfusion purpura, in which an individual in the 2% of the population that lacks the Pl^{A1} platelet antigen receives a blood transfusion containing Pl^{A1} positive platelets and, 7 to 10 days later, becomes severely thrombocytopenic. The patient forms an alloantibody to the foreign Pl^{A1} antigen that reacts, not only with the transfused platelets, but also, for an as yet unknown reason, causes the removal by the mononuclear phagocytic system of the patient's own platelets. A severe thrombocytopenia results which may last for days but which is reported to be rapidly corrected by plasmaphoresis.

(5) Neonatal thrombocytopenia, which may result from:
   (a) *Maternal platelet autoantibodies* that cross the placenta and coat the infant's platelets. This occurs in infants of mothers who have or have had idiopathic thrombocytopenic purpura.
   (b) *Maternal platelet alloantibodies* that arise when fetal platelets antigenically different from the mother's platelets immunize the mother. In a mechanism analogous to Rh hemolytic disease, the resultant maternal antibody crosses the platenta and coats the platelets of the fetus.

b. *Thrombocytopenia secondary to intravascular clotting and damage to platelets by thrombin.*

This results in a mild to moderate thrombocytopenia in which platelet counts usually do not fall below about 30,000 per μL. Thrombocytopenia following diffuse intravascular clotting may occur in:

(1) Obstetric complications in which procoagulant material enters the maternal circulation, for example, premature separation of the placenta, amniotic fluid embolism, retained dead fetus syndrome.

(2) Metastatic tumors (prostate, pancreas, stomach, and so on).

(3) Severe gram-negative bacteremia, for example, meningococcemia. (As noted below, other mechanisms also cause thrombocytopenia in infection.)

(4) Traumatic brain damage with exposure of blood to brain tissue with potent tissue factor activity.

Thrombocytopenia may also follow clotting in a local vascular bed, for example, in a massive hemangioma of the skin as seen in the Kasabach-Merritt syndrome.

c. *Thrombocytopenias related to alterations induced in platelets as blood flows through small vessels containing lose strands of fibrin:*

(1) Around tumor emboli in the microcirculation.

(2) In the glomerular capillary bed in hemolytic-uremic syndromes.

4. *Dilutional thrombocytopenia,* which develops after massive hemorrhage when blood volume and red cell mass are restored with banked blood that does not contain viable platelets.

5. *Thrombocytopenias caused by complex or poorly understood mechanisms.*

a. Thrombocytopenia resulting from infection. Patients with worsening infection, usually a gram-negative bacterial infection but occasionally a staphylococcal or other infection, may become severely thrombocytopenic. The thrombocytopenia exceeds that attributable to disseminated intravascular coagulation. Multiple other factors contribute to its pathogenesis—activation of complement, coating of platelets with immune complexes, loss of circulating platelets secondary to their adherence to damaged endothelium in the microcirculation, and suppression of platelet production.

b. Thrombotic thrombocytopenic purpura. In this poorly understood condition, platelets may be damaged by a platelet-aggregating material demonstrable in the plasma of some, but not all, patients. Thrombocytopenia results from deposition of damaged platelets in small platelet-fibrin thrombi in multiple organs and also, probably, by removal of damaged platelets by the mononuclear phagocytic system.

c. "Intensive care unit thrombocytopenia." Desperately ill patients in an intensive care unit occasionally become severely thrombocytopenic. Multiple factors may contribute to its pathogenesis—severe infection, deposition of platelets upon the damaged endothelium of the plumonary capillaries in the adult respiratory distress syndrome, and, in unusual patients, heparin-induced thrombocytopenia in patients in whom access channels have been kept open for many days with heparin.

EVALUATING THE THROMBOCYTOPENIC PATIENT

Serious in itself, thrombocytopenia may also mean serious underlying disease. Therefore, every thrombocytopenic patient requires careful study.

The History

The patient should be questioned about:

1. *Date of onset* of the thrombocytopenia and possible prior episodes. One must obtain details of past experiences that could have caused excessive bleeding if the patient were then thrombocytopenic (for example, dental extractions). In women, a careful menstrual history must be taken.
2. *Exposure to drugs and toxins.* One seeks to identify every drug or chemical agent that the patient was exposed to at the onset of the thrombocytopenia. Of particular concern are:
   a. Drugs known to cause increased platelet destruction—quinidine, antibacterial sulfa preparations, other sulfa derivatives, such as oral diuretics and oral antidiabetic agents, rifampicin, gold salts, valproic acid, and heparin.
   b. Drugs and toxins that may cause marrow aplasia (see Chapter 22).
   c. Heavy alcohol consumption.
3. *Recent infections or blood transfusions.* An acute episode of thrombocytopenia in children may follow known or presumed

viral infection. A blood transfusion within the past 14 days raises the possibility of post-transfusion purpura.

4. Possible *underlying immunologic disease*, for example, symptoms suggestive of systemic lupus erythematosus, such as skin rashes, arthralgia, Raynaud's phenomena, and unexplained fever.

5. *Sexual habits*, because of the recently noted increased frequency of thrombocytopenia in homosexual males.

Physical Examination

Important points on physical examination include:

1. The presence or absence of *fever*. Idiopathic thrombocytopenic purpura and drug-related thrombocytopenias are afebrile disorders. Fever alerts one to the possibilities of thrombocytopenia secondary to gram-negative endotoxemia, an underlying lupus erythematosus, or thrombotic thrombocytopenic purpura.

2. The extent to which petechiae and purpuric lesions are present on the skin and mucous membranes. One worries particularly about catastrophic CNS or gastrointestinal bleeding in the patient whose skin is covered with such lesions and who has purpuric bleb-like lesions in the mouth and pharynx. In contrast, an occasional severely thrombocytopenic patient has so few petichiae (usually confined to the lower legs and ankles of the ambulatory patient and to skin creases) that they can be missed if not looked for carefully.

3. *The size of the spleen.* As already noted, splenomegaly may produce a moderate thrombocytopenia due to a shift in distribution of platelets. In contrast, the spleen is not palpably enlarged in most thrombocytopenias caused by increased platelet destruction (for example, idiopathic thrombocytopenic purpura, drug-related immune thrombocytopenia, thrombotic thrombocytopenic purpura).

Laboratory Tests

Thrombocytopenia is established from a platelet count, usually obtained from an electronic blood counter, coupled with looking at a well-stained peripheral blood smear. The latter serves as a visual check of the accuracy of the platelet count. Occasional discrepancies may be found. For example,

1. Counting red cell fragments as platelets may mask the true ex-

tent of thrombocytopenia in thrombocytopenic disorders associated with red cell fragmentation (see below).
2. Clumping of platelets in vitro due to a platelet cold agglutinin may result in an artifactually reduced platelet count. This is recognized by noting the clumps of platelets on the blood smear.

THE BLOOD COUNT

Important clues to the cause for a thrombocytopenia are obtained from the blood count and blood smear. Thus,

1. In thrombocytopenias due to marrow disease, the peripheral blood will usually contain other evidence of marrow dysfunction:
   a. In thrombocytopenia secondary to leukemia, abnormal WBC can almost always be found on the blood smear.
   b. In thrombocytopenia secondary to marrow aplasia, the patient will be anemic with a depressed reticulocyte count and will be granulocytopenic. Immature WBC will not be found on the blood smear.
   c. In thrombocytopenia secondary to a megaloblastic anemia, oval macrocytes and hypersegmented granulocytes will be seen on the blood smear.
2. Discovering fragmented RBCs (schistiocytes, see Fig. 2-12) and polychromatophilic macrocytes on the blood smear may provide the first evidence of a disorder requiring urgent management in which thrombocytopenia is associated with hemolysis from mechanical damage to RBC in the microcirculation (for example, thrombotic thrombocytopenic purpura, a hemolytic-uremic syndrome complicating pre-eclampsia).
3. Normal red blood cell morphology is the expected finding in immune thrombocytopenias such as ITP, although recent substantial bleeding (for example, heavy menstrual bleeding due to the thrombocytopenia) may cause polychromatophilic macrocytes to be present on the blood smear.
4. Platelet size provides indirect evidence for the pathogenesis of the thrombocytopenia. This can be evaluated by looking for large platelets on the blood smear, which should be present in thrombocytopenias stemming from increased platelet destruction. Additional information is obtained from the mean platelet volume (MPV), a measurement provided by many electronic counters. In patients with normal marrow function, platelet production will

be stimulated as the platelet count begins to fall. Consequently, mean platelet volume rises because larger, newly made platelets will make up a higher proportion of the circulating platelets. An MPV that remains the same as the MPV for nonthrombocytopenic normal persons is not a normal finding in a thrombocytopenic patient and suggests that failure of platelet production has contributed significantly to the pathogenesis of the thrombocytopenia.

BONE MARROW EXAMINATION

The bone marrow of a thrombocytopenic patient is examined for two reasons:

1. To evaluate platelet production from the number and appearance of the megakaryocytes.
2. To confirm the impression derived from the peripheral blood smear of the presence or absence of marrow disease.

OTHER TESTS

Additional tests may be indicated after the initial evaluation, for example:

1. A bleeding time, if the platelet count is above 20,000 per μL.
2. Platelet-associated IgG (PAIgG). Methods of measuring PAIgG were developed as a hoped for means of identifying immune thrombocytopenias in which IgG binds to the platelet surface. PAIgG levels are elevated in virtually all patients with idiopathic thrombocytopenic purpura or immunologic drug-related thrombocytopenias. However, PAIgG levels are also increased in other thrombocytopenias due to increased platelet destruction, for example, in thrombocytopenia accompanying septicemia and in thrombotic thrombocytopenic purpura. (Apparently, damage to platelets may cause platelet membranes to disrupt and then reseal with resultant entrance of IgG and other plasma proteins into the platelet.) Although measuring PAIgG is thus not specific for antibody-induced thrombocytopenia, it may help in selected patients in recognizing thrombocytopenia resulting from increased peripheral destruction.
3. An APTT test to rule out an associated lupus anticoagulant (see Chapter 28).

IDIOPATHIC THROMBOCYTOPENIC PURPURA

In small children, idiopathic thrombocytopenic purpura (ITP) is usually an acute, self-limited disorder triggered by the synthesis of antibody to a viral antigen. The antibody either binds as immune complexes to platelet Fc receptors or binds by its antibody combining sites to viral antigen that has come down onto the platelets. *The ITP seen in adult male homosexuals* may also result from the binding of immune complexes to platelets, but like ITP in other adult patients is not self-limited but chronic. *ITP in most other adults* is a chronic disorder in which a patient with no recognizable underlying disease or significant drug exposure makes a platelet autoantibody.

The following observations provide convincing evidence for a pathogenetic role of antiplatelet antibodies in the latter type of adult ITP:

1. Women with ITP frequently give birth to thrombocytopenic infants. This suggests the transplacental passage of a maternal IgG antibody.
2. Plasma taken from a patient with ITP will produce temporary thrombocytopenia if given back to the patient after recovery or if transfused into a normal human volunteer. The material causing thrombocytopenia is found in the gamma globulin fraction of plasma and can be adsorbed by incubation with platelets.

However, proof that a platelet antibody is an autoantibody (that is, is directed against a normal structural component of the platelet surface membrane) requires identification of the antigen. Recently, platelet antibodies from a number of patients with ITP have been shown to react with epitopes on specific glycoproteins of the platelet surface membrane, for example, epitopes on GP IIIa or on GP Ib.

Clinical and Laboratory Manifestations

ITP is a diagnosis of exclusion. Its manifestations are:

1. The onset of easy bruising, a petechial rash, and, in women, increased menstrual bleeding. Profoundly thrombocytopenic patients may also develop gingival bleeding, epistaxis, or hematuria.
2. No history of a recognizable precipitating agent or event. (This is key, since drug-related immune thrombocytopenia and post-transfusion purpura may present with manifestations resembling ITP in all other ways.)

3. Abnormal findings on physical examination limited to petechiae and purpura on the skin and, sometimes, purpuric blebs on the mucous membranes of the mouth. The patient is afebrile and the spleen is not palpable.
4. A normal peripheral blood examination except for thrombocytopenia with large thrombocytes and, if the patient has bled recently, a mild normochromic, normocytic anemia with a scattering of polychromatophilic macrocytes on the blood smear. (If a woman has had excessive menstrual bleeding for a number of months, microcytosis and hypochromia due to iron deficiency may also be noted.)
5. A bone marrow examination showing:
   a. Morphologic evidence suggestive of increased platelet production—increased numbers of promegakaryocytes and megakaryocytes and also megakaryocytes with increased nuclear lobulation. (In unusual patients in whom an autoantibody may also impede megakaryocyte maturation, megakaryocytes may be diminished and even absent.)
   b. Mild erythroid hyperplasia if bleeding has been recent.
   c. Possible reduced or absent stainable iron stores.
6. In patients who undergo splenectomy, no evidence of an underlying disease on microscopic examination of the spleen.

Management of ITP in the Adult

The mainstays of therapy are:

1. Adrenal glucocorticoids, which act primarily:
   a. To suppress mononuclear phagocyte activity and thereby impede removal of IgG-coated platelets in the spleen and liver.
   b. To decrease binding of IgG to the platelet surface.

   When given in large doses for many days, adrenal glucocorticoids may also suppress the production of a platelet autoantibody.
2. Splenectomy, which eliminates a major site of removal of IgG-coated platelets and also may eliminate a major site of platelet antibody production.

Treatment usually begins with a high dose of adrenal steroids, that is 80 mg of prednisone in a divided dose daily. In the patient who responds, the platelet count begins to rise within several days. Some physicians reduce the steroid dose slowly, continuing a relatively high dose for a number of weeks after the platelet count has returned to normal in the hope of obtaining an added immunosuppressive effect. Other physicians reduce the steroid dose more rapidly. Regardless of the schedule used, thrombocytopenia reappears in a high percentage of patients as the dosage is reduced.

If steroids fail to correct the thrombocytopenia or if thrombocytopenia reappears as steroids are tapered, splenectomy is usually resorted to next. (Because splenectomy creates a risk of overwhelming pneumococcal infection, pneumococcal vaccine should be given before splenectomy.) Platelet levels rise promptly after splenectomy in about 75% of patients. However, in a substantial number, the platelet count falls again to between about 30,000 to 100,000 per μL within weeks to months after splenectomy. Unless the antibody inducing the thrombocytopenia also impairs the function of the circulating platelets, such patients usually have a normal bleeding time and only minimal problems with excessive bleeding. Therefore, they require no treatment, but they must scrupulously avoid using drugs that impair platelet function (aspirin, indomethacin, other nonsteroidal antiinflammatory agents). They are also at risk of developing episodes of more severe thrombocytopenia, often after an infection, that may require treatment with a high dose of adrenal steroids for a short period.

In a minority of patients, the platelet count may rise for a variable period after splenectomy but then a severe, thrombocytopenia returns and persists. A variety of agents are then usually tried, including:

1. Danazol, a synthetic impeded androgen, which apparently also suppresses mononuclear phagocytic function and so may improve the platelet count in some patients without the side effects resulting from the prolonged use of high doses of adrenal steroids.
2. Injections of the vinca alkaloids, vincristine, or vinblastine, which often causes platelet counts to rise transiently but rarely has a lasting effect.
3. Azathioprine, which after several months of therapy may induce a prolonged remission in a few patients.
4. Cyclophosphamide, which is probably best avoided until all else fails because of its leukemogenic potential.
5. Intravenous gamma globulin in very large amounts (400 mg per kg for 5 consecutive days) which, by occupying the Fc receptor sites of the cells of the mononuclear phagocytic system, may impede the removal of antibody-coated platelets and so cause the platelet count to rise temporarily. Intravenous gamma glob-

ulin may be particularly useful when one wishes to increase the platelet count briefly for a particular purpose, for example, a surgical procedure or an invasive diagnostic procedure.

Platelet concentrates have little prophylactic value in the severely thrombocytopenic patient, since transfused normal platelets will be removed from the circulation just as rapidly as the patient's own platelets. Platelet concentrates are given during an acute, life-threatening bleeding episode for whatever transient effect that they may have.

An infant born of a mother with ITP is at risk for neonatal thrombocytopenia. If the mother's platelet count is below 100,000 per μL or if she has been splenectomized (regardless of her platelet count), some physicians recommend Caesarian section to eliminate the risk of intracranial hemorrhage in a thrombocytopenic infant during the trauma of vaginal delivery. Others recommend treating the mother with adrenal steroids beginning shortly before confinement, allowing vaginal delivery, and giving steroids to the newborn infant for a brief period. A new technique for obtaining a fetal scalp vein platelet count at the onset of labor may help one to decide if a Caesarian section is warranted.

DISORDERS WITH THROMBOCYTOPENIA, HEMOLYSIS, AND FRAGMENTED RBCs

Thrombocytopenia and hemolysis caused by RBC fragmentation (see Fig. 2-12) may develop in disorders in which loose fibrin strands are laid down in small blood vessels. Possible pathogenetic mechanisms for the deposition of fibrin in multiple small vessels include:

1. Primary vascular wall injury, for example, from deposition of immune complexes leading to a vasculitis of multiple small blood vessels in which thrombin generation and secondary deposition of fibrin are part of the inflammatory response.
2. Diffuse intravascular clotting, which may cause fibrin that forms in the circulating blood to become deposited within normal small blood vessels. The fibrin is predominantly laid down in glomerular vessels with resultant renal damage out of proportion to other organ damage. (This sequence of events induced experimentally in the rabbit is called the generalized Shwartzman reaction.)
3. Multifocal clotting induced by small metastatic foci of tumor

cells within blood vessels, particularly multiple micrometastases within the pulmonary capillary bed.

4. An abnormality of the plasma that triggers the formation of platelet aggregates, which then lodge in the microcirulation and induce vessel wall damage with resultant fibrin deposition.

The first three of these processes have been clearly shown to occur in humans. The fourth is postulated to occur on the basis of in vitro evidence of a platelet aggregating factor in the plasma of patients with thrombotic thrombocytopenic purpura.

The disorders in which the combination of thrombocytopenia and hemolysis with fragmented RBCs may occur include:

1. Thrombotic thrombocytopenic purpura.
2. Systemic lupus erythematosus. In most patients with lupus, the combination of thrombocytopenia and hemolysis results from the binding of antibodies to both platelets and RBCs (Evans syndrome). However, in an infrequent patient with severe vasculitis, enough fibrin may be deposited in vessels to produce thrombocytopenia and hemolysis from mechanical damage to platelets and RBCs.
3. Metastatic carcinoma.
4. Hemolytic-uremic syndromes.

Thrombotic Thrombocytopenic Purpura

Thrombotic thrombocytopenic purpura (TTP) is an acute, potentially fatal disorder of unknown etiology affecting women more frequently than men. Its clinical manifestations are:

1. Fever, which may be minimal or promient.
2. Thrombocytopenia, which is usually severe.
3. Hemolysis, with fragmented RBCs on the blood smear.
4. Changing manifestations of damage to multiple organs, which may include:
   a. Fluctuating, bizarre CNS findings.
   b. Fluctuating jaundice, with elevation of both the direct and indirect bilirubin because of the combination of hemolysis and liver damage.
   c. Varying manifestations of renal damage, such as proteinuria, hematuria, and a mild elevation of the BUN. However, overwhelming renal damage with anuria and fulminant uremia does not occur (which helps to distinguish TTP from hemolytic-uremic syndromes).

d. Evidence of myocardial damage, such as changing rhythms and congestive heart failure.

e. Episodes of abdominal pain and elevated serum amylase suggestive of pancreatitis.

Coagulation tests usually reveal a normal prothrombin time, a normal to short activated partial thromboplastin time, and, initially, a normal or elevated fibrinogen level. The fibrinogen level reflects a balance between increased fibrinogen consumption in platelet-fibrin thrombi and increased fibrinogen synthesis in the acute phase response to illness. If a patient is given large doses of adrenal steroids, which suppress the acute phase response, the plasma fibrinogen concentration may fall to a subnormal level.

A *presumptive diagnosis* of TTP can be made in a patient with the above findings after systemic lupus erythematosus and a neoplasm have been ruled out. A *definitive diagnosis* requires the demonstration by biopsy of typical vascular lesions of TTP (Fig. 25-2). However, a biopsy is not commonly performed.

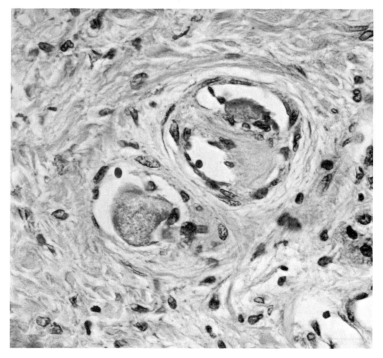

Fig. 25-2. High-power view showing two affected small blood vessels in capsule of adrenal gland from patient with thrombotic thrombocytopenic purpura.

The characteristic *autopsy findings* of TTP are:

1. Involvement of vessels in multiple organs with particularly prominent lesions in the vessels of the brain, heart, pancreas, capsule of the adrenals, and capsule of lymph nodes.
2. A predilection for localization of lesions to arteriolo-capillary junctions.
3. A "bland" vessel wall lesion without evidence of inflammatory vasculitis, that is, without infiltrations of granulocytes within and around vessel walls (see Fig. 25-2). The lesion is characterized by accumulation of material with a strongly positive periodic acid-Schiff (PAS) reaction in the vessel wall, loss of overlying endothelial cells, aneurysmal dilatations, and fibrin within the lumen of vessels at many sites of wall damage.

The *etiology* of TTP is unknown but unlikely to involve deposition of immune complexes, which, by activating complement, liberate chemoattractants that invoke an inflammatory granulocytic response. A pathogenetic mechanism must account for four observations:

1. The plasma of at least some patients with TTP contains a factor inducing the aggregation of normal platelets in vitro.
2. The IgG fraction of normal plasma contains an activity inhibiting the platelet aggregating factor of TTP plasma.
3. The plasma of a patient in remission often contains increased amounts of large multimers of von Willebrand factor, which disappear from the plasma when the patient relapses.
4. The transfusion of large amounts of normal plasma into a patient with TTP usually suppresses manifestations of disease activity.

Patients with TTP are usually treated by transfusion of large volumes of plasma and administration of adrenal steroids. Such large volumes of plasma must be given that many patients require repeated plasmaphoresis and plasma exchange. The disease remits in many but not all patients following such therapy. Some patients will relapse and repeated, prophylactic administration of plasma may be required to prevent relapses.

The Hemolytic-Uremic Syndrome

The hemolytic-uremic syndrome (HUS) occurs most often in two groups of patients:

1. In infants and small children (occasionally in older children or young adults) following a febrile illness, often associated with vomiting and diarrhea and the demonstrated presence of pathologic gastrointestinal organisms (for example, a strain of E coli producing an unusual toxin, Campylobacter, Shigella).
2. In a pregnant or postpartum woman, usually following gram-negative infection (amnionitis, pyelonephritis, septic abortion) or premature separation of the placenta, but occasionally developing several days to weeks after a seemingly uneventful delivery.

In both clinical settings, the syndrome of HUS is characterized by:

1. The sudden onset of acute, *anuric renal failure*, often with accompanying hypertension.
2. Brisk intravascular hemolysis due to red cell fragmentation, sometimes with striking hemoglobinemia.
3. Thrombocytopenia of varying severity.
4. Minimal evidence usually of damage to organs other than the kidney.

Coagulation tests at the time a patient is usually first seen reveal a normal to short APTT, a normal to slightly prolonged prothrombin time, and a normal to moderately prolonged thrombin time. Factor VIII and fibrinogen levels may be normal or elevated. Fibrin split products are usually, but not invariably, elevated in the serum.

The renal lesion of HUS is characteristically focal. Thrombi are found in glomerular arterioles and capillaries associated with glomerular lesions of varying severity, including areas of frank cortical necrosis. Fibrinoid necrosis of afferent glomerular arterioles may be prominent. In older lesions, aneurysmal dilatation and marked fibrosis of afferent glomerular arterioles may be noted. Vascular lesions are rarely found in other organs.

The lack of clear-cut evidence of ongoing disseminated intravascular coagulation when a patient is first seen in no way rules out the possibility that an earlier episode of disseminated intravascular coagulation initiated fibrin deposition in the glomerular capillary bed. The author has seen pregnant women with severe gram-negative septicemia and depleted clotting factors indicative of extensive disseminated intravascular coagulation whose clotting factor levels have quickly returned to normal with appropriate therapy and who have then gone on to develop full-blown manifestations of HUS 24 to 48 hours later. At that time, their clotting factor studies were similar to those of the usual patient with HUS, who is first seen after hemolysis and anuria have developed.

Therefore, the author believes that one important pathogenetic mechanism for HUS is as follows:

1. An infection causing gram-negative endotoxemia or some other initiating event sets off an episode of disseminated intravasacular coagulation.
2. For unknown reasons, the mononuclear phagocytic system can not clear the circulating fibrin and large amounts are deposited in the glomerular vessels.
3. Local fibrinolytic activity (which is known to be depressed in pregnancy) fails to lyse the deposited fibrin. Consequently, the deposits persist and produce glomerular damage and renal failure, RBC fragmentation and hemolysis, and thrombocytopenia.

This concept of the initiation of HUS does not preclude a role for local factors, for example, endothelial cell injury secondary to glomerular capillary thrombosis, in the progression of HUS.

With conservative management, including dialysis therapy, most infants and children recover from HUS, often with only minimal residual renal damage. Heparin is not indicated in the usual patient since the episode of disseminated intravascular coagulation that may have initiated the process is over. For an unknown reason, women who develop HUS several days to weeks after delivery have a more severe form of the disease and usually remain anuric.

SELECTED READING

1. Aster RH: Editorial retrospective. Plasma therapy for thrombotic thrombocytopenic purpura: sometimes it works, but why? N Engl J Med 312: 985, 1985.
2. Karpatkin S: Autoimmune thrombocytopenic purpura. Semin Hematol 22: 260, 1985.
3. Kelton JG: Management of the pregnant patient with idiopathic thrombocytopenic purpura. Ann Intern Med 99:796, 1983.
4. Lian EC-Y, Mui PTK, Siddiqui FA, Chiu AYY, and Chiu LLS: Inhibition of platelet-aggregating activity in thrombotic thrombocytopenic purura plasma by normal adult immunoglobulin G. J Clin Invest 73:548, 1983.
5. McMillan R: Immune thrombocytopenia. Clin Haematol 12:69, Feb 1983.
6. Rosse W: Treatment of chronic immune thrombocytopenia. Clin Haematol 12:267, Feb 1983.
7. Wilson JJ, Naeme PB, and Kelton JG: Infection-induced thrombocytopenia. Semin Thromb Haemost 8:217, 1982.

26

Disorders with a Long Bleeding Time Not Due to Thrombocytopenia

If the bleeding time is long, yet the platelet count is normal, or if the bleeding time exceeds that expected for a mild to moderate thrombocytopenia, then hemostatic plugs do not form normally for reasons other than, or in addition to, thrombocytopenia. The impairment may stem from:

1. A qualitative abnormality of the platelet itself, that is, an *intrinsic platelet defect*, such as a missing platelet surface glycoprotein.
2. An *extrinsic factor* that alters the function of normal platelets, for example, an abnormality of plasma von Willebrand factor.

Both hereditary and acquired disorders may cause long bleeding times due to platelet dysfunction. The hereditary disorders, except for von Willebrand's disease, are uncommon, yet important, because study of their mechanisms has taught us much about how platelets normally form hemostatic plugs (Table 26-1). Acquired defects of platelet function are a common cause of clinical bleeding, but their mechanisms are often complex and poorly understood.

505

Table 26-1. Mechanisms Causing Impaired Formation of Hemostatic Plugs in Hereditary Disorders

DISORDER	MECHANISM
DISORDERS AFFECTING PLATELET ADHESION TO SUBENDOTHELIUM	
1. Von Willebrand's disease	Abnormalities of plasma von Willebrand factor
2. Bernard-Soulier syndrome	Absence of platelet surface membrane GP Ib binding site for von Willebrand factor
DISORDERS OF SECRETION	
1. Platelet granule disorders	
a. Dense granule deficiency syndromes*	Decreased storage pool ADP for secretion
b. Gray platelet syndrome*	Decreased alpha granule materials for secretion (e.g., thrombospondin, factor V)
2. Disorders of thromboxane A_2	
a. Disorders affecting synthesis	Platelet cyclooxygenase or thromboxane synthetase deficiency
b. Disorders affecting function	Defective platelet surface membrane receptors for thromboxane A_2
DISORDERS OF FIBRINOGEN BINDING TO ACTIVATED PLATELETS	
1. Thrombasthenia (Glanzmann's disease)	Absence of platelet surface membrane GP IIb-IIIa binding site for fibrinogen
2. Afibrinogenemia	Absence of plasma and platelet alpha granule fibrinogen

*Combined dense body-alpha granule disorders also exist. The gray platelet syndrome without accompanying dense granule deficiency only minimally alters hemostatic function.

HEREDITARY INTRINSIC PLATELET DISORDERS

A number of disorders have now been described. Those discussed below have been particularly instructive for understanding normal platelet function.

Bernard-Soulier Syndrome

Studies of this disorder provided the clue that plasma von Willebrand factor must bind to a site on GP Ib for platelets to adhere normally to subendothelium. Patients with Bernard-Soulier syndrome have a mild to moderate thrombocytopenia, a prolonged bleeding time exceeding that expected from the thrombocytopenia, and giant platelets on a stained blood smear. Their platelets fail to adhere normally to subendothelium when blood flows over a vessel denuded of endothelium in an *ex vivo* model system. Despite normal plasma von Willebrand factor, their platelets also fail to agglutinate on exposure to ristocetin—a reaction dependent upon the binding of von Willebrand factor to platelets. Separation of solubilized platelet membrane glycoproteins reveals that GP 1b is missing from the platelet membrane.

Disorders of Platelet Secretion

These are a group of mild bleeding disorders in which patients experience easy bruising, occasional episodes of excessive mucous membrane bleeding, and inconstant mild to moderate postoperative bleeding. They result from one of the following causes for impaired platelet secretion:

1. Insufficient storage pool ADP in the dense granules (storage pool deficiency disorders).
2. Defective synthesis of or responsiveness to thromboxane A_2.

Typical laboratory findings are:

1. Normal platelet morphology on the blood smear.
2. A slightly to moderately prolonged bleeding time.
3. Normal ristocetin-induced platelet agglutination. (Platelet agglutinination—a non-physiologic, passive electrostatic adherence of platelets to each other—differs from platelet aggregation, which results from an active metabolic response to physiologic stimuli, such as collagen, ADP, or thrombin.)
4. A normal single large wave of platelet aggregation induced by a high concentration of ADP. This reflects the normal ability of the platelets to react to *extrinsic* ADP.
5. Impaired to absent aggregation following exposure to:
   a. Collagen (Fig. 26-1).
   b. Epinephrine, which gives a small primary wave of aggregation but no second wave of aggregation.
   c. A low concentration of ADP, which also gives a small primary wave of aggregation but no second wave.

Since *intrinsic ADP* mediates collagen-induced aggregation and also the second wave of aggregation induced by either epinephrine

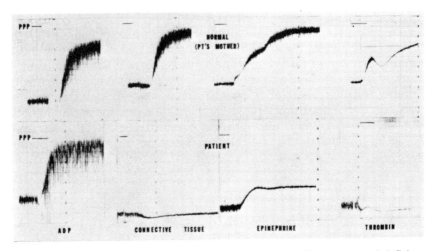

Fig. 26-1. The platelet aggregation pattern of a patient with storage pool deficiency associated with albinism (Hermansky-Pudlak syndrome) as contrasted with a normal pattern in the patient's mother. Note that the platelets in the patient's platelet-rich plasma do not exhibit a second wave of aggregation with epinephrine, do not aggregate at all with collagen, yet aggregate normally with a high concentration of extrinsic ADP. (Logan LJ, Rapaport SI, Maher BS: Albinism and abnormal platelet function. N Engl J Med 284:1340, 1971; reproduced by permission of the New England Journal of Medicine)

or a low concentration of extrinsic ADP, an impaired secretion of platelet ADP can account for all of the above abnormal findings. Special studies (for example, electron microscopy of platelets to evaluate the number of dense granules) are required to determine whether a reduced storage pool of ADP or an impaired release of a normal storage pool of ADP resulting from impaired synthesis or responsiveness to thromboxane A_2 represents the primary defect in a given patient. However, such studies are usually not pursued because they are unnecessary for a patient's clinical management.

Taking a single aspirin tablet, which inactivates platelet cyclooxygenase irreversibly, causes normal platelets to acquire an identical pattern of abnormal responses to aggregating agents. Since it persists for several days, one must know that a patient has not taken a drug containing aspirin for 1 week before attributing this pattern of platelet aggregation abnormalities to an intrinsic platelet disorder.

Moreover, whereas taking an aspirin tablet slightly lengthens the bleeding time of most normal individuals, taking an aspirin tablet strikingly prolongs (for example, to 40 minutes) the bleeding time of an occasional individual whose bleeding time before aspirin was normal. Such individuals usually have a subclinical form of a disorder of platelet secretion, whose effects become clinically significant only when worsened by aspirin's inhibition of platelet cyclooxygenase.

Bleeding in disorders of platelet secretion is seldom severe enough to require replacement therapy as long as drugs that impair platelet function, particularly drugs that contain aspirin, are scrupulously avoided. However, if serious bleeding occurs, platelet concentrates may need to be given.

Thrombasthenia

Thrombasthenia (Glanzmann's disease) is an autosomal recessive disorder characterized by *severe mucous membrane* and postoperative bleeding. Nosebleeds, which stop only after nasal packing and transfusions of platelets, may plague the patient. Bothersome gingival bleeding persists throughout a patient's lifetime, and patients must take iron to prevent iron deficiency anemia from chronic blood loss. Discovery of the defect causing thrombasthenia has significantly advanced understanding of how platelets adhere to each other in forming hemostatic plugs.

Laboratory findings are as follows:

1. Individual platelets look normal on the blood smear but smears made from blood obtained from a finger stick (that is, free of EDTA anticoagulant) fail to show the small clumps of aggregated platelets normally seen on such smears.
2. A *very long* bleeding time.
3. Absent clot retraction.
4. Failure of platelets to aggregate after exposure to all physiologic stimuli (ADP, collagen, epinephrine, thrombin). Absent aggregation after adding a high concentration of ADP to platelet-rich plasma—which bypasses the steps of thromboxane A_2 synthesis and intrinsic ADP release—is a *sine qua non* for the diagnosis.

Thrombasthenic platelets were discovered:

1. To be deficient in platelet-associated fibrinogen when it was measured in platelets isolated from plasma by techniques now known to cause partial platelet activation and, therefore, binding of plasma fibrinogen to normal platelets.
2. To lack two glycoproteins, GPIIb and GPIIIa, on electrophoresis of solubilized platelet membrane glycoproteins.

These observations stimulated further studies which established that activated normal platelets form a calcium-dependent GPIIb-IIIa complex to which fibrinogen, and also fibronectin and von Willebrand factor, can bind.

Although the functional importance of the binding of the other proteins to this site is not yet clear, fibrinogen must bind to the GPIIb-IIIa complex for normal platelet cohesion. Failure of such binding results in the profound defect in formation of hemostatic plugs and serious bleeding characteristic of thrombasthenia.

VON WILLEBRAND'S DISEASE

Von Willebrand's disease is a common hereditary bleeding disorder, perhaps even the most common, since patients with minimal disease may escape recognition. It stems from an *abnormality of von Willebrand factor itself* that results in either:

1. A quantitative plasma deficiency of all multimeric forms of von Willebrand factor. Total plasma von Willebrand antigen is usually reduced to the 15 to 60% range (type I variant). In a rare patient, it is reduced to an undetectable level (type III variant).
2. A selective deficiency affecting primarily the larger multimers of plasma von Willebrand factor (types IIa and IIb).

Type I von Willebrand's disease is more common than the type II variants.

The large multimers of plasma von Willebrand factor may also be selectively reduced in a rare hereditary platelet disorder called pseudo-von Willebrand's disease. In this disorder, von Willebrand factor itself is normal but an abnormal affinity of the platelets for von Willebrand factor enhances binding to platelets of the large multimers and so diminishes their plasma concentration.

Mechanisms responsible for abnormalities of plasma von Willebrand factor are summarized in Table 26-2.

Properties of von Willebrand Factor

Endothelial cells secrete von Willebrand factor into plasma as large multimers (see Chapter 23) which are apparently degraded into smaller multimers as the protein circulates. A hypothalamic neuro-humoral agent, probably acting through the posterior pituitary hormone vasopressin, can stimulate release into plasma of limited en-

Table 26-2. Disorders Affecting Plasma von Willebrand Factor

PRIMARY DEFECT	DISORDER	MECHANISM FOR PLASMA vWF* ABNORMALITY
Quantitative deficiency of plasma vWF	vWD*, type I	Decreased synthesis
	vWD, type III	Virtually absent synthesis
Selective deficiency of large plasma vWF multimers	vWD, type IIa	Failure to synthesize large and intermediate multimers
	vWD, type IIb	Synthesis of abnormal large multimers that rapidly disappear from the plasma
	Pseudo-vWD	Abnormal affinity of platelets for plasma vWF

*vWF stands for von Willebrand factor and vWD stands for von Willebrand's disease.

dothelial cell stores of von Willebrand factor. (As discussed later, a synthetic analogue of vasopressin, called desmopressin or DDAVP, is given to patients with type I von Willebrand's disease to raise plasma von Willebrand factor levels temporarily.)

Plasma von Willebrand factor is required for:

1. Adhesion of platelets to subendothelium (see Chapter 23). *Only the largest multimers can support platelet adhesion*; even intermediate-sized multimers are ineffective.

2. Maintenance of normal plasma levels of factor VIII. Factor VIII circulates in plasma as a complex with von Willebrand factor. Multimers of all sizes can apparently bind factor VIII, and plasma factor VIII coagulant activity is normally proportional to total plasma von Willebrand factor concentration. (One notes, therefore, that two hereditary disorders can cause a low plasma factor VIII level—hemophilia A (see Chapter 27), in which the synthesis of factor VIII itself is defective, and von Willebrand's disease.)

Why von Willebrand factor is required to maintain normal plasma factor VIII levels is unknown. It extends beyond von Willebrand factor serving as a "carrier" that stabilizes factor VIII coagulant protein in plasma. When a patient with von Willebrand's disease is transfused with a normal plasma concentrate containing both factor VIII and von Willebrand factor (cryoprecipitate), the factor VIII level may continue to rise for 24 to 36 hours after the transfusion (Fig. 26-2). This reflects release into plasma (and possibly new synthesis) of factor VIII, since the intravascular half-life of the factor VIII transfused in the cryoprecipitate is only 10 hours. Moreover, the intravascular half-life of the transfused von Willebrand factor is only 18 hours. Thus, on the day after the infusion, the plasma factor VIII concentration exceeds that accountable simply by its binding to an increased plasma concentration of von Willebrand factor.

Clinical Tests for von Willebrand Factor

The *concentration of von Willebrand protein (antigen)* in plasma is measured by electroimmunoassay, a technique in which a plasma sample is subjected to electrophoresis through agarose containing

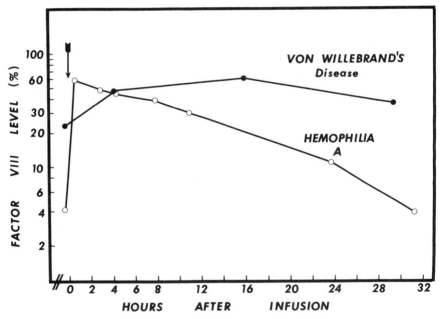

Fig. 26-2. Logarithmic plot of factor VIII levels against time after infusion showing the continuing rise in factor VIII level in a patient with von Willebrand's disease infused with cryoprecipitate and the rapid loss of factor VIII activity in a patient with hemophilia A infused with a factor VIII concentrate.

anti-von Willebrand factor antiserum. The height of the rocket obtained reflects total plasma von Willebrand factor concentration independent of its multimeric composition (Fig. 26-3).

The *multimeric composition* of von Willebrand factor in plasma is usually assessed in the clinical laboratory by crossed immunoelectrophoresis, a technique combining electrophoresis and electroimmunoassay. An arc is obtained (Fig. 26-4) whose shape reflects the proportion of multimers of different sizes in the plasma. A more sensitive method for analyzing multimers, in which plasma is subjected to large-pore agarose gel electrophoresis, is as yet available only in a few laboratories. The multimers move different distances into the gel, depending on their size. They are visualized as a series of bands by reacting the gel with purified radiolabeled anti-von Wil-

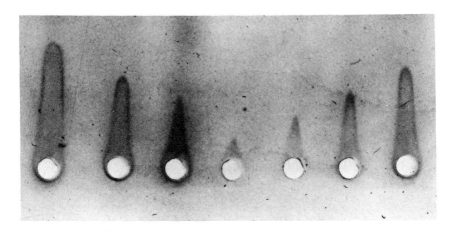

H   HC   VWD   N/8   N/4   N/2   N

Fig. 26-3. Rockets obtained by electroimmunoassay of plasma in agarose containing anti-von Willebrand factor antiserum. The height of each rocket is proportional to the concentration of von Willebrand factor in the test sample added to the well. Looking from right to left, one sees the rocket heights obtained with decreasing concentrations of a normal pooled plasma standard: N, 100%; N/2, 50%; N/4, 25%; N/8, 12.5%. The remaining wells contain test samples as follows:

    vWD—a patient with type I von Willebrand's disease with a vWF antigen of 50% (and a factor VIII coagulant activity of 56%).

    HC—a carrier for hemophilia A with a vWF antigen of 90% (and a factor VIII coagulant activity of 24%).

    H—a patient with hemophilia A with an unusually high vWF antigen of 200% (and a factor VIII coagulant activity of 6%).

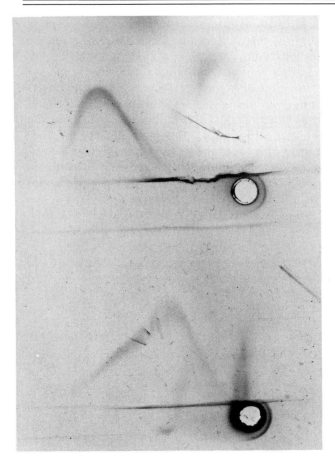

Fig. 26-4. Crossed immunoelectrophoresis of normal pooled plasma (bottom arc) and plasma from a patient with type IIa von Willebrand's disease (top arc). Note that the arc of the type IIa plasma has moved further from the well than the arc of normal plasma, which contains larger, slower moving forms not present in the type IIa plasma.

lebrand factor antibody and subjecting the gel to autoradiography (Fig. 26-5).

An in vitro test is not available to measure the *functional activity* of the largest multimers of von Willebrand factor, that is, the multimers required for normal platelet adhesion to subendothelium. One can only use the bleeding time. If a therapeutic procedure shortens the bleeding time of a patient with von Willebrand's disease, one assumes that it has increased the plasma concentration of the largest multimers.

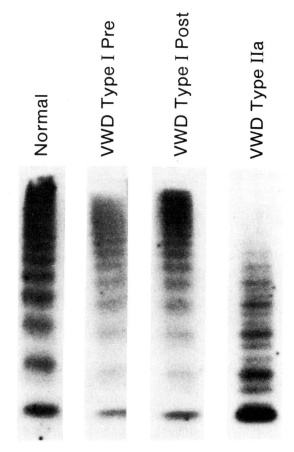

Fig. 26-5. Radioautographs prepared after SDS agarose gel electrophoresis of plasma and reaction of the gels with a radioactive antibody against von Willebrand factor. The degree of penetration of von Willebrand factor into the gel is a function of its multimer size. Thus, material at the top of the gel represents the largest multimers, and material at the bottom of the gel represents the smallest multimers. From left to right are shown a normal gel, gels from a patient with type I von Willebrand's disease before and after administration of DDAVP, and a gel from a patient with type IIa von Willebrand's disease. Note that the patient with type I von Willebrand's disease has a reduced staining of all the multimers, with an increase in predominantly large forms shortly after the administration of DDAVP. The patient with type IIa disease has a reduced amount of the large multimers but a normal to increased amount of the smaller multimers.

Adding ristocetin (a material originally developed as an antibiotic but abandoned for that purpose when it was discovered to induce thrombocytopenia) to platelet-rich plasma agglutinates the platelets in a reaction requiring the participation of the *intermediate-sized* multimers of von Willebrand factor. This test, *ristocetin-induced platelet agglutination*, is used as a screening test for von Willebrand's disease. A semi-quantitative test, *the ristocetin cofactor assay*, has also been developed. In this test, one compares the rate of ristocetin-induced agglutination of washed normal platelets obtained with dilutions of a patient's plasma and dilutions of a standard reference plasma.

Clinical Manifestations of Types I and II von Willebrand's Disease

These forms of von Willebrand's disease cause relatively mild bleeding in most patients—frequent, prolonged nosebleeds during childhood, increased menstrual bleeding, and excessive bleeding from small cuts and after dental extractions or other surgery. Massive tissue bleeding or joint hemorrhages do not occur. Occasional affected individuals discovered in family studies deny excessive bleeding. In contrast, a rare older patient may experience repeated, severe gastrointestinal hemorrhages due to a combination of von Willebrand's disease and malformations of small blood vessels in the intestinal mucosa called angiodysplasia. (The angiodysplasia could possibly result from an impaired ability of endothelial cells to secrete von Willebrand factor into vascular subendothelial matrix.)

Since the type I and type II variants of von Willebrand's disease are autosomal dominant disorders, one parent of a patient should have the disorder and each sibling and child of a patient has a 50% chance of being affected. Therefore, when a patient is identified, other members of the family should be studied.

Laboratory Manifestations of Type I von Willebrand's Disease

The typical laboratory findings of type I disease are:

1. A prolonged bleeding time.
2. A slightly prolonged APTT due to a moderate depression of factor VIII coagulant activity.
3. A reduced rocket height of von Willebrand antigen on elec-

troimmunoassay (see Fig. 26-3) as evidence of a decreased total plasma concentration of von Willebrand factor.

4. Failure of agglutination of platelets in the patient's platelet-rich plasma by ristocetin at a concentration of 1.5 mg per mL (ristocetin-induced platelet agglutination) and a reduced ristocetin cofactor activity of the patient's plasma on quantitative assay.

In type I disease, the findings are *concordant*, that is, the antigen level, the ristocetin cofactor activity, and the factor VIII coagulant activity are all depressed to the same extent. This varies from about 15 to 60% of normal and determines the severity of a patient's bleeding tendency.

Laboratory Manifestations of Type IIa von Willebrand's Disease

A type IIa variant is suspected when one finds a relatively normal level of von Willebrand antigen on electroimmunoassay, yet platelets in the patient's platelet-rich plasma fail to agglutinate with 1.5 mg per mL ristocetin. The full pattern of laboratory findings is:

1. A long bleeding time, absence of ristocetin-induced platelet agglutination, and markedly reduced ristocetin cofactor activity on quantitative assay.
2. A normal to only modestly reduced concentration of von Willebrand antigen and of factor VIII coagulant activity.
3. An abnormal arc on crossed immunoelectrophoresis due to the absence of larger, slower moving multimers (see Fig. 26-4).

Multimeric analysis of plasma von Willebrand factor by agarose gel electrophoresis (see Fig. 26-5) discloses a deficiency both of large multimers—which accounts for the prolonged bleeding time—and of intermediate multimers—which accounts for the failure of ristocetin-induced agglutination. In contrast, the smaller multimers are increased in concentration, which explains why total antigen and factor VIII coagulant activity are normal or only modestly reduced.

When the *von Willebrand factor in the platelets* of patients with the type IIa variant is subjected to multimeric analysis, a pattern similar to that of plasma von Willebrand factor is found. The multimeric composition of platelet von Willebrand factor reflects the multimeric composition of von Willebrand factor synthesized, not only by megakaryocytes, but also by endothelial cells. Therefore, the finding of reduced large and intermediate multimers in the platelets is taken as evidence that the type IIa variant stems from an inability of endothelial cells to synthesize large and intermediate-sized multimers.

Laboratory Manifestations of Type IIb von Willebrand's Disease

A paradoxically *increased* sensitivity to ristocetin-induced agglutination characterizes the type IIb variant. Whereas a 1.5 mg per mL ristocetin concentration agglutinates platelets in normal platelet-rich plasma, a ristocetin concentration of only 0.5 mg per mL agglutinates platelets in type IIb platelet-rich plasma. Other findings are a long bleeding time, a normal to modestly reduced concentration of von Willebrand antigen and factor VIII coagulant activity, and an arc indicating absence of larger, slower moving multimers on crossed immunoelectrophoresis.

Multimeric analysis reveals that the largest multimers are missing from the plasma, whereas the intermediate multimers appear to be increased. The latter apparently accounts for the ability of a lower concentration of ristocetin to agglutinate the platelets. *Platelet von Willebrand factor has a normal multimeric composition.* Apparently, therefore, endothelial cells release large multimers into the plasma, but the multimers are abnormal in some way that causes their rapid disappearance.

Pseudo-von Willebrand's Disease

The laboratory findings of pseudo-von Willebrand's disease resemble those of type IIb von Willebrand's disease. It can be distinguished from type IIb von Willebrand's disease in that adding large multimers of normal von Willebrand factor (as cryoprecipitate) to the patient's platelet-rich plasma causes platelet agglutination in the absence of ristocetin. This abnormal response reflects an abnormal affinity of the platelets for the large multimers of von Willebrand factor.

Patients with pseudo-von Willebrand's disease have episodes of mild to moderate thrombocytopenia. These are thought to stem from increased release of von Willebrand factor from endothelial cells during an acute phase reaction or after endothelial cell injury, with resultant aggregation and accelerated removal of platelets.

Thrombocytopenia has also been reported recently in patients with type IIb von Willebrand's disease given DDAVP. The plasma obtained after giving DDAVP contains material—presumably, abnormal large multimers of von Willebrand factor released from endothelial stores—which can induce aggregation in normal, platelet-rich plasma. Thus, stimulation of endothelial cell release of von Willebrand factor may cause thrombocytopenia in both pseudo-von Willebrand's disease and in type IIb von Willebrand's disease but for different reasons:

1. In pseudo-von Willebrand's disease because newly released *normal large multimers* of von Willebrand factor bind to the patient's *abnormal platelets*.
2. In type IIb von Willebrand's disease because newly released *abnormal large multimers* of von Willebrand factor bind to the patient's *normal platelets*.

Type III von Willebrand's Disease

These rare patients have essentially no measurable plasma von Willebrand antigen or ristocetin cofactor activity and a markedly reduced factor VIII coagulant activity (1% to 3% of normal). They experience serious episodes of mucous membrane bleeding and also skeletal bleeding and joint hemorrhages similar to those of patients with severe hemophilia (see Chapter 27).

Parents of type III patients have no excessive bleeding and normal bleeding times and factor VIII levels. Von Willebrand antigen and ristocetin cofactor activity may be either normal or moderately depressed. Thus, affected offspring are homozygotes (or double heterozygotes) for a recessive genetic defect (or defects), which, unlike the genetic defects causing types I and II von Willebrand disease, produce no clinical disease in the heterozygote.

Treatment of von Willebrand's Disease

One may increase plasma von Willebrand factor levels by:

1. Infusion of DDAVP which, through release of endothelial stores of von Willebrand factor, causes a rise in the plasma level of both von Willebrand factor and factor VIII that persists for several hours. Since an initial infusion depletes the stores, 24 to 48 hours must elapse before a second infusion will produce a comparable second effect. Although an important therapeutic agent for the more common type I von Willebrand's disease, DDAVP is useless in type II disorders and, by causing thrombocytopenia, may be harmful in the type IIb variant and in pseudo-

von Willebrand's disease. Therefore, one must know what type of von Willebrand's disease a patient has before giving DDAVP.

2. Replacement therapy with the single donor plasma concentrate, cryoprecipitate. Lyophilized factor VIII concentrate should not be used, both because of the risk of transmitting infection (see Chapter 27) and because different lots vary widely in their content of the large multimers of von Willebrand factor.

In a type I patient, an initial infusion of DDAVP, combined with the use of the anti-fibrinolytic agent EACA (epsilon aminocaproic acid), may suffice to allow a patient to undergo minor surgery, for example, dental surgery, without the need for replacement therapy with plasma products. If late bleeding occurs, a second infusion may be given.

Major surgery requires replacement therapy with cryoprecipitate, which may be needed over a 7- to 10-day period. Initial dosage is often selected empirically, for example, 10 bags every 12 hours, because in some patients, the bleeding time fails to shorten substantially, even though sufficient cryoprecipitate has been given to prevent excessive bleeding from the operative site. (The reason for this is unknown.) Subsequent dosage is guided by the patient's clinical response.

Distinguishing von Willebrand's Disease From Hemophilia A

Some patients with von Willebrand's disease may have a prolonged bleeding time on one examination and a borderline or even a normal bleeding time on another examination. Therefore, when a patient under investigation for a possible hereditary bleeding disorder is found to have a factor VIII coagulant activity in the 25% to 50% range and a bleeding time at the upper limit of the normal range, one must consider the following diagnostic possibilities:

1. von Willebrand's disease.
2. Mild hemophilia A, if the patient is a male.
3. The carrier state for hemophilia A, if the patient is a female.

Since a carrier for hemophilia A may bear sons with a bleeding disorder much more disabling than von Willebrand's disease, it is particularly important to distinguish between von Willebrand's disease and the carrier state. Measuring von Willebrand antigen by electroimmunoassay usually accomplishes this. A woman with the common type I form of von Willebrand's disease should have proportionately reduced levels of von Willebrand antigen and factor VIII coagulant activity, whereas a hemophilia A carrier should have a substantially higher level of von Willebrand antigen than of factor VIII coagulant activity (see Fig. 26-3).

ACQUIRED DISORDERS CAUSING DEFECTIVE PLATELET FUNCTION

Although relatively common, impaired formation of hemostatic plugs is often overlooked as an acquired cause for abnormal bleeding when the platelet count is normal. This is because the physician often checks only the platelet count and the screening tests of blood coagulation (prothrombin time, APTT). Unless the bleeding time is also measured, the patient whose platelet count is normal, but who, nevertheless, cannot form hemostatic plugs normally, will be missed.

Mechanisms disturbing formation of hemostatic plugs and the disorders in which they occur are summarized in Table 26-3.

Table 26-3. Mechanisms Impairing Platelet Function in Acquired Nonthrombocytopenic States with Long Bleeding Times

MECHANISM	STATE
Abnormal thrombopoiesis producing platelet membrane and enzymatic defects	Myeloproliferative and myelodysplastic disorders
Platelet damage induced by:	
Antibodies	ITP-related syndromes, SLE*
Mechanical events	Cardiopulmonary bypass
Coating of platelets by:	
Abnormal proteins	Macroglobulinemia, multiple myeloma
Drugs	Penicillin, cephalosporin, dextran
Adding platelet cyclooxygenase deficiency to an existing hemostatic abnormality	Giving aspirin to a patient with a platelet functional defect or a blood coagulation abnormality
Binding of FDP to GP IIb-IIIa fibrinogen receptor	Extensive fibrinolysis
Retention of unknown plasma materials	Uremia
Antibodies against plasma von Willebrand factor	Acquired von Willebrand's disease

*Abbreviations are SLE, systemic lupus erythematosus; FDP, fibrin degradation products.

Myeloproliferative and Myelodysplastic Disorders

Patients with myelofibrosis, polycythemia vera, or essential thrombocythemia frequently have prolonged bleeding times and may bruise and bleed excessively. They may also have an increased tendency for thrombosis. Those patients with very high platelet counts (over 1,000,000 per μL) have the highest risk for both bleeding and thrombosis. Reducing the platelet count with chemotherapy decreases but does not eliminate these risks, because qualitative platelet abnormalities may persist. These include:

1. Loss of platelet surface membrane alpha adrenergic receptors. (As a result, the platelets fail to aggregate with epinephrine, a finding that helps to distinguish the high platelet count of essential thrombocythemia from the high platelet count of a reactive thrombocytosis.)
2. Loss of platelet surface membrane receptors for PGD_2, a minor product of platelet arachidonic acid oxidation by the cyclooxygenase pathway that inhibits platelet aggregation (see Chapter 23).
3. Impaired oxidation of arachidonic acid by the lipoxygenase pathway with resultant impaired formation of 12-HETE.
4. An abnormality of dense granules that causes depletion of dense granule ADP as the platelet circulates.

Absence of the large multimers of plasma von Willebrand factor has also recently been reported in several patients with myeloproliferative disorders. The mechanism is not established, but one suspects that it reflects increased binding of plasma von Willebrand factor to an abnormal platelet surface membrane. To what extent each of the above abnormalities may contribute to a patient's bleeding or thrombotic tendency is not clear.

Platelet dysfunction is sometimes found in patients with myelodysplastic syndromes (see Chapter 11). In a rare patient, isolated platelet dysfunction, causing a prolonged bleedig time and excessive bruising, precedes by many months the development of acute non-lymphocytic leukemia.

Antibody-Mediated Platelet Damage

Autoantibodies causing ITP sometimes also impair the function of the platelets remaining in the circulation. One suspects this possibility when the bruising or mucosal bleeding of a patient with ITP appears excessive and the bleeding time appears disproportionately lengthened for the level of the platelet count. A rare patient may develop acquired thrombasthenia—with laboratory findings indistinguishable from Glanzmann's disease—due to an autoantibody against the GP IIb-IIIa complex that impairs its function but does not induce thrombocytopenia.

Some patients with the lupus anticoagulant (see Chapter 27) also have a prolonged bleeding time, a normal to minimally reduced platelet count, and platelet aggregation tests suggestive of depleted storage pool ADP. They are thought to have an antibody that can activate platelets with resultant secretion of granule contents. Whether this same antibody also causes the lupus anticoagulant phenomenon in this subset of patients is not clear.

Cardiopulmonary Bypass

Platelets may be activated and release their granule contents as blood circulates through a pump oxygenator during cardiac surgery. Platelet dysfunction leading to excessive intraoperative or postoperative bleeding may result. The bleeding time is prolonged disproportionately to the platelet count, which is usually moderately reduced but occasionally normal. Therefore, regardless of the platelet count, the patient should continue to receive platelet concentrates until excessive bleeding ceases. A patient should not be given aspirin for several days before cardiac surgery, because aspirin worsens bleeding due to platelet dysfunction after cardiopulmonary bypass.

Macroglobulinemia and Multiple Myeloma

A patient with a high concentration of plasma IgM due to macroglobulinemia of Waldenström will have a long bleeding time and may experience mucosal bleeding (nosebleeds, rectal bleeding, gross hematuria). This stems from a combination of hyperviscosity and platelet dysfunction. The IgM coats the platelets, interfering with platelet aggregation induced in vitro by a variety of aggregating agents. Lowering the IgM concentration by plasmaphoresis corrects the abnormal bleeding tendency.

Coating of platelets with plasma IgG or IgA may contribute to a bleeding tendency in multiple myeloma, as may hyperviscosity, particularly in the patient with IgA myeloma (because plasma IgA tends to polymerize). Thrombocytopenia and interference by a myeloma protein with fibrin polymerization are other causes for bleeding in multiple myeloma.

Drug-Induced Platelet Dysfunction

As discussed in Chapter 23, aspirin slightly prolongs the bleeding time of most normal individuals. However, aspirin may strikingly prolong the bleeding time of a thrombocytopenic patient, of a patient who has platelet dysfunction from another cause, or of a patient with a blood coagulation disorder that severely impairs the generation of thrombin. Its use must be avoided in such patients.

Carbenicillin and other penicillins given in large doses bind to the platelet surface membrane and interfere with the binding of von Willebrand factor and of platelet activating agents (for example, ADP, epinephrine) to platelet surface receptors. Patients with renal failure are particularly prone to develop penicillin-induced platelet dysfunction because of high blood levels that may result from impaired renal excretion. Penicillin-induced platelet dysfunction also enhances the risk of bleeding in thrombocytopenic patients with marrow aplasia or acute leukemia, who frequently must be given large doses of penicillin derivatives to combat life-threatening infection.

Some of the newer cephalosporin-related antibiotics also induce platelet dysfunction, presumably by a mechanism similar to that for penicillin-induced platelet dysfunction. Dextran is another drug that can coat the platelet surface, and patients given large amounts of dextran may develop a bleeding tendency associated with a prolonged bleeding time.

Platelet Dysfunction Due to Fibrin Degradation Products

Fibrinolysis induced therapeutically with streptokinase or urokinase (see Chapter 29) or after extensive disseminated intravascular coagulation may cause fibrin degradation products to accumulate in high concentration in the plasma. They can then apparently compete with fibrinogen for the GP IIb-IIIa binding site to which fibrinogen must bind for normal platelet cohesion. The resultant impaired formation of hemostatic plugs contributes to fibrinolytic bleeding.

Uremia

A uremic patient may bleed abnormally, particularly after a surgical or invasive diagnostic procedure. The bleeding time is prolonged out of proportion to the platelet count, which is usually normal or only minimally depressed. Vigorous hemodialysis or peritoneal dialysis temporarily shortens the bleeding time, which suggests that accumulation of a waste substance in plasma interferes with platelet function and impairs formation of hemostatic plugs. Plasma von Willebrand factor concentration is high in uremic patients. Therefore, it is puzzling that maneuvers increasing plasma von Willebrand factor concentration—infusion of cryoprecipitate and administration of DDAVP—have recently been shown to shorten the bleeding time of uremic patients and may have a place in the management of uremic bleeding.

Acquired von Willebrand's Disease

A rare patient with previously normal hemostatic function may develop findings of von Willebrand's disease—mucosal and postoperative bleeding, a prolonged bleeding time, and reduced plasma concentration of von Willebrand antigen, ristocetin cofactor activity, and factor VIII coagulant activity. Most such patients have had an underlying disorder that disturbs immune function—macroglobulinemia of Waldenström, other lymphomas, or systemic lupus erythematosus. In some but not all patients, adding the immunoglobulin fraction of the patient's plasma to normal plasma neutralizes the ristocetin cofactor activity of the normal plasma. This is considered evidence of an antibody in the patient's plasma against von Willebrand factor.

As mentioned, a selective decrease of the large multimers of plasma von Willebrand factor has recently been reported in several patients with myeloproliferative disorders.

SELECTED READING

1. Bellucci S, Tobelem G, and Caen JP: Inherited platelet disorders. In Brown EB (ed): Progress in Hematology. Vol. 13, New York, Grune & Stratton, 1983, pp. 223.
2. George JN, Nurden AT, and Phillips DR: Molecular defects in interactions of platelets with the vessel wall. N Engl J Med 311:1084, 1984.
3. Handin RI, Martin V, and Moloney WC: Antibody-induced von Willebrand's disease: a newly defined inhibitor syndrome. Blood 48:393, 1976.
4. Janson PA, Jubelirer SJ, Weinstein MJ, and Deykin D: Treatment of the bleeding tendency in uremia with cryoprecipitate. N Engl J Med 303: 1318, 1980.

5. Rao AK, and Holmsen H: Congenital disorders of platelet function. Semin Hematol 23:102, 1986.
6. Weiss HJ, Meyer D, Rabinowitz R, Pietu G, Girma J-P, Vicic WJ, and Rogers J: Pseudo-von Willebrand's disease: an intrinsic platelet defect with aggregation by unmodified human factor VIII/ von Willebrand factor and enhanced adsorption of its high molecular weight multimers. N Engl J Med 306:326, 1982.
7. Zimmerman TS, and Ruggeri ZM: Von Willebrand's disease. Clin Haematol 12:175, 1983.

27

Genetic Clotting Factor Disorders

Specific hereditary deficiency states have been identified for each of the plasma hemostatic factors. Each causes abnormal bleeding except:

1. Factor XII, high molecular weight kininogen, and prekallikrein deficiency, which prolong the clotting time of blood in a glass tube but do not impair coagulation in vivo.
2. Protein C deficiency, protein S deficiency, certain of the dysfibrinogenemias, and antithrombin III deficiency, which are thrombotic disorders (see Chapter 29).

As apparent from the discussion of von Willebrand's disease in Chapter 26, hereditary clotting factor disorders stem from two types of genetic defects:

1. Mutations diminishing the synthesis of a clotting factor, with resultant equally reduced levels of the functional activity of a clotting factor and of its plasma concentration measured as antigen.
2. Mutations resulting in synthesis of an abnormal clotting protein, with resultant greater reduction of the functional activity of the clotting factor than of its plasma concentration measured as antigen (which need not be reduced at all).

With some notable exceptions—von Willebrand's disease, protein C deficiency, protein S deficiency, the dysfibrinogenemias, antithrom-

527

bin III deficiency—a patient with one abnormal gene for a clotting factor and one normal gene for that clotting factor will be aysmptomatic. Therefore, the prevalence of symptomatic disease for most hereditary clotting factor disorders whose genes are located on autosomal chromosomes is very low. However, if, as in the hemophilias, a gene is located on the X chromosome (sex-linked), then a male, who has only one X chromosome, will develop clinically significant disease if he receives a single abnormal gene from his mother. This explains why hemophilia A and hemophilia B are the most common of the serious hereditary bleeding disorders but are essentially confined to males. The reported incidence of hemophilia A is 1 in 10,000 males.

HEMOPHILIA A AND HEMOPHILIA B

Hemophilia A (factor VIII deficiency) and hemophilia B (factor IX deficiency) have the same clinical and genetic findings and cause the same abnormalities in screening tests. One measures factor VIII and factor IX clotting activity in specific assays to distinguish the two disorders. This is necessary since bleeding is frequently treated with plasma concentrates that contain either factor VIII or factor IX, but not both. About 85% of hemophilic patients will have factor VIII deficiency and about 15% will have factor IX deficiency.

Genetic Manifestations

The transmission of hemophilia is illustrated in the genetic diagrams of Figure 27-1 and may be summarized as follows:

1. If a hemophilic male marries a normal woman,
   a. All daughters are obligatory carriers.
   b. All sons are normal.
2. If a normal male marries a carrier,
   a. Each son has a 50% chance of having hemophilia.
   b. Each daughter has a 50% chance of being a carrier.

About two thirds of patients will have a positive family history. When a new hemophilic patient is discovered, the following family members deserve study for the possibility of hemophilia: male siblings, sons of female siblings, the mother's brothers, the mother's sisters' sons.

The severity of hemophilia runs true in families. Affected members will have either severe hemophilia, with factor VIII or IX clotting

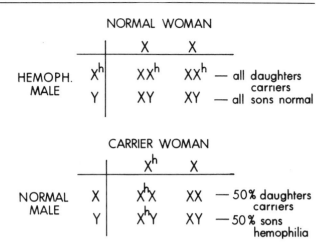

Fig. 27-1. Genetic transmission of hemophilia.

activity below 1% of normal, moderately severe hemophilia, with activity between 1% and 5% of normal, or mild hemophilia, with activity between about 5% and 30% of normal. This reflects the existence of different abnormal alleles capable of supporting different levels of factor VIII or factor IX activity.

In about 90% of patients with hemophilia A, factor VIII antigen and factor VIII coagulant activity are equivalently reduced. The remaining 10% have a higher level of antigen than of activity, that is, have immunologic evidence of an abnormal circulating factor VIII molecule. Unlike von Willebrand factor, factor VIII antigen cannot be demonstrated in plasma as a rocket on electroimmunoassay. It is usually measured in an immunoradiometric assay based upon the extent of binding of a purified human anti-factor VIII antibody to factor VIII antigen in the patient's plasma. (This test is called the VIII:Cag assay, the term "Cag" standing for coagulant antigen.)

In hemophilia B, about one third of patients have evidence of a circulating abnormal factor IX molecule, that is, of a higher concentration of factor IX antigen (usually measured by electroimmunoassay). Several different variant factor IX molecules have now been purified from the plasma of such patients and the abnormalities responsible for their defective function have been characterized at the molecular level.

Although immunologic studies provide insight into genetic mechanisms, the severity of a hemophilic patient's bleeding is independent of whether clotting factor activity is depressed because a molecule is absent or because a molecule is abnormal. The severity of bleeding depends upon the level of residual clotting factor activity.

Clinical Manifestations

In *severe hemophilia*, the patient bleeds repeatedly throughout his lifetime, particularly into joints and muscles but potentially into any organ or tissue. For an unknown reason, since neither factor VIII nor factor IX crosses the placental barrier, the infant is usually born without large bruises or a cephalohematoma, and bleeding from the umbilical stump is rare. If the mother is a known or possible carrier, a sample of cord blood should be drawn for factor VIII or IX assay; puncturing the infant's femoral or external jugular vein later to obtain blood for assay may trigger disastrous hemorrhage. Circumcision should be avoided.

A hemophilic infant should be given hepatitis B vaccine to protect against at least this type of transfusion-transmitted hepatitis. In three quarters of severely affected infants, the first major bleeding episode will occur before the age of 18 months. Bleeding into the base of the tongue or tissues of the neck is of particular concern because of the risk of airway compression and suffocation. Until plasma concentrates became available, the child frequently grew into adult life with crippling deformities secondary to major musculoskeletal hemorrhages (atrophied muscles, shortened tendons, fixed joints). Intracranial bleeding is an ever-present danger, and prophylactic replacement therapy is indicated after even a trivial blow to the head.

In *mild hemophilia*, the patient may be aware of easy bruising and of moderately excessive bleeding after trauma but often has little difficulty in daily living. Crippling musculoskeletal deformities are rare. Nevertheless, the patient will usually bleed seriously after surgery or dental extractions unless given prophylactic therapy.

Laboratory Manifestations

SCREENING TESTS

In hemophilia, one finds that:

1. *The activated partial thromboplastin time (APTT) is prolonged* because the sequence of clotting reactions triggered in vitro by contact activation of plasma requires both factor VIII and factor IX to activate factor X (see Fig. 24-1). Mixing equal parts of the patient's plasma with normal plasma shortens the APTT almost to normal because the prolongation stems from a clotting factor

deficiency and not from an inhibitor that can neutralize the factor VIII or factor IX activity of normal plasma.

2. *Other screening tests are normal:*

   a. The bleeding time, because hemostatic plugs can form adequately.

   b. The prothrombin time, because the high concentration of tissue factor used in this test results in direct tissue factor-factor VII activation of factor X, which bypasses the need for factors VIII and IX (see Fig. 24-1).

   c. The thrombin time, because the thrombin-fibrinogen reaction is normal.

DIAGNOSTIC TESTS

Quantitative assays for factors VIII and IX establish the type and severity of the hemophilia. These assays are based on the ability of a dilution of the patient's plasma to correct the prolonged APTT of known hemophilia A and hemophilia B plasmas.

If factor IX is the deficient factor, no further tests are needed. If factor VIII is the deficient factor, one often also measures the plasma level of von Willebrand antigen by electroimmunoassay to rule out any possibility of von Willebrand's disease. This is particularly important if the patient is a mild hemophilic with a factor VIII level in the 15% to 30% range, since such values can occasionally be found in type I von Willebrand's disease. However, measuring the plasma level of von Willebrand antigen is unnecessary if an unequivocal family history of sex-linked transmission has been obtained.

About 15% of patients with hemophilia A develop factor VIII inhibitors, which are antibodies that arise after the transfusion of factor VIII. This serious complication is suspected when mixing equal parts of the patient's plasma and normal plasma fails to shorten the prolonged APTT appropriately. If an inhibitor is of low titer, a more sensitive screening test—involving incubating a 4:1 mixture of the patient's and normal plasma—may be necessary to detect its presence.

Management

USE OF PLASMA PRODUCTS IN SEVERE HEMOPHILIA

The patient with severe hemophilia receives plasma products to prevent or control episodes of bleeding throughout his lifetime. The factor VIII or IX level must be raised transiently to about 30% to protect against bleeding after minor surgery, such as dental extraction, or to abort a beginning joint hemorrhage. If major joint or intramuscular bleeding is already evident, the plasma activity is raised to about 50% and often kept in the 25% to 50% range for several days. Before major surgery in hemophilia A, the plasma level of factor VIII is usually raised to 100%, and this normal peak level, with a trough level of about 50%, is maintained for 7 to 10 days after the surgery. Because of the risk of thrombosis after repeatedly giving large amounts of factor IX concentrate (see below), major surgery in hemophilia B is carried out with a peak factor IX level of about 60% and a trough level that is allowed to fall to about 30%.

Since factor VIII has a biologic intravascular half-life of about 10 hours and factor IX has a biologic intravascular half-life of about 24 hours, such therapeutic goals are unachievable without the use of plasma fractions enriched in factor VIII or factor IX.

Therapeutic Preparations. Two factor VIII preparations are available:

1. *Cryoprecipitate.* When plasma is thawed slowly, factor VIII, von Willebrand factor, fibrinogen, and factor XIII remain in the last crystals of ice to dissolve. By a simple closed-bag technique of removing the thawed plasma before the last ice crystals dissolve, one can prepare single-donor bags of cryoprecipitate for clinical use. These are stored frozen and their contents are dissolved in about 10 ml of saline just before use. Although the factor VIII content of an individual bag is unknown, each bag is assumed to contain 80 factor VIII units. (One factor VIII unit is the amount of factor VIII in 1 mL of normal plasma.)

2. *Commercial, lyophilized factor VIII concentrates.* These concentrates are prepared in lots made by pooling the plasma of 2000 to 5000 donors. The lyophilized powder is packaged in bottles supplying 250 to 1000 factor VIII units. It is dissolved in 10 to 100 mL of a sterile diluent just before use. Preparations are now heat-treated to reduce the risk of transmitting hepatitis and AIDS.

Factor IX concentrate is available as a lyophilized "prothrombin complex concentrate" that contains, not only factor IX, but all of the vitamin K-dependent clotting factors. Like lyophilized factor VIII concentrate, it is prepared from large plasma pools and is heat treated to reduce the risk of transmitting hepatitis and AIDS.

Dosage. One calculates the factor VIII units required to obtain a desired plasma concentration from knowing that the infusion of one unit of factor VIII per kg of body weight will increase plasma factor VIII concentration by 2 percentage points. Thus, to raise to 50% the factor VIII level of a severely affected adult patient who has less than 1% factor VIII and who weighs 70 kg, one would infuse:

$$50 \times 70/2 = 1750 \text{ units}$$

This would require 22 bags of cryoprecipitate ($80 \times 22 = 1760$ units). The number of vials of concentrate would be calculated from the number of units listed on the label, rounded off, if necessary, to the nearest number of vials exceeding the calculated dose. One half of the initial units of factor VIII infused would be given again every 8 to 12 hours to maintain the factor VIII level between the peak level selected and a trough level that is half of the peak level.

The factor IX units needed to achieve a given plasma factor IX concentrate is calculated similarly except that one does not divide the body weight in kg by two. This is because only one half of the factor IX units listed on the label are recovered in the patient's plasma. (Endothelium has been recently shown to possess binding sites for factor IX and the need to saturate such binding sites may account for this phenomenon.)

Factor IX concentrates contain variable amounts of activated clotting factors, and patients receiving large repeated doses of factor IX concentrate may develop laboratory evidence of intravascular coagulation. Occasional patients have developed venous thrombosis, pulmonary embolism, and even, rarely, myocardial infarction. Therefore, many physicians add 5 to 10 units of heparin to each mL of reconstituted concentrate. Moreover, if a patient must receive replacement therapy for a number of days after a surgical procedure, some physicians increase the amount of heparin to 20 U per mL of reconstituted concentrate and will also reduce the amount of concentrate used by giving the patient fresh frozen plasma as a supplemental source of factor IX.

USE OF PLASMA PRODUCTS IN MILD HEMOPHILIA

Patients with mild hemophilia usually need replacement therapy only after trauma or to prevent postoperative bleeding. Since the lifetime exposure of patients with mild hemophilia to plasma products may be limited, lyophilized concentrates made from large plasma pools are avoided to minimize the risk of transmitting hepatitis and AIDS. Cryoprecipitate should be used in hemophilia A and, if at all possible, only whole plasma in hemophilia B.

Moreover, the intravenous infusion of DDAVP (0.3 µg per kg) may obviate or reduce the need for cryoprecipitate in mild hemophilia A. In a patient whose baseline factor VIII concentration is between

10% and 20%, the factor VIII level may rise to between 40% and 80% shortly after the injection. If the baseline factor VIII level is in the 5% to 10% range, it may rise to between 15% and 25% following DDAVP. Levels fall back to baseline over about 12 hours, and 24 to 48 hours must elapse before a second injection will produce a comparable rise. (Unfortunately, DDAVP does not cause factor VIII levels to rise in patients with severe hemophilia A.)

THE PROBLEM OF AIDS

Over 75% of patients with hemophilia A treated with factor VIII concentrates in the United States before 1985 have serologic evidence of infection with HTLV-III. As of the spring of 1986, over 150 patients in the United States with hemophilia (most with hemophilia A but a few with hemophilia B) had developed AIDS, and the number will grow. Thus, a crisis exists in hemophilia care.

It is hoped that present methods of heat treatment of factor VIII and factor IX concentrates will reduce, if not eliminate, the risk of transmission of AIDS through the use of concentrates. Some early data have been encouraging, but there are reports of patients developing evidence of infection with HTLV-III after receiving only heat-treated factor VIII.

As this is written, it is recommended that adult patients who have already received large amounts of lyophilized concentrate use heat-treated concentrate as replacement therapy. Infants and children newly discovered to have severe hemophilia A are being treated only with cryoprecipitate whenever possible. The author presently does not know which is safer—multiple bags of cryoprecipitate or heat-treated factor VIII concentrate—for an adult patient who has not received large amounts of plasma products previously and in whom a need for replacement therapy over a number of days arises after severe trauma or nonelective surgery. Physicians in the United States who treat hemophilia should remain current with recommendations for management provided by the National Hemophilia Foundation and other authoritative sources. A solution to the problem through the availability of factor VIII prepared by recombinant DNA technology seems to be a number of years away.

ANTIFIBRINOLYTIC THERAPY

In some circumstances, the use of an antifibrinolytic agent can reduce the need for replacement therapy. Dental extractions are frequently carried out under cover either of an infusion of a plasma preparation (severe hemophilia A) or the adminstration of DDAVP (mild hemophilia A), followed by the use of an antifibrinolytic agent, for example, epsilon aminocaproic acid (EACA), 2.5 to 4.0 grams four times daily for 1 week. Suppressing fibrinolysis impedes lysis of the initial clot formed after raising the plasma factor VIII level. If the clot holds, then further measures to maintain an elevated plasma factor VIII concentration will not be needed. However, when a patient with hemophilia B is given factor IX concentrate prior to dental extraction, one should be cautious and wait at least 10 hours before giving EACA to allow time for clearance of activated clotting factors infused in the concentrate.

Adminstering EACA also helps in managing other causes of bleeding from the oropharynx or gastrointestinal tract. In contrast, EACA may be harmful in hematuria of renal origin because ureteral clots resistant to lysis may form with resultant acute hydronephrosis. It is also usually avoided in musculoskeletal bleeding because impeding fibrinolysis could impair resolution of large tissue hematomas.

FACTOR VIII INHIBITORS

A factor VIII inhibitor is suspected when a given dose of concentrate fails to raise plasma factor VIII to the expected level. Its presence is confirmed by the in vitro mixing tests described earlier. Its potency, which is expressed in inhibitor units, is measured by assay techniques based upon determining the dilution of the patient's plasma that neutralizes a set amount of factor VIII under standardized incubation conditions.

When first discovered, an inhibitor may be present in low or high titer. In a few patients with a low titer inhibitor, the titer does not rise after infusing further factor VIII. However, in most patients, infused factor VIII acts as an immunogen. The factor VIII antibody titer rises sharply, beginning about the fourth day after the infusion and falls back to a low level only after many months. Therefore, in a patient with a low titer inhibitor, one attempts to manage mild or moderate musculoskeletal hemorrhages without giving factor VIII. If factor VIII must be used, it is given in a large dose calculated to overcome the low titer inhibitor and allow an initial clot to form. The rise in antibody titer that usually then follows precludes continued effective administration of factor VIII.

Therefore, if the initial clot does not hold or in the patient presenting with a high titer inhibitor, one must resort to other means to control bleeding. These include:

1. Administration of the prothrombin complex concentrates used for the treatment of hemophilia B. These concentrates contain variable amounts of an activated material or materials that bypasses the need for factor VIII during hemostasis in vivo.
2. Administration of prothrombin complex concentrates especially prepared to contain large amounts of activated material. (The extreme expense of these concentrates usually limits their use to truly life-threatening circumstances.)
3. Administration of porcine factor VIII. In contrast to its potency against human factor VIII, a factor VIII antibody may only minimally inhibit porcine factor VIII. A porcine factor VIII product, recently licensed for use in the United States, may well prove valuable in the management of factor VIII inhibitors.

Unlike hemophilia A, the development of an inhibitor in hemophilia B is an uncommon event.

OTHER POINTS IN MANAGEMENT

Patients with hemophilia should avoid drugs interfering with platelet function, particularly *aspirin*. Acetaminophen is used for analgesia. If this does not control chronic, disabling musculoskeletal pain and one must give one of the nonsteroidal anti-inflammatory agents that impair platelet arachidonic acid metabolism, ibuprofen may be the drug of choice. It reportedly does not prolong the hemophilic patient's bleeding time.

Any patient with a serious bleeding tendency who needs medications should receive them either orally or intravenously. Intramuscular injections are avoided because they can cause large, painful hematomas.

Detection of Carriers

The daughter of a hemophilic father is an obligatory carrier. The sister of a hemophilic or of a known carrier has an equal chance of being either a carrier or normal. Since factor VIII circulates in plasma complexed with von Willebrand factor, comparing the plasma factor VIII coagulant activity level with the plasma von Willebrand antigen level (see Fig. 26-3) will usually identify the carrier of hemophilia A. The ratio of factor VIII coagulant activity to von Willebrand antigen will cluster around 1.0 for normal women and around 0.5 for carriers. However, since inactivation of one X chromosome in the female during embryonic development is random, an occasional carrier will have inactivated primarily the abnormal X chromosome in the cells that produce factor VIII and so will have a factor VIII:von Willebrand antigen ratio that falls within the range for normal women.

In hemophilia B, one is limited to measuring factor IX coagulant activity. If it is below 50% of normal, the probability of a potential carrier being a true carrier exceeds 90%. If the level is 100% or more, a potential carrier has a high probability but no absolute guarantee of being normal.

One anticipates that molecular genetic techniques will become generally available within the foreseeable future that will allow the diagnosis of hemophilia A or B to be made in utero from analysis of the DNA of amniotic fluid cells.

FACTOR XI DEFICIENCY

Factor XI (PTA) deficiency is much less common than hemophilia and occurs most often (but not exclusively) in patients of Ashkenazic Jewish descent. The same screening test pattern is found as in hemophilia—an abnormal APTT with other screening tests being normal. The diagnosis is established by measuring factor XI activity in a quantitative assay.

Since factor XI deficiency is an autosomal recessive disorder, it affects both men and women. A sibling of the patient has a 25% chance of also having the disease. The children of the patient should be heterozygotes and free of clinically significant bleeding.

Factor XI deficiency is a milder bleeding disease than hemophilia. Musculoskeletal bleeding and joint hemorrhages do not occur. Postoperative bleeding may be troublesome but rarely life-threatening. For an unknown reason, occasional patients have not bled abnormally despite repeated hemostatic challenges, including surgery. However, one is never sure that such a patient will not bleed abnormally after the next surgical procedure. Bleeding is treated with fresh or frozen plasma and with supplemental EACA as described for hemophilia.

DEFICIENCIES OF OTHER CONTACT ACTIVATION FACTORS

Individuals with factor XII, prekallikrein, or high molecular weight kininogen deficiency are discovered accidentally, usually as a result of an APTT being performed prior to elective surgery. Again, the screening pattern is identical to that of the hemophilias and the diagnosis is established by specific assays. As mentioned earlier, a deficiency of factor XII, prekallikrein, or high molecular weight kininogen strikingly prolongs the clotting of plasma by the contact activation pathway in vitro but does not impair blood coagulation in vivo. All concerned should be reassured that the patient will not bleed abnormally. A high prevalence of partial deficiency of factor XII (30% to 50% of normal) has been noted in the United States in recent immigrants from southeast Asia.

DISORDERS PROLONGING THE PROTHROMBIN TIME

The disorders discussed so far in this chapter all have the coagulation screening test pattern of the hemophilias—a long APTT with a normal prothrombin time. Hereditary deficiencies of the other factors required for thrombin generation—factors VII, X, V, and prothrombin—prolong the prothrombin time. In factor VII deficiency, only the prothrombin time is prolonged (see Fig. 24-1), whereas in the other disorders, both the prothrombin time and the APTT are prolonged. A diagnosis is established by specific factor assays based upon the ability of a test plasma to correct the delayed clotting of plasma from a patient with an established deficiency of a specific factor.

A patient with *hereditary factor VII deficiency* may have a substantially depressed factor VII level, for example, 3% to 15% of normal, and experience only minimal or even no excessive bleeding. Such reduced levels may still provide enough factor VII molecules to react effectively with the limited number of tissue factor molecules to which the blood is usually exposed during a hemostatic challenge. In contrast, a patient with hereditary factor VII deficiency and plasma factor VII activity in the 1% of normal range may experience repeated serious episodes of bleeding or may die in infancy from fatal intracerebral hemorrhage. As discussed in Chapter 23, such patients establish the importance of the tissue factor pathway of blood coagulation for normal hemostasis.

Hereditary factor V deficiency is also a disorder of variable severity. Patients in whom both plasma and platelet factor V activity are markedly reduced have more severe bleeding than patients with markedly reduced plasma factor V but substantial amounts of residual platelet factor V activity. Moreover, a family with serious bleeding has been described in which affected members have very low platelet factor V levels but only moderately depressed plasma factor V activity. Thus, the extent of bleeding in hereditary disorders of factor V seems to depend primarily upon the amount of residual platelet factor V activity.

Patients with hereditary prothrombin deficiency or hereditary factor X deficiency usually experience serious episodes of bleeding.

DISORDERS OF FIBRINOGEN AND FIBRINOGEN STABILIZATION

Hereditary Afibrinogenemia

In this rare, autosomal recessive disorder, only traces of fibrinogen are present in the blood. The blood fails to clot in all coagulation screening tests; the bleeding time may also be prolonged because of insufficient fibrinogen in the plasma and in the platelet alpha granules to support platelet cohesion (see Chapter 23). Patients may have surprisingly little spontaneous bleeding but bleed heavily after surgery. Cryoprecipitate provides a ready source of fibrinogen for replacement therapy. In some patients, antibodies to fibrinogen are formed after replacement therapy. These may cause serious reactions after subsequent replacement therapy due to the intravascular precipitation of fibrinogen-fibrinogen antibody complexes.

A heterozygote for hereditary afibrinogenemia has a plasma fibrinogen level in the 80 to 120 mg per dL range, which is borderline for effective postoperative hemostasis. Some patients have experienced mildly excessive intraoperative or early postoperative bleeding. However, within about 24 hours after surgery, fibrinogen levels rise temporarily to the 150 to 250 mg per dL range. This reflects the ability of the hepatocyte to increase basal fibrinogen production as part of the acute phase response.

Dysfibrinogenemias

The dysfibrinogenemias are rare hereditary autosomal dominant disorders in which the plasma fibrinogen consists of a mixture of normal fibrinogen and a qualitatively abnormal fibrinogen. The latter, by interfering with fibrinopeptide release, fibrin polymerization, or both processes, prolongs the thrombin time test, which is usually the screening test clue to the existence of the disorder. Depending upon the molecular abnormality, the patient may experience abnormal bleeding, no symptoms, or, in a few instances, an increased tendency for thrombosis.

Factor XIII Deficiency

The patient with this rare disorder frequently has a history of:

1. Bleeding from the umbilical stump at birth and throughout life after trauma or surgery.
2. Poor wound healing.
3. Cessation of bleeding following transfusion of a single unit of blood or plasma.

In addition, women with factor XIII deficiency may have a history of repeated spontaneous abortions.

Screening coagulation tests will be normal except for dissolution of the recalcified plasma clot on incubation overnight in 5 M urea solution. Because of the long intravascular half-life of factor XIII and the ability of low plasma levels to support fibrin crosslinking, prophylactic transfusion of a unit of plasma every 4 to 6 weeks will prevent abnormal bleeding.

SELECTED READING

1. Beck EA: Congenital disorders of fibrin formation and stabilization. *In* Colman RW, Hirsh J, Marder VJ, and Salzman EW (eds): Hemostasis and Thrombosis. Basic Principles amd Clinical Practice. Philadelphia, JB Lippincott, 1982.
2. Kasper CK and Dietrich SL: Comprehensive management of hemophilia. Clin Haematol 14:489, 1985.
3. Roberts HR and Foster PA: Inherited disorders of prothrombin conversion. *In* Colman RW, Hirsh J, Marder VJ, and Salzman EW (eds): Hemostasis and Thrombosis. Basic Principles and Clinical Practice. Ed. 2. Philadelphia, JB Lippincott, 1987.

28

Acquired Coagulation Disorders

The common acquired coagulation disorders result from:

1. Vitamin K deficiency.
2. Liver disease.
3. Disseminated intravascular clotting with secondary fibrinolysis.
4. Antibodies to hemostatic factors.

Blood coagulation is also purposefully impaired when patients are given heparin or coumarin anticoagulants and is impaired as an unwanted side effect of the administration of the fibrinolytic agents streptokinase and urokinase.

VITAMIN K DEFICIENCY

Humans must absorb about 2 μg of vitamin K per kg of body weight daily to maintain normal vitamin K body stores. The vitamin K comes from two sources—the diet and bacterial synthesis of vitamin K in the intestine. A normal diet in the United States provides about 300 to 500 μg of vitamin K per day, principally in leafy green vegetables but also in other vegetables, cheese, bacon, liver, and some cereal and grain products.

541

Causes of Vitamin K Deficiency

The activity of the vitamin K-dependent clotting factors falls when:

1. The *supply* of vitamin K is inadequate. Tissue stores of vitamin K are limited. Therefore, patients maintained on intravenous fluids (and so deprived of a dietary source of vitamin K) and given broad-spectrum antibiotics that sterilize the gut (and so deprived of a bacterial source of vitamin K) may develop a bleeding tendency due to vitamin K deficiency within 7 to 10 days. The usual setting is a very ill patient in an intensive care unit who is not given supplemental vitamin K.

   It takes several days for intestinal bacteria to colonize the gut of the newborn infant and human breast milk is a poor source of vitamin K. Therefore, newborn infants in the United States are routinely given 100 μg to 1 mg of vitamin K at birth to prevent hemorrhagic disease of the newborn due to vitamin K deficiency.

2. The *absorption* of vitamin K is impaired. Vitamin K is fat soluble, and disorders interfering with fat absorption impair vitamin K absorption. For example:
   a. Obstructive jaundice, in which bile salts necessary for fat absorption fail to reach the gut.
   b. Abnormalities of the intestinal wall producing steatorrhea (for example, sprue, regional ileitis). A patient with underlying malabsorption is particularly prone to develop vitamin K deficiency when given a broad-spectrum antibiotic.

3. The *function* of vitamin K is inhibited by coumarin anticoagulants. In a patient presenting with a "mysterious bleeding disease" associated with a prolonged prothrombin time, one needs to consider possible surreptitious use of coumarin anticoagulants.

Laboratory Manifestations

The vitamin K-dependent clotting factors—prothrombin and factors VII, IX and X—are required to generate thrombin (see Fig. 23-6). Vitamin K deficiency produces the following pattern of screening coagulation test results:

1. *A prothrombin time that is always prolonged*, because this test is sensitive to deficiencies of factor VII, factor X, and prothrombin. A normal prothrombin time rules out vitamin K deficiency. (Giving vitamin K to a patient who is bleeding from an unknown cause but whose prothrombin time is normal will not affect the bleeding.)

2. An activated partial thromboplastin time (APTT) that may be either normal or prolonged. As a patient becomes vitamin K deficient, plasma factor VII activity, whose intravascular half-life is only 5 hours, falls more rapidly than does the plasma activities of factor IX, factor X, and prothrombin, whose intravascular half-lives exceed 24 hours. Since factor VII participates in clotting initiated by tissue factor but not in clotting initiated by contact activation of plasma, the prothrombin time lengthens in early vitamin K deficiency, while the APTT remains within the normal range. Furthermore, sick patients often have a high plasma factor VIII level, which compensates for the effect of a begining fall of plasma factor IX, X, and prothrombin activity upon the APTT and so maintains the test result within the normal range. However, when vitamin K deficiency is established and severe, the APTT will be prolonged.

3. A normal thrombin time, because the exogenous thrombin added to plasma in this test bypasses the defects in thrombin generation that vitamin K deficiency induces.

To establish that a moderately prolonged prothrombin time stems from vitamin K deficiency, one gives the patient 15 mg of vitamin K_1 (Aqua-Mephyton) subcutaneously and repeats the test 24 hours later. The prothrombin time should return almost to normal. A chemical test for coumarin anticoagulants in plasma is available and is used to confirm suspected surreptitious use of these drugs.

Treatment of Vitamin K Deficiency

If a patient with vitamin K deficiency develops *life-threatening bleeding*, he or she should be given 25 mg of vitamin K_1 intravenously *very slowly* (1 mg per minute). Since hemostatically effective levels of all of the vitamin K-dependent clotting factors will not be achieved for 12 to 16 hours, plasma transfusions to replace vitamin K-dependent clotting factors should also be given.

LIVER DISEASE

Liver disease may impair hemostasis because of:

1. *Impaired synthesis of clotting factors.* All of the plasma clotting factors, except factor VIII, are made primarily by hepatic parenchymal cells. Therefore, the levels of all factors except factor VIII fall in parenchymal liver disease. The extent of the fall reflects the extent of hepatic cell damage.

2. *Increased fibrinolysis.* Plasminogen activators released from vascular endothelium into the blood (see Chapter 23) are normally cleared from the blood as it flows through the liver. The hepatocyte also makes alpha$_2$ antiplasmin, the primary inhibitor of plasmin. Impairment of both processes may increase fibrinolytic activity in chronic liver disease. (Patients with cirrhosis occasionally develop unexpected generalized oozing during portal shunt surgery, which may stop after the administration of epsilon aminocaproic acid.)

3. *Thrombocytopenia.* Congestive splenomegaly develops as cirrhosis worsens and results in a moderate thrombocytopenia due to an increased sequestration of platelets in the spleen. Rare patients with acute hepatitis may develop an unexplained profound thrombocytopenia.

4. *Increased consumption of clotting factors in intravascular coagulation.* Patients with fulminant hepatitis or with the acute fatty liver of pregnancy may develop laboratory findings indicative of intravascular coagulation, for example, increased levels of fibrin degradation products, a positive plasma protamine paracoagulation test, and a virtual disappearance of plasma antithrombin III activity. The marked fall in antithrombin III reflects increased use and impaired synthesis by the damaged hepatocyte. The clotting may occur primarily within the sinusoids of the liver itself, presumably from release of procoagulant material from severely injured liver cells. (One attempts to replace antithrombin III with fresh plasma or an antithrombin III concentrate but should not give heparin to such patients because of the high risk of inducing life-threatening bleeding.)

The typical patient with acute viral hepatitis has a slightly to moderately prolonged prothrombin time but no serious bleeding. A sudden, marked fall in the prothrombin time represents an ominous sign of increasing hepatic necrosis. The patient may then develop large ecchymoses and bleed from sites of injections.

The response of the prothrombin time to vitamin K occasionally helps in the diagnosis of a jaundiced patient. A long prothrombin time caused by obstructive jaundice shortens after vitamin K therapy, whereas a long prothrombin time caused by liver cell injury does not.

Patients with advanced cirrhosis may bleed uncontrollably from esophageal varices or a peptic ulcer because of impaired hemostasis. One gives fresh frozen plasma, cryoprecipitate (as a source of fibrinogen if the fibrinogen concentration is low), and platelet concentrates in an attempt to stop the bleeding. One avoids giving prothrombin complex concentrates to replace the vitamin K-dependent factors because activated clotting intermediates in these concentrates may trigger substantial intravascular coagulation and secondary fibrinolysis in patients with advanced liver disease.

DISSEMINATED INTRAVASCULAR CLOTTING

Exposure of the circulating blood to procoagulant activity capable of initiating blood coagulation may cause:

1. No recognizable clinical manifestations.
2. Venous thrombosis, if the blood coagulations reactions progress to formation of fibrin in a local area of vascular stasis with resultant formation of a venous thrombus (see Chapter 29).
3. Disseminated intravascular coagulation, that is, the formation of fibrin in the flowing blood. This usually requires a substantial exposure of the blood to material with tissue factor activity.

Causes of Disseminated Intravascular Coagulation

Disseminated intravascular coagulation is usually seen in one of three clinical settings:

1. *Severe infection*, particularly gram-negative infection (for example, meningococcemia, Pseudomonas septicemia). Gram-negative endotoxin damages platelets and vascular endothelium and also activates factor XII, all of which could initiate coagulation. However, gram-negative endotoxin also sets off reactions involving activation of complement that generate tissue factor activity on the surface membrane of monocytes. Depletion of blood monocytes prevents disseminated intravascular coagulation after the intravenous injection of endotoxin in experimental animals. Therefore, the generation of monocyte tissue factor activity is thought to represent the primary mechanism whereby gram-negative endotoxin initiates disseminated intravasacular coagulation in human gram-negative infections.
2. *Complications of pregnancy.*
   a. Premature separation of the placenta, in which placental material with tissue factor activity is presumably discharged into the circulation.
   b. Amniotic fluid embolism, in which amniotic fluid enters the circulation and triggers intravascular clotting followed by powerful fibrinolysis.

c. Retained dead fetus in which intrauterine material with tissue factor activity may be absorbed into the maternal circulation over a number of days.

d. Abortion induced by the intra-amniotic infusion of hypertonic saline, which produces subclinical intravascular coagulation in most patients and striking disseminated intravascular coagulation in a rare patient.

e. Gram-negative endotoxemia complicating a septic abortion or amnionitis.

3. *Malignancies*, in which procoagulant tumor products possessing tissue factor activity gain access to the blood. Disseminated intravascular coagulation has been noted particularly in:

a. Mucin-secreting carcinomas (pancreas, prostate, stomach, bowel, lung).

b. Acute promyelocytic leukemia.

In addition, disseminated intravascular coagulation may occur in a variety of less common clinical circumstances. These include:

1. Head trauma with brain tissue destruction (for example, a gunshot wound to the head) in which the blood may be exposed to brain tissue with potent tissue factor activity.

2. Complications of transuretheral prostatic resection that result in procoagulant prostatic material entering the circulation.

3. A hemolytic transfusion reaction. The mechanism initiating intravascular coagulation is unknown but may be related both to the release of RBC stroma into the circulation and the activation of complement by the antigen-antibody reaction initiating the hemolysis.

4. Venomous snake bite. Different venoms initiate coagulation at different steps in the coagulation sequence, for example, by activating factor X, by activating prothrombin, or by splitting fibrinopeptide A from fibrinogen and so directly converting fibrinogen to fibrin.

5. Purpura fulminans (see below).

When evidence of disseminated intravascular coagulation is found, one must always establish and seek to correct its underlying cause.

Laboratory Manifestations of Extensive Disseminated Intravascular Coagulation

Acute, extensive disseminated intravascular clotting causes the following:

1. Thrombocytopenia and the consumption of plasma coagulation factors.
2. Appearance in the plasma of:
   a. Products of the activation of blood coagulation—fibrin monomer, fibrinopeptides, prothrombin fragments. Fibrin monomer can be readily demonstrated by a paracoagulation test (see Chapter 24). Fibrinopeptides and prothrombin fragments are measured by radioimmunoassays not generally available for clinical use.
   b. Fibrin degradation products, as a consequence of fibrin deposition in the microcirculation and secondary fibrinolysis.

Therefore, *massive intravascular coagulation* produces the following pattern of laboratory test abnormalitites:

1. Thrombocytopenia, as demonstrated by a platelet count and examination of the blood smear. (The blood smear must always be examined, even though the platelets are counted, to look for fragmented RBCs suggestive of deposition of fibrin in small vessels.)
2. A small clot—sometimes no clot—when 2 mL of blood is placed in a glass tube. *Whatever clot does form, does not lyse on standing.* A plasma clot also does not lyse when incubated in saline.
3. A long prothrombin time, APTT, and thrombin time. (Sometimes the plasma contains insufficient fibrinogen to trigger the sensor on an automatic machine used for prothrombin time and APTT tests. Clotting times are then reported as greater than a certain number of seconds, for example, greater than 200 seconds.)
4. A reduced plasma fibrinogen concentration.
5. A positive plasma protamine paracoagulation test for fibrin monomer.
6. A positive test for fibrin degradation products in serum (see Chapter 24).

Massive hepatic necrosis can produce screening test results sometimes difficult to distinguish from those of extensive intravascular coagulation. An assay for factor VIII helps to distinguish these conditions. Factor VIII is high in massive hepatic necrosis because hepatic parenchymal cells are not its site of synthesis. In contrast, factor VIII levels are low in extensive intravascular coagulation, presumably because of activation of factor VIII during clotting to factor

VIIIa and the subsequent inactivation of factor VIIIa by activated protein C (see Chapter 23).

A critically ill patient occasionally becomes thrombocytopenic for reasons that may be difficult to ascertain (see Chapter 25). He or she may also develop a prolonged prothrombin time and APTT because of vitamin K deficiency. Particularly if the patient has an infection or a malignancy, this combination of findings may initially arouse suspicion of disseminated intravascular coagulation. However, the abnormal coagulation tests are corrected after giving the patient vitamin K.

Very rarely, usually as a complication of liver disease or a malignancy, circulating plasminogen may be activated to plasmin with consequent lysis of circulating fibrinogen. The test findings resulting from such *primary fibrinogenolysis* differ from those of extensive intravascular coagulation in that:

1. Whole blood and diluted plasma clots lyse rapidly.
2. Thrombocytopenia and a positive plasma protamine paracoagulation test are not found.

Clinical Manifestations

Disseminated intravascular coagulation may lead to:

1. *Bleeding.* Massive intravascular coagulation obviously produces a serious potential bleeding tendency resulting from thrombocytopenia, depleted plasma clotting factors, and the deleterious hemostatic effects of fibrin degradation products. However, whether the patient actually bleeds depends on other clinical circumstances. Thus, the woman with premature separation of the placenta may bleed heavily from the placental site if the uterus fails to contract well after delivery. In contrast, a patient with disseminated intravascular clotting secondary to severe gram-negative bacteremia may not bleed at all unless some invasive procedure is undertaken that initiates the bleeding.

2. *Hemorrhagic tissue necrosis.* Although fortunately uncommon, occlusion of multiple small blood vessels with fibrin after disseminated intravascular coagulation may result in hemorrhagic necrosis of tissues. Ischemic necrosis occurs most often in the kidney, where it may lead to acute anuric renal failure. This may be reversible or irreversible (renal cortical necrosis). Hemorrhagic necrosis occurring in the adrenal glands and in the skin produces the pathologic findings characteristic of the Water-

house-Friderichsen syndrome. Thrombi in the vessels of the fingers and toes may cause gangrene and loss of digits. Whether or not a patient with disseminated intravascular clotting develops serious sequelae from fibrin deposition in small blood vessels depends upon several factors:

a. The ability of the mononuclear phagocytic system in the liver, spleen, and bone marrow to remove circulating fibrin.

b. Alterations in blood flow through tissues. (The author saw a patient with diffuse intravascular clotting who developed gangrene of fingers and toes after cooling measures to reduce high fever diminished blood flow to the hands and feet.)

c. Local tissue changes that prepare a microcirculatory bed to retain fibrin. In the rabbit, an injection into the skin of a variety of materials that cause granulocytes to accumulate and release their lysosomal enzymes "prepares" that skin site to undergo hemorrhagic necrosis when the animal is given an intravavenous injection of gram-negative endotoxin 24 hours later (local Shwartzman reaction). A similar sequence of events may be responsible for some instances of hemorrhagic skin necrosis complicating infection in humans.

d. The adequacy of local fibrinolysis. When fibrin is deposited in the microcirculation, plasminogen activator is released from endothelial cells and initiates secondary fibrinolysis. If such secondary fibrinolysis fails to dissolve occluding fibrin thrombi, ischemic tissue necrosis may result. The increased susceptibility for ischemic necrosis of the kidneys after gram-negative bacteremia in pregnancy may reflect the known depressed fibrinolysis associated with pregnancy.

3. *Hemolytic anemia.* As blood flows through small vessels containing loose fibrin strands, the RBCs may undergo mechanical damage, with resultant intravascular hemolysis and the appearance of fragmented RBCs on the peripheral blood smear (see Fig. 2-12). Such fragmentation hemolysis is sometimes called microangiopathic hemolytic anemia. Confusion has existed about the relation between fragmented RBCs on a blood smear and disseminated intravascular coagulation. One should understand that:

a. Hemolysis with fragmented RBCs on the blood smear is an important but *uncommon* complication of disseminated intravascular coagulation. Most patients with disseminated intravascular coagulation do not have fragmented RBCs on the blood smear.

b. Finding fragmented RBCs on a blood smear is not evidence, in itself, that a patient has undergone disseminated intravascular coagulation. Other causes for fibrin deposition in small vessels (for example, multifocal clotting around tumor emboli in small vessels) are more commonly responsible for this morphologic abnormality.

When hemolysis with fragmented RBCs does occur after an episode of intravascular coagulation, fibrin has usually been deposited in the glomerular capillary bed. The patient then also develops acute anuric renal failure with a resultant hemolytic-uremic syndrome (see Chapter 25).

Subacute Intravascular Coagulation

Patients with slower, subacute disseminated intravascular coagulation may have the following pattern of hemostatic test results:

1. Thrombocytopenia.
2. A normal to slightly prolonged prothrombin time. The prolongation is artifactual. It reflects the inability of automated coagulation instruments to adjust for the smaller clot resulting from a moderately depressed fibrinogen level within the 12 seconds of a normal prothrombin time test.
3. A normal to *short* APTT. The short APTT probably stems from the presence in the plasma of activated clotting intermediates.
4. A fibrinogen level that may be normal or depressed. Since fibrinogen levels should rise in sick patients, a "normal" level may reflect increased fibrinogen consumption in intravascular clotting.
5. A positive paracoagulation test (protamine paracoagulation test or ethanol gel test) for circulating fibrin monomer.
6. A positive test for fibrin degradation products.

Many, but not all, patients with these findings are discovered to have a malignancy. In such patients, one should be alert for serious manifestations of malignant disease attributable to hypercoagulability—venous thrombosis, thrombotic vegetations on the aortic heart valve, and arterial emboli from such vegetations.

A similar pattern of hemostatic test results may stem, not from slow *disseminated* intravascular clotting, but from continuing slow clotting in a *large local site*, for example, in a large aortic aneurysm or in a giant hemangioma (Kasabach-Merritt syndrome).

Purpura Fulminans

In purpura fulminans, the patient, usually a small child, develops hemorrhagic necrosis in the skin and underlying tissues following an illness that usually involves the skin (for example, scarlatina, varicella). At 1 to 4 weeks after the onset of the preparatory illness, the child develops painful, gradually enlarging, confluent purplish-black areas of hemorrhagic necrosis of the skin. The lesions are surrounded by a bright red border; the skin between areas of involvement looks normal. Examination of the blood in some, but not all, patients reveals thrombocytopenia, low fibrinogen levels, and low factor V and VIII levels. The disease tends to progress in a wave-like fashion. Unless checked by the vigorous and prolonged use of heparin, often followed by a further period of administration of a coumarin anticoagulant, purpura fulminans may end fatally. The pathogenesis of the syndrome is unknown. Laboratory evidence of defibrination does not necessarily mean that disseminated intravascular coagulation plays a pathogenetic role; rather, defibrination could be an epiphenomenon reflecting increased consumption of these factors in an expanding localized area of hemorrhagic necrosis. The discovery that the syndrome of neonatal purpura fulminans can result from homozygous hereditary protein C deficiency and the resemblance of purpura fulminans to the syndrome of coumarin-induced skin necrosis (see Chapter 29) suggest that an acquired abnormality affecting thrombomodulin, protein C, or protein S could be one cause for the disorder.

ANTIBODIES TO HEMOSTATIC FACTORS

Antibodies to hemostatic factors may arise:

1. After replacement therapy in a small proportion of patients with a hereditary deficiency of a clotting factor. The patient's immune system reacts to the administered clotting factor as if it were a foreign protein and makes antibodies against it.
2. As an autoimmune reaction in patients with previously normal hemostatic factors. Immunogic tolerance for "self" breaks down and the immune system makes antibodies to an antigenic determinant or determinants present on an endogenous hemostatic factor.

Antibodies to a clotting factor usually neutralize the coagulant activity of the clotting factor. Thus, the vast majority of antibodies to clotting factors act as *circulating anticoagulants* identifiable in vitro by relatively simple experiments in which mixing the patient's plasma with a source of the clotting factor inhibits the coagulant activity of the added clotting factor.

However, unusual antibodies to clotting factors may bind to a clotting factor without neutralizing its coagulant activity. They produce an in vivo deficiency of the clotting factor because of rapid clearance of antibody-clotting factor immune complex by the mononuclear phagocytic system. Demonstrating the presence of such antibodies, which give negative test results in in vitro mixing systems measuring the residual coagulant activity of an added clotting factor, requires showing that binding to antibody has altered a physical property of the clotting factor, for example, has slowed its mobility on crossed immunoelectrophoresis. Such antibodies have now been recognized as a cause for acute acquired hypoprothrombinemia in unusual patients and acute factor X deficiency in rare patients.

Factor VIII Antibodies

Antibodies that inhibit factor VIII clotting activity may develop in the following types of patients:

1. Patients with hemophilia A after replacement therapy.
2. Postpartum women. In this rare complication of pregnancy, the antibody is recognized immediately or soon after delivery, disappears gradually over months, and, surprisingly, seems not to recur after a subsequent delivery.
3. Patients with underlying immunogic disorders—rheumatoid arthritis, ulcerative colitis, immunologic skin diseases.
4. Patients, usually older persons, with no known underlying disease or precipitating cause.

Factor VIII antibodies produce a severe, potentially fatal bleeding diathesis. Screening test findings resemble those of hemophilia A in that the APTT is prolonged, but the bleeding time, prothrombin time, and thrombin time are normal. However, normal plasma fails to correct the patient's prolonged APTT. When a source of factor VIII is added to the patient's plasma, the mixture immediately (high titer antibodies) or progressively (low titer antibodies) loses its factor VIII activity. The antibodies are, with rare exception, of the IgG class.

With some of the antibodies that develop in nonhemophilic patients, a value of 5% to 20% factor VIII activity may be obtained in a factor VIII assay, even though the plasma contains excess antibody capable of reducing the activity of added factor VIII to this level of residual activity. This phenomenon probably reflects partial activity in the assay system of a factor VIII antigen-factor VIII antibody complex. It does not mean that the patient will behave like a mild hemophilic, who rarely has serious spontaneous hemorrhages. The patient will behave like a severe hemophilic, that is, like a patient with essentially no functional factor VIII activity *in vivo.*

Hemophilic and nonhemophilic patients with a factor VIII anticoagulant respond differently to therapy. Immunosuppressive agents, for example, a combination of adrenal steroids and cyclophosphamide, are without effect in the hemophilic patient. In contrast, they may cause a factor VIII antibody to disappear in the nonhemophilic patient, particularly in the older patient who develops an antibody with no evidence of underlying disease.

The Lupus Anticoagulant

Between 5% and 10% of patients with systemic lupus erythematosus develop plasma antibodies that inhibit the procoagulant functions of the phospholipid used in APTT test systems. These antibodies also may cause a biologic false-positive test for syphilis (VDRL) because they can react with cardiolipin, the phospholipid antigen used in the test. (One can demonstrate antibodies against cardiolipin in almost all patients with the lupus anticoagulant if one uses a more sensitive radioimmunoassay technique.)

An increased incidence of mild thrombocytopenia, usually between 100,000 and 150,000 platelets per μL, has also been noted in patients with systemic lupus erythematosus who have the anticoagulant. Moreover, the platelets of some patients with the lupus anticoagulant behave in platelet function studies as if they were "exhausted platelets" that have released their granule contents as a result of activation in vivo. These findings may well result from reactions between antiphospholipid plasma antibodies and phospholipids of the platelet membrane.

The term "lupus anticoagulant" is a misnomer, since this anticoagulant is also found in patients who do not have systemic lupus erythematosus, including:

1. Patients with other types of immunologic disorders.
2. Patients taking certain drugs, such as chlorpromazine, procainamide, or quinidine. (A surprisingly high prevalence of the lupus anticoagulant of about 30% was reported in psychiatric pa-

tients treated for long periods with high doses of
chlorpromazine.)
3. Patients with a variety of other disorders in which the association is probably coincidental.

The immunglobulin class of the antibodies differs. In patients
taking chlorpromazine, the antibodies are IgM, in other patients, the
antibodies are IgG, and in still others, the antibodies are both IgM
and IgG.

LABORATORY MANIFESTATIONS

The lupus anticoagulant typically produces the following pattern
of coagulation test abnormalities:

1. Screening tests.
   a. A prolonged APTT that fails to correct on mixing the patient's
   plasma with an equal amount of normal plasma.
   b. A normal to slightly prolonged prothrombin time and a normal thrombin time.
2. Specific assays.
   a. Low values in one-stage assays for factors XII, XI, IX, and
   VIII. These assays are based on the APTT technique and the
   patient's anticoagulant, by interfering with the function of the
   phospholipid reagent, can prolong assay clotting times. These
   prolonged times are then reported as low values for the specific factors measured.
   b. Higher values for these specific factors when a greater dilution of the patient's plasma is used in the assay systems, since
   this weakens the effect of the patient's antiphospholipid antibody upon the assay systems.
3. Special tests.
   a. Adding supplemental phospholipid, either as a synthetic
   phospholipid mixture or as frozen and thawed platelets, to an
   APTT system shortens the prolonged clotting time. Reducing
   the phospholipid of the APTT system or adding no phospholipid, as in the recalcification time test or the kaolin clotting
   time test, sensitizes the test system and makes possible detection of weaker lupus anticoagulants.
   b. Diluting the tissue factor reagent of the prothrombin time test
   lengthens the patient's clotting time substantially more than it

lengthens the clotting time of normal plasma. This is called a positive dilute thromboplastin inhibition test result.

For an unknown reason, a small number of patients with the lupus anticoagulant also develop non-neutralizing antibodies to prothrombin with resultant acquired hypoprothrombinemia due to rapid removal of prothrombin-prothrombin antibody complexes by the mononuclear phagocytic system. Associated hypoprothrombinemia is suspected when the prothrombin time with full-strength tissue factor is substantially prolonged and is confirmed by demonstrating a reduced plasma prothrombin concentration in a specific prothrombin assay. Since the antibody is a non-neutralizing antibody, it does not cause loss of prothrombin activity from a mixture of the patient's plasma and a prothrombin source (for example, normal plasma). One can establish its presence by adding a source of prothrombin to the patient's plasma in vitro and demonstrating a reduced mobility of prothrombin on crossed immunoelectrophoresis due to formation of a prothrombin-prothrombin antibody complex.

CLINICAL MANIFESTATIONS

Despite their abnormal laboratory test results, patients who have only the lupus anticoagulant do not appear to bleed abnormally. The reason for the lack of clinical bleeding is not yet clear. It may reflect an inability of the antibodies to interfere with the function of procoagulant phospholipids as they are present on the surface of activated platelets or other cells.

However, whenever the lupus anticoagulant is discovered in a routine preoperative screening evaluation of hemostasis, one should check for possible associated abnormalities that could cause bleeding. Only after thrombocytopenia, a prolonged bleeding time due to a qualitative platelet abnormality, or associated acquired hypoprothrombinemia have been ruled out, can one conclude that the patient has no increased risk of postoperative bleeding.

Paradoxically, a growing body of clinical evidence indicates that patients with the lupus anticoagulant are at increased risk for major *thrombotic episodes*. The reason for the association is unknown, but it is very real. Anticoagulant therapy effectively prevents extension or recurrence of thrombosis. Therefore, if a patient with the lupus anticoagulant develops a thrombosis, he or she should probably receive anticoagulant therapy for as long as evidence of the lupus anticoagulant persists.

An association between the lupus anticoagulant and repeated early spontaneous abortions has also recently been reported. Placental insufficiency due to thrombosis of placental vessels is the suspected cause for the abortions.

Antibodies to Other Clotting Factors

Antibodies to factor IX occasionally develop after replacement therapy in hemophilia B but virtually never develop spontaneously in nonhemophilic patients. A small number of patients have developed antibodies to factor V. These are often transient and usually have been discovered in postoperative patients. Some patients with factor V antibodies have bled extensively, whereas other patients have experienced little or no excessive bleeding. Possibly, the extent of bleeding depends on whether the antibody can also effectively inactivate platelet factor V.

A patient with transient acute factor X deficiency has been described recently whose plasma contains antibodies that bind factor X but do not neutralize its coagulant activity in vitro. A few patients have also been reported with antibodies that inhibit fibrin polymerization or fibrin stabilization. In some, the antibodies have reacted with antigenic determinants on fibrinogen, whereas in others, the antibodies have been directed against factor XIII.

UNUSUAL CAUSES OF ACQUIRED COAGULATION DISORDERS

A small number of patients with amyloidosis develop an acquired deficiency of factor X. Their plasma does not contain antibodies against factor X. However, factor X activity disappears from the patient's plasma abnormally rapidly after transfusion because it binds to amyloid in the tissues.

The monoclonal plasma immunoglobulin of a patient with multiple myeloma sometimes strikingly impedes fibrin polymerization in vitro when calcium ions are absent. This phenomenon probably does not impair hemostasis in the presence of calcium ions in vivo. Patients with plasma cell dyscrasias have also been described in whom clinical bleeding has resulted from a circulating proteoglycan possessing heparin-like anticoagulant properties.

SELECTED READING

1. Feinstein DI: Acquired inhibitors against factor VIII and other clotting proteins. *In* Colman RW, Hirsh J, Marder VJ, and Salzman EW (eds): Hemostasis and Thrombosis. Basic Principles and Clinical Practice. Ed 2. Philadelphia, JB Lippincott, 1987.
2. Savage D, and Lindenbaum J: Clinical and experimental human vitamin K deficiency. *In* Lindenbaum J (ed): Nutrition in Hematology. New York, Churchill Livingstone, 1983.

29

Thrombotic Mechanisms and Antithrombotic Therapy

Disabling or fatal disease may result from formation of thrombi within arteries (for example, coronary thrombosis with myocardial infarction), within veins (for example, deep venous thrombosis of leg veins leading to pulmonary emboli), within the chambers or on the valves of the heart (for example, cerebral embolism from a thrombotic vegetation on a prosthetic heart valve), or within the microcirculation of an organ or tissue (for example, glomerular capillary thrombosis after disseminated intravascular coagulation with resultant renal cortical necrosis).

PATHOGENESIS OF ARTERIAL THROMBOSIS

In the pathogenesis of arterial thrombosis, one should note that:

1. Thrombi form only at sites of *underlying arterial wall disease.*
2. Local alteration of the vessel wall, for example, rupture of an atherosclerotic plaque with exposure of the blood to tissue factor in the vessel wall, rather than a change in platelet reactivity or in the coagulability of the circulating blood usually triggers formation of the thrombus.
3. Stasis plays a variable role. It is not required for a clinically significant nonoccluding thrombus to form at an ulcerated site

in the wall of a minimally stenotic large artery, for example, a carotid artery. In contrast, a critical degree of stenosis is required in medium-sized arteries, for example, a coronary artery, for a local change in the vessel wall, such as the rupture of an atherosclerotic plaque, to precipitate an occluding thrombosis.

4. A *platelet nidus*, made up of platelets adhering to the damaged vessel wall and to each other, forms initially and anchors the developing thrombus to the vessel wall. This is particularly important in the pathogenesis of nonoccluding thrombi in larger vessels. Small platelet masses may break away from the growing thrombus. Held together by fibrin strands, they form emboli that may occlude smaller, distal arteries with serious ischemic consequences.

5. An occluding clot in a stenotic medium-sized vessel is *small*, often only a millimeter or two in diameter, and so presumably requires only transient, limited activation of blood coagulation.

Preventing arterial thrombotic disease requires preventing atheroslcerosis, the major cause of arterial wall disease. Atherosclerotic plaques are thought to form at sites of hemodynamic vessel wall stress as a result of repeated episodes of minimal endothelial injury. Deposition of platelets at the site of endothelial cell injury has been postulated as important in the pathogenesis of atherosclerosis because:

1. Release from activated platelets of platelet-derived growth factor (PDGF) can stimulate the proliferation and migration into the intima of smooth muscle cells and fibroblasts.

2. Platelet-fibrin thrombi may be incorporated into the arterial wall as new endothelium overgrows a site of wall injury.

Experimental thrombocytopenia in rabbits diminishes the size of plaques formed after mechanical injury to the aorta. Moreover, pigs with severe homozygous von Willebrand's disease reportedly develop less atherosclerosis of the abdominal aorta than do normal control pigs. However, no evidence exists that impaired platelet reactivity can impede the development of atherosclerosis in humans. Patients with the common type I form of von Willebrand's disease (von Willebrand factor levels in the 15% to 60% of normal range) are not protected from developing severe atherosclerosis.

A patient the author has seen has two hereditary disorders—a disorder of lipid metabolism leading to hypercholesterolemia and a hereditary disorder of platelet function limiting release of ADP from platelets. She developed very severe coronary atherosclerosis secondary to hypercholesterolemia despite life-long impaired platelet function that prolongs the bleeding time to over 20 minutes. Such an experiment of nature dampens one's enthusiasm for long-term administration of drugs inhibiting platelet function as prophylaxis against progression of atherosclerosis in humans. Moreover, it is difficult to believe that giving an antiplatelet agent or an anticoagulant to a patient who has a critical degree of stenosis in a coronary artery can protect substantially against a local event triggering formation of the tiny thrombus that can occlude the lumen and precipitate a myocardial infarction.

PATHOGENESIS OF VENOUS THROMBOSIS

Venous thrombosis differs in its pathogenesis from arterial thrombosis. In the formation of a venous thrombus:

1. *Underlying vessel wall damage is not required.* A hemophilic patient infused with large amounts of a prothrombin complex concentrate containing activated clotting factors may develop a venous thrombosis in previously normal veins.
2. As the above example illustrates, *increased systemic coagulability* usually plays a key pathogenetic role. Postoperative deep venous thrombosis, a major cause of surgical morbidity and mortality, begins with the exposure of blood to procoagulant tissue materials at the time of surgery.
3. Formation of a platelet nidus is not an initiating event. Aggregates of platelets (the so-called lines of Zahn) do form in a growing venous thrombus, but the sequence is not, as in an arterial thrombus, vessel wall injury followed by platelet adhesion and aggregation and then fibrin clot formation. Rather, the venous thrombus begins with altered coagulability leading to the formation of a fibrin clot loosely adherent to a previously undamaged vein wall. Platelets accumulate secondarily as a result of generation of thrombin and contribute to further growth of the thrombus by supplying procoagulant phospholipid, a surface on which enzyme-cofactor complexes of blood coagulation can form, and a localized, high concentration of factor V derived from platelet granules.
4. *Stasis* is important since it allows the blood coagulation reactions, once initiated, to continue to formation of fibrin at a local site. Otherwise, in the absence of wall damage and an anchor-

ing platelet nidus, activated clotting intermediates would be swept away in the flowing blood. Therefore, venous thrombi form primarily in the leg veins of patients at bed rest, beginning behind a valve pocket or in stagnant blood in the arcades of the deep veins of the calf.

5. Clinically significant venous thrombi are large thrombi that have usually progressively increased in size over several days. When radiolabeled fibrinogen is injected immediately after surgery and the legs are scanned for radioactivity with an external counter 24 hours later, "hot spots" representing small subclinical venous thrombi may be found in up to 40% of older postoperative patients. However, in only a few patients do such thrombi grow into large, clinically significant lesions. Their growth usually requires a continuing generation of thrombin over several days at the expanding borders of the thrombus.

From the above, one can readily understand why impairing blood coagulation with anticoagulant drugs can prevent both initiation and propagation of venous thrombi. Thrombi forming within the chambers of the heart (mural thrombi) are also large thrombi with continuing activation of the blood coagulation reactions at their borders. Anticoagulants can also prevent their formation and extension.

EVALUATION OF INCREASED THROMBOTIC RISK

A thrombotic event in an apparently healthy young adult, thrombosis at an unusual site (for example, mesenteric vein thrombosis), recurrent unexplained episodes of venous thrombosis, or a strong family history of thrombosis alerts one to the possibility of an underlying disorder increasing a patient's risk for thrombosis (Table 29-1). Some of the conditions listed in Table 29-1 will be readily apparent from the patient's general examination, but others require special tests for their diagnosis.

In evaluating screening laboratory tests, one checks particularly for:

1. An elevated hematocrit or platelet count.
2. Clues on the blood smear to a myeloproliferative disorder—macrocytosis and teardrop-shaped RBCs, "shift reticulocytes," rare nucleated RBCs, immature WBCs, and large platelets.
3. A prolonged APTT that is not corrected by mixing the patient's plasma with an equal quantity of normal plasma, which raises the possibility of the lupus anticoagulant.

Table 29-1. Conditions Associated with an Increased Risk of Thrombosis

CONDITION	MECHANISM
HEREDITARY	
1. Antithrombin III deficiency	Impaired neutralization of serine proteases: thrombin, Xa, IXa
2. Protein C deficiency or protein S deficiency	Failure of proteolytic inhibition of the cofactors VIIIa and Va. Impaired activation of fibrinolysis?
3. Rare disorders of fibrinogen and fibrinolysis	
a. Certain dysfibrinogenemias	Unknown, possible impaired neutralization of thrombin by adsorption to fibrin, impaired binding of plasminogen
b. Abnormal plasminogen	Impaired formation of plasmin
ACQUIRED	
1. Carcinoma	Exposure of blood to tumor cells or tumor products with tissue factor activity
2. Hematologic proliferative disorders	
a. Acute promyelocytic leukemia	Release of tissue factor from WBC granules
b. Myeloproliferative disorders (polycythemia, essential thrombocythemia)	Elevated blood viscosity, thrombocytosis, altered platelet membrane receptors and platelet responses
c. Paroxysmal nocturnal hemoglobinuria (PNH)	Unknown, possibly intravascular release of RBC products plus blockade of clearance of activated factors by mononuclear phagocytic system loaded with RBC breakdown products
3. Behçet's syndrome (oral and genital ulcers, ocular inflammation)	Unknown
4. Lupus anticoagulant	Unknown, related to antibodies reacting with membrane phospholipids
5. Nephrosis	Multiple factors: markedly elevated fibrinogen, factor VIII; low antithrombin III from urinary loss; effects of hyperlipidemia on platelet function
6. Complications of therapy	
a. Oral contraceptives	Unknown, related to estrogen effects upon vessel wall and hemostatic factors
b. Infusion of prothrombin complex concentrates	Infusion of activated clotting intermediates
c. Heparin-induced thrombocytopenia	Unknown, related to intravascular aggregation of platelets

4. A long thrombin time suggestive of a possible dysfibrinogene-
mia.

If the screening tests provide no clue to an underlying diagnosis,
one frequently then:

1. Tests for platelet hyper-responsiveness by looking for aggregation of platelets in platelet-rich plasma on stirring without addition of an aggregating agent.
2. Measures antithrombin III by a functional assay testing the ability of heparin to enhance the reactivity of antithrombin III. Immunologic assays measuring antithrombin III antigen are insufficient because hereditary antithrombin III deficiency is a
heterogenous disorder that may stem from either decreased production of a normal molecule or from normal production of a
defective molecule.
3. Measures protein C antigen and protein S antigen by an immunologic technique, for example, electroimmunoassay. Functional
assays for protein C activity are now also available in some centers.
4. Evaluates adequacy of fibrinolysis by:
   a. Measuring plasminogen concentration.
   b. Determining the euglobulin lysis time before and after venous stasis (cuff on arm between systolic and diastolic pressure for 5 minutes and sample drawn from vein just before
   cuff pressure lowered). Plasminogen activator release from
   vascular endothelium during stasis should substantially
   shorten the post-stasis euglobulin lysis time.
   c. Measuring the rate of inactivation of plasmin added to the patient's plasma (as is done in an alpha$_2$ antiplasma assay) to
   screen for abnormal inhibition of plasmin activity.
5. Performs a sucrose hemolysis test for paroxysmal nocturnal hemoglobinuria (in patients with intra-abdominal thrombosis).

Despite this systematic evaluation, a cause for an increased tendency for thrombosis will be discovered in only about one quarter of
patients in whom its existence is suspected.

ANTITHROMBOTIC THERAPY

Antiplatelet Agents

Antiplatelet therapy has been used primarily in arterial thromboembolic disease or in patients with vascular shunts or prosthetic heart
valves. The two drugs that have been most widely used are:

1. Aspirin, which interferes with platelet function by inhibiting oxidation of arachidonic acid by cyclooxygenase (see Chapter 23).
2. Dipyridamole (Persantin), a phosphodiesterase inhibitor thought to elevate cyclic AMP levels in circulating platelets and so decrease their responsiveness to activating stimuli.

Other platelet inhibitors being studied experimentally include thromboxane synthetase inhibitors, which not only block conversion of endoperoxides to thromboxane A_2 in platelets but may make more platelet endoperoxide available to endothelium for synthesis of prostacyclin (see Fig. 23-3).

Aspirin has been used in several clinical settings:

1. In the secondary prevention of myocardial infarction, that is, to prevent new infarction or sudden death in patients who have had an initial myocardial infarction. Six randomized clinical trials have each failed to yield conclusive evidence of benefit; their data must be pooled to demonstrate a modest reduction in new infarction and mortality rates in the aspirin-treated patients. This is not surprising since a subset of patients benefiting from aspirin might well disappear statistically within a population in which many factors influence prognosis, for example, the extent of existing vessel wall disease, the presence of risk factors such as diabetes or hypertension that accelerate progression of atherosclerosis, and the presence of serious arrhythmias or congestive failure as sequelae of the initial infarct. Giving an 80-mg dose of aspirin (one "baby aspirin") is now known to suppress platelet thromboxane A_2 synthesis while avoiding the gastric side effects of the large doses of aspirin used in the clinical trials. Therefore, despite lack of clear-cut evidence of its benefit, many physicians give a small daily dose of aspirin to patients who have had a myocardial infarction.
2. To prevent early occlusion of coronary artery bypass grafts. In the most encouraging study to date, aspirin was combined with dipyridamole. Dipyridamole was started before surgery and aspirin was started several hours after surgery in order to suppress platelet function as quickly as possible yet not increase post-pump bleeding (see Chapter 26).
3. To prevent formation of thrombi on prosthetic heart valves in unusual patients who develop such thrombi, despite well-regulated oral anticoagulant therapy. Either aspirin plus dipyridamole or dipyridamole alone has been added to the anticoagulant therapy. (Before giving aspirin to a patient receiving

μ

warfarin, one must have concluded that its potential benefit exceeds the increased risk of upper gastrointestinal tract bleeding that results from the combined use of these drugs.)

4. In patients with transient focal episodes of neurologic dysfunction of vascular origin (transient ischemic attacks or TIAs) to prevent new episodes and, more importantly, to prevent permanent neurologic residuals due to a subsequent stroke. Many TIAs result from platelet-fibrin emboli from mural thrombi in proximal vessels feeding the cerebral circulation. When such lesions are not surgically correctable, patients are frequently treated with an oral anticoagulant for several months (the period of greatest risk of stroke) and then treatment is continued indefinitely with aspirin.

Anticoagulants

Anticoagulant therapy is indicated:

1. To prevent or treat venous thrombosis and pulmonary embolism.
2. To prevent or treat mural thrombi in certain cardiac disorders —anterior wall transmural myocardial infarction, cardiomyopathies with dilated cardiac chambers, mitral valvular disease with left atrial dilatation and atrial fibrillation.
3. To prevent thrombosis on prosthetic heart valves.
4. To prevent further embolic episodes or occluding thrombotic disease in patients with TIAs stemming from lesions that are not surgically correctable. As noted above, in some patients, aspirin is substituted for anticoagulant therapy after an initial several month period.

Despite many clinical trials over a 30-year period, the role, if any, of long-term anticoagulant therapy in the secondary prevention of myocardial infarction remains unsettled. As suggested for aspirin, long-term anticoagulant therapy may possibly benefit a subset of patients, not yet clearly defined, within a larger population of patients who derive no benefit from their use.

HEPARIN

Structure and Mechanism of Action. Proteoglycans are compounds found in the ground substance of connective tissue, on cell surfaces, and within cells that consist of a protein core to which are attached multiple long polysaccharide side chains called glycosaminoglycans.

The glycosaminoglycans are made up of disaccharide repeating units in which one sugar of the repeating unit is a derivative of an amino sugar, either glucosamine or galactosamine. The properties of different glycosaminoglycans depend on the pattern of disaccharides in the repeating units and their degree and type of sulfation. One glycosaminoglycan, heparin, contains a number of tetrasaccharide sequences of the correct structure and charge to bind antithrombin III. This binding converts antithrombin III from a slow inactivator of thrombin, factor Xa, and factor IXa into an extremely rapid inactivator of these serine proteases. Antithrombin III functions as a physiologic regulator of blood coagulation after binding to heparin present on the luminal surface of vascular endothelium. When exogenous therapeutic heparin is given, much more antithrombin III can bind to heparin circulating in the plasma with a resultant immediate pharmacologic anticoagulant effect.

Mast cells are rich in heparin, and therapeutic heparin is extracted from tissues rich in mast cells (for example, intestinal mucosa). Such preparations are relatively crude mixtures of fragments of heparin glycosaminoglycan of differing anticoagulant activity. Therefore, dosage is expressed as units of anticoagulant activity and not milligrams of heparin. The negative charges on heparin are required for its binding to antithrombin III. Positively charged materials can neutralize the anticoagulant activity of heparin, and one such material, protamine sulfate, is used therapeutically when one must rapidly reverse anticoagulation with heparin.

Absorption and Metabolism. Heparin is ineffective orally and must be given either subcutaneously or intravenously (but never intramuscularly because of the risk of forming a large hematoma at the injection site). The intravascular half-time of heparin varies with its plasma concentration; for usual clinical doses, the half-time is 90 minutes. Thus, it takes 6 hours (four half-times) to reduce plasma heparin to 6% of the amount present immediately after an intravenous injection. An enzyme in the liver, heparinase, converts heparin into an inactive metabolic product.

Materials in plasma compete with antithrombin III for binding to heparin and so reduce its anticoagulant effect. The most important of these are the cationic platelet protein, platelet factor 4, and histidine-rich glycoprotein. Others proteins that can bind heparin include thrombospondin, fibronectin, and vitronectin.

More heparin is frequently needed right after a thrombotic episode than later to obtain adequate anticoagulation. This may reflect release of platelet factor 4 from aggregating platelets at the time of a thrombotic episode and also release induced by an initial dose of heparin of a limited amount of platelet factor 4 bound to endothelial cells.

Effects on Hemostatic Test Results. As mentioned, heparin functions as an immediate anticoagulant. After a large intravenous bolus of heparin, a patient will have:

1. A markedly prolonged APTT (for example, greater than 150 seconds).
2. A substantially prolonged prothrombin time (18 to 20 second range).
3. Absent clotting in the thrombin time test.

At a lesser plasma concentration—that obtained when heparin is given therapeutically by intravenous drip to keep the APTT between one and one half and two times normal—heparin only minimally prolongs the prothrombin time. Consequently, one can use the APTT to monitor the anticoagulant effect of heparin and the prothrombin time to monitor the anticoagulant effect of warfarin (see below) in the patient who is receiving both continuous intravenous heparin and warfarin.

Because of the powerful antithrombic activity of heparin, the thrombin time test (in which plasma is clotted with a fixed, small amount of exogenous thrombin) is exquisitely sensitive to heparin. *The thrombin time is the best screen for residual heparin in blood.* A normal thrombin time rules out the presence of even trace amounts of heparin in blood.

In usual clinical doses, heparin does not prolong the bleeding time. However, if a patient receiving heparin is given aspirin or other drugs interfering with collagen-induced platelet activation, then formation of hemostatic plugs is seriously impaired (see Chapter 23). The bleeding time lengthens and the risk of serious bleeding is enhanced.

Administration. Heparin is used for two purposes:

1. *Prophylactically,* in low doses to prevent a thrombus from begginning. The heparin is given subcutaneously, 5000 units every 8 hours or every 12 hours. These doses usually prolong the APTT only minimally.
2. *Therapeutically,* in higher doses to stop growth of a thrombus

that has already formed. The heparin is given intravenously, either by continuous infusion or by bolus injections at 4- to 6-hour intervals. Since continuous infusion requires less heparin and results in a more even anticoagulant effect, it is usually the preferred method of administration.

For continuous infusion, one often begins with an initial bolus of 5000 or 10,000 units and then sets a drip to deliver 1000 units per hour. The APTT is measured 4 to 6 hours later, and the drip is adjusted to maintain the APTT between one and one-half and two times normal. The APTT must be monitored at least once daily. If an intermittent intravenous schedule is used, one frequently begins with 5000 units every 4 hours. An APTT 4 hours after the first dose and occasionally thereafter allows one to decide if the dose needs modification.

In a patient in whom venous thrombosis is suspected but not established, one must not "waffle" and give low-dose heparin, assuming it will do some good should a thrombus be present while minimizing the risk of bleeding. *Low-dose heparin will not prevent propagation of an existing thrombus.* Instead, one should protect the patient with bolus intravenous injections of heparin while gathering the evidence (by impedence plethysmography, venography, or lung scans for pulmonary emboli) needed to reach a definitive diagnosis.

Complications. The bleeding complications of heparin therapy may be minimized by avoiding:

1. Overdosage of heparin. (When the APTT in a patient receiving continuous intravenous heparin exceeds 100 seconds, the dose should be reduced.)
2. Intramuscular injections of any kind (for example, if a patient needs parenteral antibiotics, they should be given intravenously).
3. Invasive procedures, for example, spinal tap, paracentesis.
4. Drugs that interfere with platelet function, particularly aspirin and aspirin-containing medicines.

Thrombocytopenia occasionally develops in a patient who has been receiving heparin for several days. Therefore, if one plans to continue heparin beyond 1 week, platelets should be counted initially and again after 5 to 7 days. The patient who becomes thrombocytopenic makes an antibody to heparin that causes platelet aggregation. Recent evidence suggest that the antibody interacts with heparin at a site on glycoprotein Ib of the platelet membrane. Paradoxically, the patient with heparin-induced thrombocytopenia may simultaneously experience a thromboembolic event. One mechanism for this could be the deposition of aggregated platelets upon arterial atherosclerotic plaques with consequent formation of platelet-fibrin thrombi that break off to occlude down stream vessels.

ORAL ANTICOAGULANTS

Mechanism of Action. The oral anticoagulants are coumarin derivatives; warfarin (Coumadin) is the drug primarily used today. Warfarin has no direct effect upon the blood clotting reactions. It interferes with the function of vitamin K in post-translational carboxylation of selected glutamic acid residues to form γ-carboxyglutamic acid (GLA) residues in six plasma proteins of blood coagulation—prothrombin, factors VII, IX, and X, and protein C and protein S. As a consequence, the plasma activity of these factors falls. The concentration of these factors measured by immunologic assays also falls, but to a lesser degree. Variable amounts of abnormal, partially carboxylated factors circulate.

The full anticoagulant effect of warfarin develops gradually over several days as the activities of the normal vitamin K-dependent procoagulant clotting factors fall according to their different rates of biologic decay. Factor VII has an intravascular half-time of only 5 hours, whereas the half-times of factors IX, X, and prothrombin are between 1 and 3 days. Therefore, when warfarin is started, the initial lengthening of the prothrombin time stems almost exclusively from a fall in factor VII activity. However, the antithrombotic effectiveness of the oral anticoagulants results primarily from depression of factor X activity. Consequently, regardless of the value for the prothrombin time test, oral anticoagulants do not protect against thrombosis until about 5 days after they are started. Moreover, protein C, which is a key physiologic anticoagulant, has an intravascular half-time of only 8 to 10 hours. The rapid fall in its activity creates a period of potential hypercoagulability until the activity of factor X falls to a comparable level. Therefore, when a patient with an acute thrombosis, who has been started upon heparin for its immediate anticoagulant effect, is switched to warfarin for longer term maintenance therapy, the heparin should be continued for about 5 days to allow the antithrombotic effect of warfarin to become established. (Heparin dosage is still reliably monitored by the APTT, which is insensitive to the warfarin-induced fall in factor VII.)

Monitoring Warfarin Therapy. After the levels of factors IX, X, and prothrombin fall, warfarin prolongs both the prothrombin time and the APTT. However, only "prothrombin time" tests of one type or another, that is, tests in which tissue factor is added to plasma, are used to monitor warfarin therapy. The APTT is not used—both for historical reasons and because variation in factor VIII, an acute phase protein whose level may rise sharply in an ill patient, substantially affects the prolongation of the APTT obtained with warfarin.

The original prothrombin time method of Quick is the principal test used for monitoring warfarin therapy. In this test, the patient's plasma is recalcified in the presence of a potent tissue factor reagent. The clotting time is reported, along with a value for a normal control plasma. A prothrombin ratio is calculated from the patient's time in seconds divided by the control time in seconds.

With the commercial tissue factor preparations in current use in the United States, the author aims for a therapeutic prothrombin time ratio in different types of patients as follows:

1. For a patient with an acute episode of deep venous thrombosis in whom one begins treatment with heparin and warfarin simultaneously and plans to discontinue the heparin 3 to 5 days after achieving a therapeutic prothombin time ratio—a ratio of 1.7 with an acceptable range of 1.5 to 2.0.
2. For a patient with an acute episode of deep venous thrombosis who has been treated as above for the first 3 weeks of the episode and who is then to be maintained on prophylactic anticoagulant therapy to prevent recurrance of venous thrombosis for a total period of 3 months—a ratio of 1.5 with an acceptable range of 1.3 to 1.7.
3. For a cardiac patient in whom the goal is to prevent or treat a mural thrombus, for example, a patient with an anterior wall transmural myocardial infarction or a patient with atrial fibrillation being prepared for cardioversion—a ratio of 1.5 with an acceptable range of 1.3 to 1.7.
4. For a patient who has had replacement of a heart valve:
   a. In the mitral position with a prosthetic valve—a ratio of 2.0 with an acceptable range of 1.8 to 2.2.
   b. In the mitral position with a porcine tissue valve—a ratio of 1.5 with an acceptable range of 1.3 to 1.7.
   c. In the aortic position with a prosthetic valve—a ratio of 1.7 with an acceptable range of 1.5 to 2.0.

The World Health Organization has developed an International Reference Preparation of tissue factor to promote the worldwide standardization of oral anticoagulant control. This reference tissue factor, which is prepared from human brain, is more sensitive to the reduced activity of the vitamin K dependent clotting factors induced by warfarin than are the commercial thromboplastins used in the United States, which are prepared from rabbit brain. The following approximate relations exist between an International Normalized Ratio (obtained with the human brain preparation and referred to as the INR) and a ratio obtained with commercial tissue factor preparations used in the United States (CTFR):

INR	CTFR
2.0	1.3
2.5	1.5
3.5	1.7
4.5	2.0

Modified prothrombin time methods (the P&P test or the Thrombotest) are used in a few countries. In these tests the patient's plasma is diluted 1:10 and an adsorbed ox plasma reagent is added to the clotting mixture to supply a constant amount of factor V and fibrinogen. Results are reported in percent of normal activity from a dilution curve made by plotting the clotting times obtained with increasing dilutions of a normal plasma standard. The therapeutic ranges are for the P&P test, 10% to 20%; for the Thrombotest, 7% to 15%.

Absorption and Metabolism. Warfarin is completely absorbed from the gastrointestinal tract. It circulates primarily bound to plasma albumin with a half-life of about 35 hours. Drugs that complete with warfarin for binding sites on albumin increase warfarin's free plasma concentration and, therefore, a patient's sensitivity to warfarin. Warfarin is taken up from the plasma by the hepatocyte, wherein it inhibits formation of GLA residues on the vitamin K-dependent clotting factors. Hepatocellular injury sensitizes a patient to warfarin. Hepatic microsomal enzymes metabolize warfarin, and drugs that induce increased hepatic microsomal enzyme synthesis decrease the hypoprothrombinemic effect of a given dose of warfarin.

Vitamin K stores influence a patient's sensitivity to warfarin. The prothrombin time of a patient with subclinical intestinal malabsorption, and therefore limited vitamin K stores, may prolong strikingly after only a small dose of warfarin. Conversely, a patient given a large dose of vitamin K_1, for example, 25 mg, develops an increased resistance to the hypoprothrombinemic effect of warfarin that may persist for 4 to 6 weeks.

Administration. One often starts warfarin therapy with 10 mg daily for 3 days. The prothrombin time is measured each day; from the test result on the fourth morning, the approximate maintenance dose can usually be predicted. For most patients, this will be between 4.0 and 8.0 mg daily, but occasional patients may require as little as 1 mg or as much as 15 mg daily.

One starts with a smaller dose of warfarin when:

1. Unexplained thrombosis in a young person raises the possibility of heterozygote protein C or protein S deficiency (see later).
2. Hepatocyte function may be impaired, for example, as in a patient with a congested liver secondary to right-sided congestive heart failure.
3. Vitamin K stores may be reduced, for example, as in a patient who has eaten poorly or who has been receiving broad-spectrum antibiotics.

Management of Maintenance Warfarin Therapy. For patients on maintenance therapy, dosage should be calculated on a weekly basis; small changes in the weekly dose may be needed for precise regulation— for example, from 52.5 mg weekly (7.5 mg daily) to 56 mg weekly (8 mg daily). In patients on long-term therapy, prothrombin times are repeated weekly until the exact maintenance dose is established. Then, prothrombin times at monthly intervals usually suffice unless events altering dosage requirements are anticipated.

When the *prothrombin ratio rises* above the therapeutic range in a patient previously stable on a given dose of warfarin, one considers the following possibilities:

1. Increased alcohol intake. Small amounts of alcohol, such as a glass of wine with dinner, will not affect the prothrombin time. However, larger amounts, particularly in a patient with marginal liver function due to previous heavy alcohol consumption, can markedly prolong the prothrombin time.
2. Deteriorating liver function in a cardiac patient due to increasing right-sided congestive heart failure and hepatic congestion.
3. Administration of a drug increasing warfarin's hypoprothrombinemic effect. The most common of such drugs in the author's experience are cimetidine and trimethoprim-sulfamethoxazole (Septra^R, Bactrim^R). Additional drugs include: phenytoin

(Dilantin[R]), the tricyclic antidepressants, nonsteroidal anti-inflammatory agents such as phenylbutazone, indomethacin, and sulindac, metronidazole (Flagyl[R]), disulfiram (Antabuse[R]), androgens, and large doses of vitamin E (usually self-prescribed). Other drugs may affect one patient but not another. Oral antibiotics that alter the bacterial flora of the gut (for example, ampicillin, tetracycline) may strikingly lengthen the prothrombin time of a patient with minimally impaired intestinal absorption in whom bacterial synthesis of vitamin K may serve as an important supplement to dietary vitamin K intake. One suspects any newly started drug when a patient's prothrombin time is found to be unexpectedly prolonged and no other reason is apparent.

When the *prothrombin ratio falls* below the therapeutic range in a patient previously stable on a given warfarin dose, one considers the following possibilities:

1. Failure of compliance, for example, an elderly patient forgets to take the warfarin tablets.
2. Increased intake of vitamin K. Unexpected sources of vitamin K include proprietary reducing diet formulations supplemented with vitamin K and pills purchased in health food stores that contain alfalfa. Patients with backyard vegetable gardens may seasonally increase their consumption of leafy green vegetables and need an increase in warfarin dosage to compensate for this. If a patient is given vitamin K_1 to reverse warfarin anticoagulation temporarily before surgery, he or she may require a larger maintenance dose than previously for several weeks after warfarin is started again.
3. Improved liver function, for example, as congestive heart failure is corrected.
4. Administration of a drug decreasing the hypoprothrombinemic effect of warfarin. Such drugs include carbamazepine (Tegretol[R]), rifampin, and barbiturates.

Patients taking warfarin should use acetaminophen for analgesia and avoid aspirin or other nonsteroidal anti-inflammatory agents affecting prostaglandin synthesis. If presistent musculoskeletal pain unrelieved by acetaminophen (for example, persisting severe hip pain due to osteoarthritis) forces one to prescribe one of these agents, the author prefers to prescribe ibuprofen. However, all of these agents increase the risk of upper gastrointestinal tract bleeding because:

1. They may cause erosive gastritis or peptic ulcer in susceptible individuals.
2. They impede formation of hemostatic plugs consequent to impaired platelet synthesis of thromboxane A_2.

Complications. *Bleeding* is the major complication of warfarin therapy. It may present as:

1. *Heavy menstrual bleeding.* A substantial number of women experience menorrhagia, even when the prothrombin ratio is in the therapeutic range.
2. *Hematemesis or melena.* When these occur while the prothrombin ratio is in the therapeutic range, it means that an ulcerated mucosal lesion is present. The concomitant use of a nonsteroidal anti-inflammatory agent should be suspected.
3. *Hematuria.* When this occurs while the prothrombin ratio is in the therapeutic range, one must rule out a local cause. In contrast, when hematuria occurs in a patient whose prothrombin ratio substantially exceeds the therapeutic range, one usually attributes it to overanticoagulation and does not subject the patient to a search for an underlying local lesion.
4. *Sudden, unexplained abdominal pain.* When this develops in an overanticoagulated patient, one must consider two possible hemorrhagic complications:
   a. Adrenal hemorrhage.
   b. Bleeding into the wall of the intestine (intramural hemorrhage).
5. *Pericardial tamponade*, which may develop in a patient given warfarin despite evidence of pericarditis.
6. *Signs of increased intracranial pressure or meningeal irritation* suggestive of CNS bleeding. This is the most feared complication of warfarin therapy and is of particular concern when anticoagulants are given to hypertensive patients with evidence on funduscopic examination of advanced small vessel disease.

Warfarin-induced skin necrosis is a rare, paradoxical thrombotic complication of warfarin therapy that is encountered within several days after beginning therapy. Patients with this complication have often received a large, initial loading dose of warfarin. Thrombi form in venules of the skin and subcutaneous tissues, usually in a region of increased subcutaneous fat, such as the breast or buttock, with resultant development of a spreading area of hemorrhagic necrosis resembling purpura fulminans. Several patients with this lesion have been discovered to be heterozygotes for hereditary protein C deficiency. Initial doses of warfarin in such a patient could well cause protein C activity to fall to very low levels with consequent triggering of thrombosis in venules of subcutaneous tissue before factor X activity can fall to protective, antithrombotic levels.

Warfarin has a substantial risk of inducing chondrodysplastic and CNS abnormalities in a fetus, and pregnant women should not be given warfarin except under unusual circumstances in which management with heparin through the pregnancy is impossible.

Thrombolytic Therapy

Thrombolytic therapy has been advocated for venous thrombosis and acute pulmonary embolism, for acute arterial thrombosis, and for lysis of clots occluding access shunts and intravascular or cavity catheters. In patients with extensive venous thrombosis of the legs, dissolving thrombi with thrombolytic therapy is said to preserve the anatomy and function of the venous valves and so reduce postphlebitic complications. However, rare patients with venous thrombotic disease have experienced pulmonary emboli after beginning thrombolytic therapy.

Infusion of streptokinase by an arterial catheter positioned adjacent to a thrombus has been used to lyse arterial thrombi. It is currently used in many centers as emergency therapy for acute coronary artery thrombosis. If lysis of the clot is obtained but coronary angiography shows an area of critical stenosis, the patient may then be subjected to immediate angioplasty.

Two plasminogen activators, streptokinase and urokinase, are currently generally available as thrombolytic agents. Because streptokinase is a foreign bacterial protein, febrile reactions due to reactions with naturally occurring anti-streptokinase antibodies complicate its administration. Moreover, the development of a high titer of antibodies after its initial use precludes a second use of streptokinase for 6 to 12 months thereafter. Nevertheless, because it is much less expensive than urokinase, streptokinase is the primary agent in clinical use today.

Both streptokinase and urokinase are potent activators of circulating plasminogen. When either is infused into a patient, circulating plasmin is formed, and the plasma levels of the plasmin inhibitors alpha$_2$ antiplasmin and alpha$_2$ macroglobulin fall. Following this, plasmin can attack the fibrin of the thrombus but it also can attack circulating fibrinogen, factors V and VIII, and other plasma proteins. Large amounts of fibrinogen-fibrin degradation products are formed, which inhibits platelet aggregation and fibrin polymerization. This creates a potentially hazardous bleeding tendency and invasive procedures must be scrupulously avoided in such patients. Moreover, thrombolytic agents can dissolve recently formed hemostatic seals, and, therefore, thrombolytic therapy is contraindicated in patients who have had surgery or trauma within the preceding 10 days. It is also contraindicated in patients with a cerebrovascular accident or other evidence of CNS damage within the preceding 3 months.

When streptokinase or urokinase are given intravenously in standard therapeutic doses, laboratory monitoring is usually limited to demonstrating that a systemic fibrinolytic effect has been obtained. This can be done by measuring one or more of the following: the APTT, the thrombin time, the euglobulin lysis time, or the fibrinogen concentration. When fibrinolytic therapy is discontinued, anticoagulant therapy is started with heparin, usually after delay of an hour or two to allow clearance of residual activator and the return of the APTT into a range of one and one half to two times control value. In venous thrombotic disease, anticoagulant therapy is continued in the same schedule as would have been used had fibrinolytic therapy not been given.

Tissue plasminogen activator, which is a weak activator of circulating plasminogen but a potent activator of plasminogen bound to fibrin, can generate plasmin in a thrombus with only minimal generation of circulating plasmin that attacks fibrinogen and other plasma clotting factors. Therefore, its use should diminish the risk of bleeding with fibrinolytic therapy. Cloned bacterial synthesis of tissue plasminogen activator has recently made tissue plasminogen activator available for clinical trials as a thrombolytic agent.

SELECTED READING

1. Collen D, Stassen JM, and Verstraete M: Thrombolysis with human extrinsic (tissue-type) plasminogen activator in rabbits with experimental jugular vein thrombosis. Effect of molecular form and dose of activator, age of the thrombus, and rate of administration. J Clin Invest 71:368, 1983.
2. Frishman W: Antiplatelet therapy in coronary heart disease. Hosp Pract 17:73, 1982.

3. Kelton JG, and Hirsh J: Bleeding associated with antithrombotic therapy. Semin Hematol 17:259, 1980.
4. Poller L: Oral anticoagulant therapy. *In* Bloom AL, and Thomas DP (eds): Haemostasis and Thrombosis. New York, Churchill Livingstone, 1981.
5. Sharma GVRK, Cella G, Parisi AF, and Sasahara AA: Thrombolytic therapy. N Engl J Med 306:1268, 1982.
6. Thaler E, and Lechner K: Antithrombin III deficiency and thromboembolism. Clin Haematol 10:369, 1981.
7. Vermylen J, Blockmans D, Spitz B, and Deckmyn H: Thrombosis and immune disorders. Clin Haematol 15:509, 1986.

30

Transfusion Therapy

Transfusion of blood components has largely replaced transfusion of whole blood, which should be used only to replace loss of whole blood (for example, during a massive gastrointestinal hemorrhage). Use of whole blood for other purposes is wasteful and increases the risk of circulatory overload.

CELLULAR BLOOD COMPONENTS

RBC Preparations

Major blood banks can generally provide three types of preparations for RBC component therapy:

1. *Packed or sedimented RBCs*, which is the usual preparation used for transfusions primarily given to replace RBC mass. The RBCs are concentrated (hematocrit, 60 to 70%) by gravity sedimentation or centrifugation, which removes about 80% of the plasma.
2. *Leukocyte, platelet, and plasma-poor RBCs* prepared by a machine-washing technique for washing red cells. Such washed RBCs are used in the following circumstances:
   a. To prevent febrile reactions in occasional patients who have developed antibodies to WBCs after earlier transfusions or pregnancy.
   b. To avoid sensitization to HLA antigens on WBCs and platelets in patients who may require repeated transfusions over months to years and in young patients with aplastic anemia who may be candidates for bone marrow transplantation.

c. To avoid transfusion of plasma proteins into patients:
   (1) With hemolytic anemias in which the complement proteins play a major role in the mechanism of hemolysis (for example, paroxysmal nocturnal hemoglobinuria, cold agglutinin disease).
   (2) Who have developed alloantibodies to plasma proteins (particularly anti-IgA) that induce urticarial and bronchospastic reactions after transfusion of components containing plasma proteins.
3. *Frozen blood.* Freezing blood provides a way to maintain an inventory of rare blood types. It also allows a patient who will need elective surgery requiring transfusions to store his or her own RBCs for use at the time of surgery (autotransfusion). Frozen blood is another (but more expensive) source of leukocyte and platelet-poor RBCs, because the extensive washing required to remove the cryoprotective agent also removes leukocytes and platelets.

Platelet Concentrates

Platelet concentrates are used to prevent or control thrombocytopenic bleeding. They are prepared from units of whole blood by a closed-bag differential centrifugation technique. One donor unit yields about 5×10^{10} platelets in 50 mL of plasma. When prepared and stored optimally, platelet concentrates retain hemostatic effectiveness up to 5 days. However, one feels more confident of efficacy when using concentrates that have been stored for less than 24 hours. Moreover, because they are stored at room temperature, the risk of bacterial contamination increases as the storage interval increases.

Platelets possess ABO, HL-A, and platelet-specific antigens but do not possess Rh antigens. Nevertheless, one tries to obtain both ABO and Rh-matched platelet concentrates to prevent Rh sensitization by RBCs contaminating platelet concentrates. If, in an emergency, platelets from an Rh-positive donor are given to an Rh-negative woman of reproductive age, she should be given Rh immunoglobulin (Rhogam) to prevent immunization to the Rho (D) antigen.

In an adult patient whose thrombocytopenia stems solely from diminished platelet production, the administration of 10 units should increase the platelet count by about 100,000 per μL (and also provide 500 mL of fresh plasma). However, if the patient is bleeding or has an infection with high fever, the platelet count may rise by only 10,000 to 40,000 per μL. In a patient with antiplatelet antibodies, for example, a patient with idiopathic thrombocytopenic purpura or a patient who has developed alloantibodies after previous platelet transfusions, the platelet count may not rise at all following platelet transfusion.

A patient who has become refractory to random donor platelets because of platelet alloantibodies sometimes still responds to HLA-matched platelets. By "platelet pheresis" using an automated cell separator, one may harvest enough platelets from a single HLA-matched donor to equal the platelets provided by six units of standard platelet concentrates. When repeated platelet transfusions are anticipated over a prolonged period, one may attempt to obtain HLA-matched donors from the beginning. However, an HLA-matched sibling should not be used as a donor if that sibling may later serve as a donor for bone marrow transplantation.

Granulocyte Concentrates

Granulocyte concentrates are prepared by leukopheresis of single donors, who may experience some discomfort from the procedure. Donor and recipient must be ABO compatible with a negative RBC cross match, and the recipient's serum should not contain leukoagglutinins reacting with the donor's WBC. The importance of HL-A typing remains to be established.

Administration of granulocyte concentrates may improve the chance for survival of an infected, severely neutropenic patient (less than 500 granulocytes per μL) with a positive blood culture who has failed to respond to antibiotic therapy alone and in whom endogenous granulocyte production is not anticipated to return for several days. From 1 to 4 × 10^{10} granulocytes are given during a granulocyte transfusion. Their effect lasts for less than 24 hours, and repeated transfusions are usually needed for at least several days. Reactions have occurred in which high fever and radiographic evidence of pulmonary infiltrates probably result from aggregation of transfused WBCs and their deposition in the pulmonary capillary bed.

Granulocyte transfusions are also currently used in neonates during the first week of life with the combination of:

1. Bacterial sepsis, either proved by positive blood culture or presumed on the basis of strong clinical evidence.
2. Depletion of the marrow granulocyte storage pool as evidenced by an absolute neutrophilic granulocyte count of less than 3000 per μL, with bands or more immature forms making up over 70% of the circulating granulocytes.

At least 1×10^9 granulocyte per kg of body weight are given. Donors should have negative cytomegalovirus serology. Irradiation of the concentrate is recommended to prevent graft-versus-host disease (see later).

PLASMA COMPONENTS

Plasma products available for component therapy include the following:

1. *Five per cent albumin solution,* which is used to replace plasma volume in patients with shock caused predominantly by leakage of plasma from the intravascular compartment (for example, in patients with burns, abdominal emergencies, or extensive tissue trauma). Preparations are heated at 60°C for 10 hours and do not transmit hepatitis.
2. *Fresh frozen plasma,* which is used to replace plasma volume when one also wants to replace plasma coagulation factors (other than factor VIII or fibrinogen, see below) or antithrombin III. Fresh frozen plasma is also used to treat thrombotic thrombocytopenic purpura and to replace plasma removed by therapeutic pheresis in other disorders. Because a unit of fresh frozen plasma is prepared from a single donor, it has a relatively low risk of transmitting hepatitis or other infections.
3. *Cryoprecipitate,* a plasma concentrate made from single donors, which contains factor VIII (80 to 100 units per bag), von Willebrand factor, factor XIII, fibronectin, and fibrinogen. Originally prepared for use in hemophilia A, cryoprecipitate has proved equally useful for replacement therapy in von Willebrand's disease and as a source of fibrinogen for a bleeding patient with acute defibrination. Sixteen bags of cryoprecipitate provide about 4 grams of fibrinogen, which should raise the plasma fibrinogen concentration of a normal-sized adult by more than 100 mg per dL.
4. *Lyophilized factor VIII concentrate,* a preparation made for replacement therapy in hemophilia A from pools of thousands of donors. Preparations are heat treated, which reduces the risk of transmission of HTLV-III and of hepatitis.
5. *Lyophilized prothrombin complex concentrate,* a pooled plasma concentrate of prothrombin and factors VII, IX, and X that has been used primarily to treat serious bleeding in hemophilia B. It

has also been used to replace the vitamin K-dependent clotting factors in patients receiving oral anticoagulant therapy who have developed truly *life-threatening* bleeding, for example, an intracerebral hemorrhage. As with factor VIII concentrates, preparations are heat treated to reduce the risk of transmission of HTLV-III and of hepatitis. Prothrombin complex concentrate may contain variable amounts of activated clotting factors, and occasional patients have developed venous thrombosis after receiving large amounts of concentrate (see Chapter 27).

6. **Gamma globulin.** Preparations are available for different purposes:

   a. Immune gamma globulin, a pooled plasma preparation used for replacement of gamma globulin in patients with immunologic deficiency diseases associated with severe hypogammaglobulinemia.

   b. Hyperimmune gamma globulin, which is made from individuals hyperimmunized to specific antigens (for example, hepatitis B surface antigen, tetanus) and is used to prevent or modify disease following exposure to specific infectious agents.

   c. Rh immune globulin, which is used to prevent sensitization to the Rho (D) antigen in Rh-negative women (see Chapter 9).

ROUTINE BLOOD TRANSFUSION PROCEDURE

Although 21 different blood group systems have been identified on the RBC membrane, the antigens of only two of these blood group systems—the ABO system and the Rh system—are typed prior to a blood transfusion. The ABO system is typed because each person has naturally occurring plasma antibodies to antigens of the ABO system that he or she does not possess. The Rh system is typed to determine the presence (Rh positive) or absence (Rh-negative) of the D antigen, which is highly immunogenic. Donor and recipient RBCs should be of the same type in these two systems.

The antigenic composition of the other, less immunogenic blood group systems is not routinely determined, since this would involve an impossible commitment of time, personnel, and scarce reagents. Instead, one establishes that the recipient's serum contains no antibodies that react in vitro with antigens on the donor RBCs. Although this protects against an acute hemolytic transfusion reaction, it does not prevent immunization of occasional patients to foreign antigens on donor cells, with formation of serum antibodies that then increase the difficulty of obtaining compatible blood for later transfusion.

Tests Performed on Donor Blood

Donor blood is subjected to the following tests:

1. *ABO and Rh typing of the RBCs.* If the RBCs appear to be Rh (D) negative, a further Rh typing procedure is carried out to rule out a weakly reactive Rh-positive variant known as D_u. Otherwise, one could sensitize an Rh-negative recipient by mistakingly giving Rh-positive donor cells of the D_u variant that had been mistyped as Rh negative.
2. *An antibody screen of the donor's serum.* The donor's serum is incubated with suspensions of two commercially available RBC suspensions that, between them, contain the major RBC antigens. This test detects antibodies in the donor's plasma capable of reacting after transfusion with any of the clinically important antigens the recipient's RBCs might possess.
3. *Serologic tests for transmittable infection:* AIDS (antibodies against HTLV-III virus), hepatitis (hepatitis B surface antigen), syphilis (VDLR test), and, in some circumstances, tests for antibodies against cytomegalovirus.

Tests Performed on Recipient Blood

The following tests are performed on the blood of a patient who is to receive a transfusion:

1. *ABO and Rh typing of the RBCs.* A test for the D_u variant is not essential, since giving Rh-negative blood to an Rh-positive recipient mistakenly identified as Rh negative does not cause sensitization.
2. *A "major side" crossmatch.* The recipient's serum is incubated with potential donor RBCs to detect antibodies in the recipient's serum that could react with the donor RBCs. (The antibody screen of the donor's serum described above makes unnecessary a "minor side" crossmatch, in which the recipient's RBCs are incubated with the donor's serum.)
3. *An antibody screen of the recipient's serum.* Performing an antibody screen of the recipient's serum in addition to the "major side" crossmatch may seem like duplication. However, the specially selected RBCs used for the antibody screen will occasionally detect an antibody in the recipient's serum that fails to react in the crossmatch test with weak antigen sites on the donor RBCs but which could nevertheless lead to a clinically significant reaction after transfusion.

Technique of Performing the Crossmatch and Antibody Screen

The crossmatch and antibody screen must be carried out under conditions that will detect IgM antibodies, IgG antibodies, and cell bound complement components. The tests are carried out as follows:

1. An approximately 5% suspension of RBCs in saline is incubated with serum at both room temperature and 37°C and examined for agglutination. Agglutination means that an IgM antibody has reacted with the RBCs. This may occur if:
   a. An error of ABO typing has been made.
   b. The serum contains a cold agglutinin with a thermal amplitude that extends to temperatures of clinical significance.
2. The above incubations are repeated but with the addition of two drops of a concentrated albumin solution to the mixtures. The increased protein concentration reduces the electrostatic forces separating the RBCs, which facilitates the agglutination of RBCs that have become coated with an IgG antibody.
3. An indirect anti-human globulin (Coombs') test is performed. A 5% suspension of RBCs is incubated with the serum, separated by centrifugation, washed thoroughly, and then reacted with a "broad-spectrum" anti-human globulin (Coombs') serum. The anti-human globulin serum will agglutinate the RBCs if IgG, complement, or both have bound to the RBCs during their initial incubation with the serum.

RISKS OF TRANSFUSION

The benefit of a transfusion must clearly outweigh its risk before a transfusion is indicated. The hazards of transfusion include:

1. *Immediate reactions.*
   a. Acute hemolytic reaction due to lysis of donor RBCs by antibodies in the recipient's plasma.
   b. Febrile reaction due to WBC or platelet antibodies.
   c. Pulmonary hypersensitivity reaction, another manifestation of WBC antibodies.
   d. Allergic-anaphylactoid reaction to a protein antigen in transfused plasma.

e. Endotoxemia due to transfusion of blood contaminated with gram-negative bacteria.
f. Pulmonary edema from volume overload.
2. *Delayed reactions.*
    a. Transmission of infection—hepatitis, AIDS, cytomegalovirus infection, malaria.
    b. Delayed hemolytic transfusion reaction.
    c. Graft-verus-host disease.

The risk of alloimmunization to RBC, WBC, platelet, and plasma protein antigens that can cause subsequent transfusion reactions increases with the number of times a patient must be transfused. Moreover, since each unit of blood contains about 225 mg of iron within hemoglobin, patients repeatedly transfused for conditions other than blood loss accumulate large amounts of iron in their tissues. Eventually, such iron overload may cause organ damage, for example, myocardial damage resulting in heart failure.

Hemolytic Reactions Due to Blood Group Incompatibility

Acute hemolysis is a serious complication of blood transfusion because the resultant hemoglobinuria may precipitate anuric renal failure. Manifestations may include back pain, tightness in the chest, breathlessness, chills and fever, hypotension, and dark urine (due to hemoglobinuria). After some hours, the patient may become jaundiced. If a hemolytic reaction occurs in an anesthetized patient during surgery, the sudden oozing of blood from cut surfaces may be its sole warning.

When a hemolytic reaction is suspected, one should:

1. Immediately stop the transfusion; damage is dose dependent.
2. Draw a blood sample from the patient and;
    a. Add anticoagulant to a portion, centrifuge, and examine the color of the supernatant plasma. A pink to red color indicates that the plasma contains hemoglobin; a brown color suggests that the plasma contains methemalbumin (see Chapter 2).
    b. Allow the remainder of the blood to clot in two tubes and:
        (1) Send one tube to the blood bank for serologic tests.
        (2) Send the second tube to the chemistry laboratory for pigment studies: hemoglobin, bilirubin, methemalbumin.

3. Return the remainder of the donor unit to the blood bank in its original bag and any other units that were issued with the unit that produced the reaction.
4. Examine the urine for hemoglobinuria (dark color with a positive occult blood test but a negative urinary sediment for RBCs).
5. After 8 to 10 hours, draw a second blood sample for bilirubin and methemalbumin determinations.

In the blood bank, the following serologic tests are carried out:

1. ABO and Rh typing are checked again:
   a. On the donor blood using blood from the pilot tube and from the unit given.
   b. On the recipient's blood using the pretransfusion blood sample on which the original typing was done and the blood sample drawn after the suspected reaction.
2. Crossmatches are repeated using:
   a. The patient's pretransfusion serum plus cells from the unit.
   b. The patient's post-transfusion serum plus cells from the unit.
   c. Donor plasma from the unit and the patient's pretransfusion cells.
3. Antibody screens are repeated on the patient's pretransfusion serum and on plasma from the donor unit. An antibody screen is also performed on the patient's post-transfusion serum.
4. A direct anti-human globulin (Coombs') test is performed on the RBCs drawn from the patient after the suspected reaction. This is done because all of the patient's antibody causing the reaction may have become bound to the donor cells during the transfusion and, therefore, may not be detectable in the patient's post-transfusion serum.

Most acute hemolytic transfusion reactions result from errors of identification. If such errors are to be eliminated, each step of the process, from the drawing of the initial blood sample from the recipient to the infusion of the donor unit, must be checked compulsively for accuracy of identification.

Delayed hemolytic reactions occur in patients who have been sensitized to red cell antigens by previous transfusion or pregnancy, but in whom antibody levels are too low to be detected by the pretransfusion antibody screen. Typically, the transfusion itself is uneventful, but 4 to 14 days later, manifestations of red cell destruction are found—a drop in hematocrit, jaundice, or even hemoglobinuria. Antibodies are readily detectable in the patient's serum at this time because renewed exposure to the RBC antigen has stimulated an anamnestic response.

Reactions Caused by WBC Agglutinins

Patients who have developed WBC agglutinins as the result of previous transfusions or pregnancies may develop a reaction characterized by headache, generalized malaise, and a rapid rise in temperature. Fever may develop during the transfusion or several hours afterwards and may persist for 24 to 48 hours. An occasional patient develops respiratory symptoms and radiographic evidence of pulmonary infiltrates. These stem from activation of complement, aggregation of WBC by C5a, and the deposition of WBC aggregates within the pulmonary capillaries. As mentioned, the use of leukocyte-poor RBC preparations can prevent such reactions.

Allergic-Anaphylactoid Reactions

Occasional patients, usually patients who have received many previous blood or plasma transfusions, may develop an alarming reaction, with urticaria, bronchoconstriction, and wheezing, while receiving blood or plasma. The reaction stems from an antigen-antibody reaction between a protein in the plasma being transfused and antibodies to that protein in the patient's plasma. Some of these anaphylactoid reactions have been traced to antibodies to IgA, which may form after transfusion in a patient who is IgA deficient or who has an unusual allotype of IgA. If such a patient requires only replacement of RBCs, further anaphylactoid reactions can usually be prevented by using frozen blood, from which virtually all of the plasma is removed during its processing for administration.

Endotoxemia

In this rare reaction, the donor blood is infected with large numbers of gram-negative bacteria, and, therefore, the patient receives a large intravenous injection of endotoxin. The patient develops chills, fever, diarrhea, and severe shock. When this serious reaction is suspected, a sample of blood from the original container should be centrifuged without delay and the pellet stained with Gram stain and examined for organisms. Since the manifestations of endotoxemia may sometimes resemble those of a hemolytic reaction, the serologic studies described above are also indicated.

A few gram-negative organisms can grow at 4°C, while the blood is stored in the blood bank. However, most gram-negative organisms multiply only after the blood has been warmed to room temperature. Therefore, blood should not be allowed to stand at room temperature for more than 30 minutes before it is given.

Transmission of Infection

HEPATITIS

All blood products except five per cent albumin solution and gamma globulin can transmit hepatitis. Pooled plasma products have an obviously higher risk than products prepared from single donors. The usual incubation period for transfusion-induced hepatitis is 50 to 60 days, with a range of from 2 weeks to 6 months.

At least four types of hepatitis viruses have been recognized—type A, type B, a type referred to as non-A, non-B, and the delta virus. Cytomegalovirus may also cause hepatitis (and accounts for 1% to 5% of post-transfusion hepatitis).

Type A hepatitis is rarely transmitted by transfusion because viremia in type A hepatitis is so brief that the chance of an asymptomatic viremic individual donating blood is exceedingly small. Hepatitis B formerly made up a substantial fraction of post-transfusion hepatitis; however, the mandatory use of sensitive screening tests for hepatitis B surface antigen in donor blood has reduced the percentage of post-transfusion hepatitis caused by type B virus to about 2%. The vast majority of post-transfusion hepatitis today is of the non-A, non-B type. No test is presently available to detect the carrier of non-A, non-B hepatitis virus. The delta virus is a defective virus that requires the helper function of the hepatitis B virus to replicate. When a patient positive for hepatitis B surface antigen is infected with delta virus, the superinfection can convert a previously mild hepatitis B carrier state into a severe, progressive hepatitis.

A patient has a 1% risk of developing non-A, non-B hepatitis for each unit of blood administered. Most patients developing hepatitis do not become jaundiced and escape notice unless transaminase values are measured. Nevertheless, in 20% of the patients the hepatitis will progress to cirrhosis. Thus, non-A, non-B hepatitis is a major risk of transfusion therapy. Measuring levels of alanine aminotransferase (ALT) and antibody to hepatitis B core antigen in donor units has recently been introduced as surrogate tests to identify units at high risk of transmitting non-A, non-B hepatitis.

ACQUIRED IMMUNODEFICIENCY SYNDROME

At this writing about 2% of all reported cases of AIDS in the United States have been associated with the administration of blood or blood products. The disease may be transmitted by blood or blood products prepared from asymptomatic donors, who may not develop the disease themselves for months or years thereafter or who may possibly remain asymptomatic carriers indefinitely. Apparently, HTLV-III virus will be present in the blood of about 85% of individuals who are seropositive in a recently developed ELISA test for antibodies to HTLV-III virus. The widespread application of this test should reduce the risk of transmission of AIDS by blood and blood products. However, several asymptomatic individuals infected with HTLV-III virus have been identified who do not have detectable plasma antibodies. The full impact of the transmission of this deadly infection by blood products upon the future practice of transfusion therapy cannot be assessed at this time.

CYTOMEGALOVIRUS INFECTION

Latent cytomegalovirus is present in circulating WBCs of a substantial proportion of donors, and cytomegaloviral infection is readily transmitted by blood transfusion. Serum cytomegaloviral antibody titer rises at least fourfold in about 30% of postoperative patients given a large number of transfusions during surgery. A few patients develop an infectious mononucleosis-like syndrome. Immunocompromised patients may develop severe or even fatal post-transfusion cytomegalovirus infection. Therefore, as discussed in Chapter 21, one attempts to prevent transmission of cytomegalovirus infection by the use of blood from seronegative donors or by the use of RBCs carefully washed to remove WBCs in certain groups of patients.

Graft-Versus-Host Disease

Graft-verus-host disease has been reported after blood transfusions in children with various primary immunodeficiency diseases, after intrauterine or exchange transfusions of neonates with hemolytic disease of the newborn, and after transfusion of adults with myelosuppression and immunodeficiency secondary to chemotherapy for hematologic malignancies. Irradiating blood with doses of 1500 to 3000 rads before administration prevents graft-versus-host disease by inactivating lymphocytes without impairing the function of RBCs, granulocytes, or platelets.

SELECTED READING

1. Barton JC: Nonhemolytic, noninfectious transfusion reactions. Semin Hematol 18:95, 1983.
2. Bove JR: Transfusion-transmitted diseases: current problems and challenges. Prog Hematol 16:123, 1986.
3. Curran JW and others: Acquired immunodeficiency syndrome (AIDS) associated with transfusions. N Engl J Med 320:69, 1984.
4. Menitove JE, and Aster RH: Transfusion of platelets and plasma products. Clin Haematol 12:239, 1983.
5. Mollison PL: Blood Transfusion in Clinical Medicine. Ed 3. Boston, Blackwell Scientific Publications, 1983.
6. Rosina F, Saracco G, and Rizetto M: Risk of post-transfusion infection with the hepatitis delta virus. A multicenter study. N Engl J Med 312:1488, 1985.

Index

Entries followed by "t" denote tables; entries followed by "f" denote figures.